Respiratory Critical Care

Respiratory Critical Care

Edited by

Craig Davidson

Consultant Physician in Intensive Care and Respiratory Medicine, Guy's and St Thomas' Hospital Trust and GKT School of Medicine, London, UK

and

David Treacher

Consultant Physician in Intensive Care and Respiratory Medicine, Guy's and St Thomas' Hospital Trust and GKT School of Medicine, London, UK

A member of the Hodder Headline Group
LONDON

First published in Great Britain in 2002 by
Arnold, a member of the Hodder Headline Group,
338 Euston Road, London NW1 3BH

http://www.arnoldpublishers.com

Distributed in the United States of America by
Oxford University Press Inc.,
198 Madison Avenue, New York, NY10016
Oxford is a registered trademark of Oxford University Press

Whilst the advice and information in this book are believed to be true and
accurate at the date of going to press, neither the authors nor the publisher
can accept any legal responsibility or liability for any errors or omissions that
may be made. In particular (but without limiting the generality of the
preceding disclaimer) every effort has been made to check drug dosages;
however it is still possible that errors have been missed. Furthermore, dosage
schedules are constantly being revised and new side-effects recognized. For
these reasons the reader is strongly urged to consult the drug companies'
printed instructions before administering any of the drugs recommended in
this book.

British Library Cataloguing in Publication Data
A catalogue record for this book is available from the British Library

Library of Congress Cataloging-in-Publication Data
A catalog record for this book is available from the Library of Congress

ISBN 0 340 76289 6

1 2 3 4 5 6 7 8 9 10

Commissioning Editor: Joanna Koster
Production Editor: James Rabson
Production Controller: Martin Kerans
Cover Designer: Mouse Mat Design

Typeset in 10/12 Minion and Ocean Sans by
Integra Software Services Pvt. Ltd, Pondicherry, India
Printed and bound in Italy by Giunti

Contents

Contributors

Michael Barker
Physiotherapy Department, Guy's and St Thomas' Hospital Trust and GKT School of Medicine, London, UK

Torsten T Bauer
Abteilung für Pneumologie, Allergologie und Schlafmedizin, Medizinische Klinik und Poliklinik, Bergmannsheil Klinikum der Ruhr-Universität, Bochum, Germany

Richard Beale
Intensive Care Medicine, Guy's and St Thomas' Hospital Trust and GKT School of Medicine, London, UK

Andrew Bersten
Department of Critical Care Medicine, Flinders Medical Centre, South Australia, Australia

Hilmar Burchardi
Zentrum Anaesthesiologie, Rettungs- und Intensivmedizin, University Hospital, Göttingen, Germany

Baudouin Byl
Infectious Diseases Clinic, Erasme University Hospital, Brussels, Belgium

Jean Carlet
Réanimation Polyvalente, St Joseph Hospital, Paris, France

Annalisa Carlucci
Respiratory Intensive Care Unit, Centro Medico di Pavia IRCCS, Fondazione S. Maugeri, Pavia, Italy

A Craig Davidson
Intensive Care and Respiratory Medicine, Guy's and St Thomas' Hospital Trust and GKT School of Medicine, London, UK

Sheric G Ellum
Physiotherapy Department, Guy's and St Thomas' Hospital Trust and GKT School of Medicine, London, UK

Tim W Evans
Royal Brompton Hospital, London, UK

Wolfgang Frank

Klinik III, Johanniter Krankenhaus im Fläming, Treuenbrietzen, Germany

David Ghez

Réanimation Polyvalente, St Joseph Hospital, Paris, France

John C Goldstone

The Centre for Anaesthesia, The Middlesex Hospital, London, UK

Keith G Hickling

Goldcoast Hospital, Southport, Queensland, Australia

Russell D Hull

Department of Medicine, Thrombosis Research Unit, Foothills Hospital, Calgary, Alberta, Canada

Sean P Keenan

Royal Columbian Hospital, New Westminster, British Columbia, Canada

Sarah EJ Keilty

Physiotherapy Department, Guy's and St Thomas' Hospital Trust and GKT School of Medicine, London, UK

Richard M Leach

Intensive Care Medicine, Guy's and St Thomas' Hospital Trust and GKT School of Medicine, London, UK

Wei Shen Lim

Respiratory Infection Research Group, Respiratory Medicine, Nottingham City Hospital, Nottingham, UK

Robert Loddenkemper

Lungenklinik Heckeshorn, Berlin, Germany

John T Macfarlane

Respiratory Medicine, Nottingham City Hospital, Nottingham, UK

Richard Marshall

Centre for Respiratory Research, University College London, Rayne Institute, London, UK

Stefano Nava

Respiratory Intensive Care Unit, Centro Medico di Pavia IRCCS, Fondazione S. Maugeri, Pavia, Italy

Annabel H Nickol

Respiratory Muscle Laboratory, Royal Brompton Hospital, London, UK

Daliana Peres Bota

Department of Intensive Care, Erasme University Hospital, Brussels, Belgium

Graham F Pineo

Department of Medicine, Thrombosis Research Unit, Foothills Hospital, Calgary, Alberta, Canada

Michael I Polkey
Royal Brompton Hospital, London, UK

Gary E Raskob
Departments of Biostatistics and Epidemiology, and Medicine, University of Oklahoma Health Sciences Center, Oklahoma City, Oklahoma, USA

Bernd Schönhofer
Krankenhaus Kloster Grafschaft, Zentrum für Pneumologie, Beatmungs- und Schlafmedizin, Schmallenberg-Grafschaft, Germany

William J Sibbald
Department of Medicine, Sunnybrook and Women's Health Sciences Centre, Toronto, Ontario, Canada

Jean-François Timsit
Réanimation médicale et infectieuse, Bichat Hospital, Paris, France

Antoni Torres
Hospital Clinic i Provincial, Servei de Pneumologia i Allèrgia Respiratoria, Barcelona, Spain

David F Treacher
Intensive Care and Respiratory Medicine, Guy's and St Thomas' Hospital Trust and GKT School of Medicine, London, UK

Jean-Louis Vincent
Department of Intensive Care, Erasme University Hospital, Brussels, Belgium

Michele Vitacca
Respiratory Intensive Care Unit, Istituto Scientifico di Gussago, Fondazione S. Maugeri, Pavia, Italy

David A Waller
Glenfield Hospital, Leicester, UK

Adrian J Williams
Lane-Fox Respiratory Unit, Guy's and St Thomas' Hospital Trust and GKT School of Medicine, London, UK

S John Wort
Royal Brompton Hospital, London, UK

Foreword

Intensive care is increasingly being recognized on a worldwide basis as a specialty within its own right, and the appropriate training programmes and diplomas have now been introduced in many countries. It is quite clear to many of us within the intensive care community that a multi-disciplinary approach to the care of the critically ill patient provides better care in every sense of the word.

Organ dysfunction is, of course, the major problem with most intensive care patients, and pulmonary dysfunction is particularly common. Patients range from those with severe obstructive airway disease, where the prime objective might be to try and prevent intubation and ventilation, to those with severe acute respiratory distress syndrome who are profoundly hypoxic and require urgent ventilation using the most up-to-date techniques. Within this spectrum lies a large number of complex issues which require very considerable expertise.

This book covers these issues with particular conciseness but without losing anything in clarity. The authors are internationally recognized as experts in their fields and have produced an authoritative text that can and should be used by all physicians who are interested in the management of patients with acute respiratory problems in the intensive and high dependency environments.

David Bennett
Professor of Intensive Care Medicine
St George's Hospital, London, UK

Preface

Major developments in respiratory critical care have occurred in the past decade. These have resulted in important changes in the management of acute respiratory problems, both within the intensive care unit and in other acute care areas. The improved understanding of patient – ventilator interactions, advances in ventilator technology and respiratory monitoring and the recognition of ventilator-induced lung injury have all produced significant changes in clinical practice. Non-invasive ventilation has become established as the preferred option in respiratory failure resulting from chronic obstructive pulmonary disease (COPD) and can be used to speed weaning from invasive ventilation in this condition. Its use has been extended to the management of non-COPD respiratory failure and it should now be used, at least initially, in immunocompromised patients presenting with acute respiratory failure.

Other areas of change include new strategies for ventilation in acute lung injury and weaning from mechanical ventilation following critical illness. Using more precise classification of patient populations and definition of ventilatory strategies, randomized trials have resulted in important changes in practice in both these areas. The science of aerosol delivery has also become established. New therapies have come, others have gone and others have yet to find wide application. The initial hopes for extracorporeal membrane oxygenation and nitric oxide in refractory hypoxaemia have not been realized, and prone positioning, although increasingly practised, was not shown to provide any outcome benefit in a multicentre study. Simpler, less dramatic strategies, such as nursing intensive care unit patients in the semi-recumbent position, have been shown to reduce the incidence of nosocomial pneumonia. Finally, cost-effectiveness and ethical dilemmas are being more widely debated and, in certain cases, will influence decisions concerning the appropriateness of admission to the high dependency or intensive care unit as institutions attempt to justify, and governments to quantify, the cost of caring for these patients.

Against this exciting background of clinical progress, the training and provision of critical care medicine is changing. Historically, in the USA, its development has been linked to respiratory medicine and more than 80% of trainees opt for dual accreditation with critical care. In Australia, on the other hand, it has emerged as a separate specialty and is increasingly recognized as such in Europe. In the UK, intensive care has traditionally been dominated in number by anaesthetists, who often have, in addition, a full anaesthetic practice with relatively few formal sessions available for intensive care. There is now recognition that intensive care should be a separate specialty, with sufficient dedicated sessions to ensure quality of care and to permit training of junior doctors from other medical disciplines. In America and many European countries, intensive care is organized by specialty rather than by having general or mixed intensive care units. The re-creation of respiratory intensive care units, in which both intubated and non-invasively ventilated patients are managed, has seen greater involvement of respiratory physicians in the delivery of care. These changes have broadened the appeal of critical care and, in Europe and in the UK, respiratory physicians are becoming more involved.

For all these reasons, there is now a need for the major developments in respiratory critical care to be reviewed and for a text that provides a balanced clinical approach with state-of-the-art commentary. The contributors to this book are both acknowledged experts and practising clinicians, with a wide spread of cultural backgrounds to reflect the international nature of medicine in the twenty-first century. Excessive referencing has been avoided in favour of readability and, inevitably, some readers will feel that important topics have been either omitted or dealt with superficially. Standard textbooks already provide excellent reviews of cardiopulmonary physiology, the management of the difficult airway or the finer details of blood-gas analysis. By omitting these subjects, we have been able to focus on the areas in which new evidence is driving changes in clinical practice. We hope that this book will appeal to all those working or training in critical care, whatever their background or interests. Most particularly, this book is addressed to respiratory physicians, who, we believe, are now recognized as increasingly important and necessary contributors to the practice and development of critical care medicine.

Craig Davidson and David Treacher

July 2002

Respiratory muscles, pulmonary mechanics and ventilatory control

ANNABEL H NICKOL AND MICHAEL I POLKEY

INTRODUCTION

Passage of air into and out of the lungs is essential for the maintenance of O_2 and CO_2 homeostasis. In spontaneously breathing humans this is achieved by contraction of the respiratory muscles. The activity of these muscles is governed at both a voluntary and an involuntary level by specific areas of the brain, and disease processes that interfere with either ventilatory control or the respiratory muscle pump (Fig. 1.1) may cause ventilatory failure or difficulty in weaning from mechanical ventilation. Similarly, if the load placed on the respiratory muscle pump exceeds its capacity (even if the pump is normal), ventilatory failure results (Fig. 1.2). Different diseases impose different types of load on the respiratory muscle pump and understanding these differences is important.

In this chapter, the respiratory muscle pump, the control of breathing, respiratory muscle fatigue and interactions with sleep are reviewed in both normal subjects and patients with respiratory failure. Methods for testing the function of the respiratory muscle pump and the influences of various conditions on pulmonary mechanics are considered and critical care conditions that affect the respiratory muscle pump are also reviewed.

THE RESPIRATORY MUSCLE PUMP

Anatomically, the muscles forming the respiratory muscle pump may be considered as either inspiratory (diaphragm and extradiaphragmatic inspiratory muscles) or expiratory, of which the abdominal muscles are the most important. Histologically, the respiratory muscles are similar to skeletal muscle, with approximately 50% Type I 'slow' fibres and 25% each of Type IIa and Type IIb, and are therefore susceptible to the same physiological processes, including the development of fatigue. Similarly, diseases that affect skeletal muscle or its innervation may also involve the diaphragm and occasionally patients with these diseases present with respiratory failure.

The diaphragm deserves special consideration because it is the most important respiratory muscle, accounting for approximately 70% of resting ventilation. Moreover, because the phrenic nerves that supply it have a long course from their origin in the neck from the 3rd, 4th and 5th cervical roots, the nerves may be damaged by a variety of diseases, trauma or iatrogenically. As well as being uniquely vulnerable, the diaphragm is the only respiratory muscle that has a nerve supply, with surface landmarks allowing it to be stimulated in isolation and in which tension

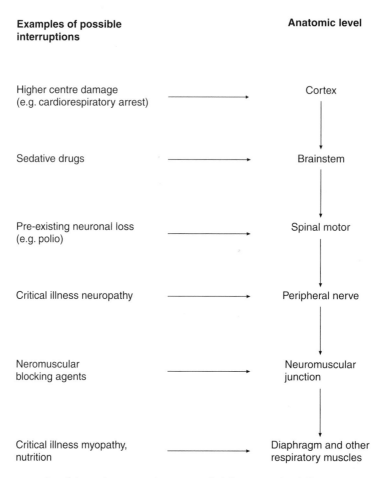

Examples of possible interruptions	Anatomic level

Higher centre damage (e.g. cardiorespiratory arrest)   →   Cortex

Sedative drugs   →   Brainstem

Pre-existing neuronal loss (e.g. polio)   →   Spinal motor

Critical illness neuropathy   →   Peripheral nerve

Neromuscular blocking agents   →   Neuromuscular junction

Critical illness myopathy, nutrition   →   Diaphragm and other respiratory muscles

Figure 1.1 *Schematic representation of the respiratory muscle pump. On the left are examples of disease processes that occur in critically ill patients and can compromise the pump. (Adapted from reference 37.)*

generation can be estimated (as transdiaphragmatic pressure, Pdi). When the diaphragm contracts, it moves caudally, creating a negative intrathoracic pressure and a positive abdominal pressure. This pressure is transmitted laterally through the zone of apposition to the lower ribcage, causing outward displacement of the lower ribs. The function of the extradiaphragmatic inspiratory muscles (for example the scalenes and parasternal intercostals) during respiration in normal humans is to prevent collapse of the upper ribcage. Consequently, in patients with unopposed diaphragm activity, such as high tetraplegics fitted with diaphragm pacers, diaphragm contraction results in an inward, expiratory movement of the upper ribcage.

The abdominal muscles have important functions in relation to coughing, laughing and speaking. In particular, an effective cough depends on achieving dynamic airway closure, which, in turn, depends on the development of a gastric pressure greater than 50 cmH_2O.[1] The contribution of the abdominal muscles to ventilation is more controversial; in spontaneously ventilated subjects without airflow limitation, these muscles are recruited during movement from the supine to the erect posture and when minute ventilation is increased for any reason, for example during exercise. The mechanism of action is thought to be that expiratory muscle activity drives the diaphragm to a lower lung volume and functional residual capacity (FRC); this in turn assists the subsequent inspiration because gravity assists the inspiratory descent of the diaphragm, thereby increasing its length and the force it generates.[2] However, this mechanism cannot operate in patients who are supine or in those who are flow limited at rest, as are the majority of patients with chronic obstructive pulmonary disease

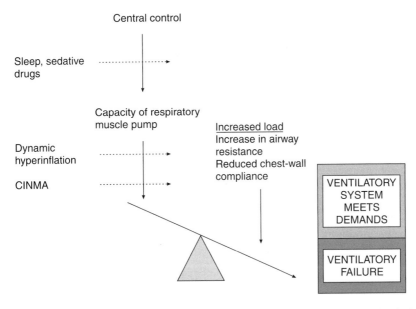

Figure 1.2 *Load–capacity imbalance of the respiratory muscle pump results in ventilatory failure or, if the patient is already receiving ventilatory support, difficulty weaning. CINMA, critical illness neuropathy and myopathy.*

(COPD) requiring mechanical ventilation. In these circumstances, abdominal muscle action may be counterproductive, both because the energy expended is wasted and because it may contribute to patient–ventilator asynchrony.[3]

Pathophysiological processes affecting the respiratory muscle pump

DISEASE PROCESSES

Respiratory muscle dysfunction due to neurological disease may precipitate respiratory failure;[4]

important causes are shown in Table 1.1. Many of these conditions can be excluded by clinical history or simple measurements. Myasthenia gravis merits particular review. In addition to therapeutic approaches to modify disease activity (such as thymectomy or steroid therapy), patients with myasthenia gravis are usually treated with anticholinesterases. This therapy affects muscle groups differentially and patients with apparently optimally controlled myasthenia gravis may have significant respiratory muscle weakness.[5] Such patients are predisposed to acute ventilatory failure if the dose of anticholinesterase is either too low or too high.

Table 1.1 *Neurological causes of acute respiratory failure*

Spinal cord or higher	Nerve	Neuromuscular junction	Muscle
Trauma to nerve or high cervical spine	Guillain–Barré	Botulism	Biochemical disturbance, e.g hypokalaemia
Sedative drugs – prescribed	Organophosphate poisoning	Envenomation/shellfish poison	Periodic paralysis
Overdose (narcotic or other)		Drugs with neuromuscular blocking effects (as main or side effect)	
		Myasthenia gravis	
		Lambert–Eaton syndrome	

MUSCLE SHORTENING

Like all skeletal muscles, the diaphragm and other respiratory muscles have an optimum length, defined by the length at which a given stimulus generates the greatest tension. For the human diaphragm, the optimum length (usually measured as lung volume) has not been determined *in vivo*, but it must be below FRC because numerous studies have established that the pressure-generating capacity of the diaphragm increases between total lung capacity (TLC) and FRC (Fig. 1.3). Importantly, in both normal subjects and patients with COPD,[6] the reduction is primarily in the capacity of the diaphragm to lower intrathoracic pressure. As well as pre-existing COPD, lung volume is increased in the intensive care unit (ICU) by acquired obstructive defects and the application of extrinsic positive end expiratory pressure/continuous positive airway pressure (PEEP/CPAP).

MUSCLE FATIGUE

If skeletal muscle is subjected to increased load, a reduction in tension generation occurs, which resolves with rest; this process is termed fatigue. Failure of neural output is termed central fatigue, but this is impossible to differentiate *in vivo* from lack of motivation. Fatigue may also result from defects arising at the neuromuscular junction, e.g. myasthenia gravis or neuromuscular blockade. However, the form of fatigue thought to be of greatest relevance to the critically ill patient is low-frequency fatigue, because it is long lasting (24 hours or more) and

in-vivo respiratory motoneurons discharge at low frequencies. For skeletal muscle, the tension generated increases with increasing stimulation frequency, reaching a plateau at around 100 Hz. In low-frequency fatigue, the tension generated at low-frequency stimulation (10–20 Hz) is reduced, but there is little reduction at higher frequencies. Low-frequency diaphragm fatigue has been demonstrated in normal subjects after voluntary hyperventilation and exhaustive treadmill exercise. However, evidence that low-frequency diaphragm fatigue contributes to ventilatory failure in clinical practice is thus far lacking and attempts to produce it in stable patients with COPD have failed.

Does the respiratory muscle pump really fail?

There are no clear-cut 'markers' of respiratory muscle pump failure, although failure is suggested by a rise in $PaCO_2$ without a fall in PaO_2. There have as yet been no serial studies that have demonstrated a decrease in strength as a patient develops respiratory failure, or that respiratory muscle strength *per se* distinguishes patients failing and succeeding in a weaning trial. Measurable changes in respiratory muscle physiology such as slowing of the maximal relaxation rate or a decrease in the ratio of high-frequency to low-frequency electromyogram (EMG) signal merely reflect the fact that the muscle is loaded. Respiratory failure occurs as the result of an unfavourable load:capacity ratio,[7] an increase in respiratory load being the more

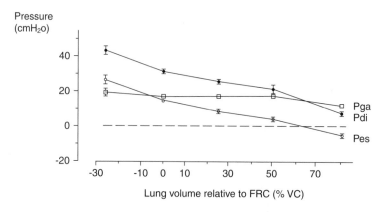

Figure 1.3 *Effect of lung volume change (VC) relative to functional residual capacity (FRC) on the pressure generated in response to a single bilateral supramaximal stimulation of the phrenic nerves. Mean data from eight subjects are shown. Pga, gastric pressure; Pdi, transdiaphragmatic pressure; Pes, oesophageal pressure. (Modified from reference 38.)*

usual reason for ICU admission or the need for continuing ventilation. Indeed, laboratory studies involving inspiratory loading have demonstrated that respiratory muscle fatigue develops when the mean inspiratory capacity during each breath becomes a high proportion (>15–20%) of maximum inspiratory pressure. Similarly in the ICU, long-term ventilator patients have been shown to fail a weaning trial when the oesophageal pressure required to achieve adequate ventilation is a large fraction of maximum inspiratory pressure.

Sleep

The normal physiological changes that occur in sleep have particular relevance in those with significant weakness of the diaphragm, in obstructive lung disease, congestive cardiac failure and in the profoundly obese. In the context of the acutely unwell, who may have incipient respiratory failure, it may be a critically important time as respiratory failure may worsen, with episodes of severe hypoxaemia and the potential for cardiac arrhythmias or even cardiorespiratory arrest. Sleep will be also important during the weaning period, not only because of the sleep fragmentation that often occurs in the ICU,[8] but also because it is a risk period for the recently extubated. Inadequate alveolar ventilation may occur during weaning, when spontaneous modes of ventilatory support may provide insufficient ventilatory control.

The features of sleep-disordered breathing (SDB) include hypoventilation, with resulting respiratory acidosis, hypoxaemia and recurrent arousal.[9] Arousal will, at times, also produce, profound sympathetic and parasympathetic activation. SDB results from both obstructive and non-obstructive (central) sleep apnoea, a mixture of the two or a greater than normal diminution in alveolar ventilation, particularly during rapid eye movement (REM) sleep. Alveolar hypoventilation results from either chest-wall or neuromuscular disease, when there is a reduction in the 'power' of the respiratory pump, or when the load is increased, e.g. COPD. It is a consequence of the normal reduction in striated muscle activity at sleep onset, with a further reduction during REM, which leads to significant hypoventilation with the loss of the accessory muscles' contribution to ventilation. A reduction in tone of the pharyngeal muscles may also promote obstructive events. Additional changes in chest or abdominal wall compliance, only partially explained by body position, may also affect V̇Q and lead to hypoxaemia. Arousal, which is typically recurrent in OSA, results in sympathetic stimulation, the importance of which is increasingly being recognized in congestive cardiac failure as contributing to sympathetic activation. Monitoring of respiratory function during sleep is therefore important in several risk groups: the acutely unwell, non-ventilated patient; the at-risk neuromuscular or COPD patient, especially during weaning; and recently extubated patients who may be at more risk of upper airway obstruction.

Acquired damage to the respiratory muscle pump

CRITICAL ILLNESS NEUROMUSCULAR ABNORMALITIES

Neurological abnormalities are common in patients in whom weaning is difficult. Spitzer et al., for example, concluded that, in 'difficult to wean' patients, 62% had neuromuscular disease sufficiently severe to account for ventilator dependency.[10] The identification of previously unsuspected neurological disease is therefore important. Full neurological examination of the ICU patient is difficult, but it should still be possible to identify muscle wasting, fasciculation and the presence or absence of tendon jerks. Preservation of tendon reflexes is important as it demonstrates retained motor nerve function.[11] In some cases, a demyelinating neuropathy occurs, which may be considered an acquired Guillain–Barré syndrome. An EMG may be helpful, although myopathy can be difficult or impossible to distinguish on electrophysiological grounds from an axonal neuropathy. That myopathy, rather than neuropathy, occurs in some patients is supported by histological and biochemical data.[12]

Only a few studies have investigated the electrophysiology of the respiratory muscles in ICU and none has systematically assessed respiratory muscle strength. The frequency of reported abnormalities is high and does not have a straightforward relationship with the frequency of abnormalities of the peripheral nervous system. Neuromuscular abnormalities of the respiratory muscles and peripheral muscles frequently co-exist. Moreover, patients with critical illness axonal polyneuropathy involving non-respiratory nerves are likely to require longer periods of ventilatory support than those without.[13]

The causes of critical illness neuromuscular abnormalities (CINMA) are not well established (for a fuller discussion, see references 14 and 15), but multiple organ dysfunction is a recognized risk factor. Both neuromuscular blocking agents and corticosteroids have been implicated in the aetiology, but CINMA commonly occurs without exposure to these drugs.[12] In renal failure, the accumulation of active drug or metabolite such as 3-desacetyl-vecuronium can occur, leading to persistent neuromuscular failure.

IATROGENIC DAMAGE TO THE RESPIRATORY MUSCLE PUMP

Phrenic nerve injury is a recognized complication of surgery to the heart, liver or upper gastrointestinal (GI) tract and central venous cannulation. Chest-wall pain and upper GI surgery may also impair diaphragm function.

Assessment of the respiratory muscle pump in the intensive care unit

The function of the inspiratory muscles is to produce an intrathoracic pressure below atmospheric pressure so that inspiration occurs. Theoretically, the pump can be assessed at any level from the cortex to flow in the respiratory airways. Although measurements of tidal volume and vital capacity broadly indicate whether a patient has sufficient respiratory function to avoid progressive ventilatory failure, their value in the detailed assessment of pump function is limited because they are influenced by lung mechanics. However, in patients with isolated respiratory muscle disease, changes in vital capacity are useful in predicting the need for ventilation and in evaluating recovery.

PRESSURE MEASUREMENTS

In ambulant patients, the pressure developed at the mouth or in the oesophagus during a maximal voluntary effort is often used as a measure of inspiratory muscle strength. This method has been adapted for use in the ICU by using a valve that only permits expiration, but the test fails to predict weaning outcome, presumably because patients in the ICU are seldom able to make a truly maximal voluntary effort. Clearly, patients who can generate a high pressure do not have respiratory muscle weakness, but this seldom applies to ICU patients.

To measure respiratory muscle strength independent of patient effort, it is necessary to stimulate the nerve supplying the muscle artificially, using electrical or magnetic stimulation, and measure the force output. The only muscle in which this can be performed *in vivo* is the diaphragm, but because it accounts for approximately 70% of resting ventilation in humans, this is useful when respiratory muscle weakness is suspected.

Phrenic nerve stimulation allows the force output of the diaphragm to be measured independently of patient effort. It is quantified by the transdiaphragmatic or mouth/endotracheal tube pressure (Pdi or Pm/P_{ET}, respectively) generated in response to a single supramaximal stimulus applied to both phrenic nerves, a 'twitch' (Tw). The measurement of Tw Pdi requires the use of oesophageal and gastric balloons, which is not always possible in intubated patients. An alternative is to measure the Tw P_{ET} by occluding the endotracheal tube at end-expiration. Although this approach has clear attractions, Tw P_{ET} is similar to oesophageal rather than to transdiaphragmatic pressure and, being 50–60% smaller, may be harder to measure accurately because the 'noise-to-signal' ratio will be large. Similarly, increases in lung volume, for example with PEEP, disproportionately influence the value.

Magnetic nerve stimulation is a novel technique with advantages over direct electrical stimulation. Either bilateral anterior magnetic stimulation (Fig. 1.4) or a single circular coil anteriorly over the upper mediastinum can be employed to confirm or refute a clinical diagnosis of respiratory muscle weakness. The use of both techniques requires experience.[16]

ELECTROPHYSIOLOGICAL MEASUREMENTS

These have the disadvantage that they do not give information regarding the force-generating capacity of the muscle. Nevertheless, investigation of the integrity of the phrenic nerve may be indicated in the following situations.

- To determine prognosis if weakness related to medical intervention is demonstrated. For example, if hemidiaphragm paralysis follows cardiac surgery, one would expect the prognosis to be

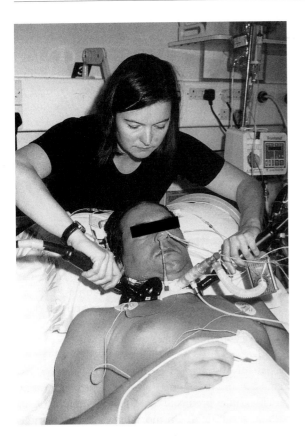

Figure 1.4 *Bilateral anterior magnetic stimulation of the phrenic nerves in a patient with chronic obstructive pulmonary disease with difficulty weaning from mechanical ventilation.*

better if an action potential is still demonstrable. This distinction can occasionally be of medico-legal importance.

- Occasionally where it is considered necessary to distinguish axonal from demyelinating neuropathies. In the former, the amplitude of the action potential is diminished, whereas in the latter, the conduction time is prolonged.

The basic measurement of phrenic nerve electrophysiology is conduction time (PNCT). For this measurement, it is critical that the action potential measured originates from the diaphragm. The probability that this is so can be increased by selectively stimulating the phrenic nerve with electrical stimulation or, alternatively, using an oesophageal electrode to record selectively from the diaphragm. PNCT is only mildly influenced by stimulus intensity, so the simplest practical option is to use electrical stimulation in conjunction with surface electrodes, though care must be taken to avoid brachial plexus contamination. An example of an action potential is shown in Figure 1.5.

Quantification of the action potential requires supramaximal stimulation to ensure that all axons are recruited; this is difficult with electrical stimulation, and the combination of magnetic stimulation and an oesophageal electrode is preferred.[17] This technique does, however, require specialist expertise, as do other techniques such as needle electromyography. Neither of these techniques is routinely used in European ICUs.

PULMONARY MECHANICS

To obtain optimal mechanical ventilatory support requires an understanding of pulmonary mechanics. Interventions within the ICU often aim to achieve this by increasing pulmonary compliance and decreasing both airway resistance and intrinsic PEEP, thus reducing the work of breathing.

Lung volumes

Lung volume is often reduced in the critically ill by a variety of factors: underlying lung disease, e.g. atelectasis, or reduced muscle strength from critical illness myopathy or factors that affect diaphragm function such as abdominal distension.

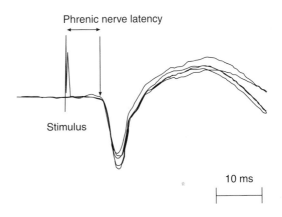

Figure 1.5 *Example of an action potential recorded from an oesophageal electrode using unilateral electrical stimulation. (Figure courtesy of Dr YM Luo, Kings College Hospital, London UK.)*

VITAL CAPACITY AND FORCED EXPIRATORY VOLUME

The measurement of vital capacity is most commonly used to monitor progress in conditions in which there is acute respiratory muscle weakness. It is of use in predicting the need for ventilatory support in Guillain–Barré syndrome but not in myasthenia gravis,[18] possibly reflecting the tendency for acute deterioration in the latter condition. In general terms, a vital capacity of more than 10 mL kg appears to be required to sustain adequate spontaneous ventilation. Vital capactiy has not been shown to be of use in predicting the requirement for ventilatory support in conditions other than respiratory muscle weakness.

Portable spirometers permit the bedside measurement of vital capacity and forced expiratory volume (FEV_1) in the non-intubated, spontaneously breathing subject. Accurate vital capacity measurements require patient co-operation and may be difficult to undertake in the ICU setting if patients are confused or sedated.

FUNCTIONAL RESIDUAL CAPACITY

Functional residual capacity is the lung volume in the neutral position with complete respiratory muscle relaxation. At this point, the inward elastic recoil pressure of the lung is equal to the outward recoil pressure of the chest wall and corresponds to lung volume at end-expiration. Measurement of FRC is not commonly carried out in the ICU. The two techniques most commonly used are helium dilution and the nitrogen wash-out method.[19] Both methods only measure the volume of gas in ventilated parts of the lung and will underestimate gas volume in lung units with long time constants.

Helium dilution
The technique relies on measuring the differences in helium concentration before and after the subject is switched into a closed-circuit rebreathing system when they are at FRC. By knowing the volume of the circuit and helium concentrations, FRC can then be calculated.

Nitrogen wash-out technique
The patient is ventilated with air before being switched to a ventilator at end-expiration (FRC) and ventilated with 100% O_2 at the end of expiration (i.e. at FRC). Breath by breath N_2 concentration and flow measurements are made until the concentration of N_2 is less than 1%. FRC is then given by the total volume of N_2 washed out divided by the fall in the percentage of N_2 from the start to the end of the test.

A theoretical disadvantage of the helium dilution technique is that the value of FRC is determined at the *end* of the test when expiratory resistance due to the rebreathing circuit may have artificially increased FRC; whereas in the nitrogen wash-out technique the value of FRC is determined at the *start* of the test. In fact, comparison of the two methods has shown them to produce similar results.

Breathing pattern

In many critically ill patients, breathing *pattern* is of greater interest than lung volumes *per se*. Abnormalities of respiratory frequency and tidal volume are common and in several studies an elevated respiratory frequency has been shown to predict an adverse outcome. In a case-controlled study of patients discharged from the ICU, respiratory frequency and haematocrit were the only continuous variables that predicted re-admission to the ICU, with a resulting high mortality.[20] Tidal volume, respiratory frequency and minute volume are easy to measure in intubated patients and the values are continuously displayed on all modern ventilators.

Compliance

Compliance of the respiratory system (C_{rs}) is reduced (made stiffer) in conditions such as pulmonary fibrosis that affect the lungs or respiratory muscle weakness, where the change is more in chest-wall elasticity (the reciprocal of compliance). Of particular relevance in the ICU, is the fact that compliance is reduced by increases in pulmonary venous pressure or in alveolar oedema, acute respiratory distress syndrome (ARDS) and pneumonia. Total respiratory system compliance is made up of lung, chest-wall and abdominal components and, in some conditions, such as intra-abdominal sepsis, the fall in abdominal compliance is very significant.

C_{rs} is the change in lung volume (ΔV) produced per unit change in recoil pressure across the respiratory system (ΔP_{rs}): $C_{rs} = \Delta V/\Delta P_{rs}$. The measurement of compliance may be useful, particularly when assessing the response to therapeutic interventions, and several methods exist.

MEASUREMENT OF STATIC COMPLIANCE DURING MECHANICAL VENTILATION

Compliance is measured at zero airflow so that changes in pressure reflect changes in elastic recoil of the lung and chest wall and are not influenced by airway resistance, which will increase the driving pressure required to generate a given airflow. Accurate compliance measurements require total relaxation of the inspiratory and expiratory muscles, making it one of the few tests that is more readily performed in the ICU than in the lung function laboratory! It should be noted that distensible ventilator tubing may contribute significantly to the measured compliance, particularly in those with abnormally stiff lungs.

Rapid airway occlusion technique

After ensuring that the patient is relaxed and only occasionally triggering the ventilator, a series of end-inspiratory airway occlusions is made at different inflation volumes from end-expiratory lung volumes (EELV) to EELV + 1000 mL. Between each test breath, normal ventilation is resumed. Different inflation volumes may be achieved by changing the respiratory frequency, with the inflation volume being derived from integration of the flow signal using a pneumotachograph connected to a differential pressure transducer inserted between the ventilator circuit and the endotracheal tube. When the airway is occluded (by pressing the expiratory hold button on the ventilator at end inflation), the pressure at the airway opening (Pao) rises to a peak and then plateaus at a pressure equal to alveolar pressure P2, as shown in Figure 1.6. This plateau pressure less the sum of intrinsic and extrinsic PEEP represents the elastic recoil of the respiratory system at end inflation, Prs. Equilibration is usually complete within 3 s, although it may take longer with airflow limitation. This method is derived from the 'super-syringe' method, in which lung inflation is carried out in 100-mL increments using a large, calibrated syringe during a prolonged apnoea, and Prs is determined in the same way.

The inspiratory pressure–volume curve can then be constructed by plotting volume against the corresponding static Pao (see the inspiratory limb of

Fig. 1.9). Compliance is given by the gradient of the *linear* portion of the curve, which tends to be between FRC and FRC + 500 mL in normal patients. Within this range (expanding pressure of about −2 to −10 cmH$_2$O), the lung is remarkably distensible (very compliant) at around 0.2 L/cmH$_2$O. At extremes of lung volume, compliance is reduced, as reflected by flattening of the pressure–volume curve. At high lung volume this is due to increased inwards elastic recoil and at volumes below FRC it is attributed to increased outwards elastic recoil of the chest wall and increased airway closure. It is over the linear portion of the pressure–volume curve that most efficient ventilation takes place, with the greatest change in lung volume for a given applied pressure.

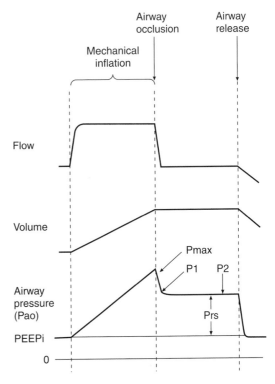

Figure 1.6 *Representation of flow, volume and airway opening pressure (Pao) for determination of compliance and resistance in a mechanically ventilated patient using the rapid airway occlusion technique. Following a constant inspiratory flow, the airway is occluded at end-inspiration. Pao falls rapidly from a peak (Pmax) to P1, and more slowly to a plateau, P2. The elastic recoil of the respiratory system is given by (P2 − PEEP). Prs, respiratory system pressure.*

Pulse method[21]

As with the rapid occlusion method, flow is measured using a pneumotachograph positioned either attached to the ETT or integral to the ventilator. Transthoracic pressure is taken as the difference between mouth pressure measured at the proximal pneumotachograph port and atmospheric pressure (Pao). The ventilator is adjusted to deliver a constant rate of airflow, $\dot{V}$. When inflation begins, the pressure tracing shows an initial step rise related to the flow resistance of the subject, followed by a section with a slower rise and a constant slope, $(Pao)_{slope}$. Compliance is then given by $C_{rs} = \dot{V}/(Pao)_{slope}$ where $\dot{V}$ is measured in L/s and $(Pao)_{slope}$ in cmH$_2$O/s. This method has several advantages, the most important of which is its ability to be used in patients in assist modes of ventilation. The patient's respiratory effort is detected as an irregular flow tracing, and these breaths may be discarded from the analysis. Some ventilators have this method incorporated into the monitoring options. It is a method that has been shown to correlate well with values of C_{rs} obtained using the rapid airway occlusion method.

MEASUREMENT OF DYNAMIC COMPLIANCE

During spontaneous breathing, measurement of static compliance requires patient co-operation with a difficult technique and the equipment is not very portable. Measurement of *dynamic* compliance, C_{Dyn}, may, however, be carried out. The patient breathes either via a pneumotachograph to give volume or via a spirometer so that tidal volume (V_T) may be determined breath by breath. Continuous measurement of oesophageal pressure (P_{es}) as an estimate of pleural pressure is made using an oesophageal balloon. ΔP_{es} between points of zero airflow is determined breath by breath from end-inspiration to end-expiration, as an assumption is made that at these points there is complete respiratory muscle relaxation and that no airflow is present. Values are averaged over 10–15 breaths and dynamic compliance determined: $C_{Dyn} = V_T/\Delta P_{oes}$. For any given measurement of pleural pressure, the associated lung volume will be greater during expiration than during inspiration due to the hysteresis of the pressure–volume curve (see Fig. 1.7). This is due to the pressure required to overcome surface tension forces within the alveoli during inspiration. Dynamic compliance measurements should therefore be made during the expiratory phase. Dynamic compliance is unreliable in airflow obstruction, especially at higher respiratory frequencies, as airflow within the lungs may be present even when the airway is occluded.

TECHNIQUES USED TO DETERMINE COMPLIANCE

Super-syringe

Provides full pressure–volume curve during inflation and deflation, but:

(i) the patient is temporarily disconnected from the ventilator, changing both the previous volume history and the end-expiratory lung volume,

(ii) it is time consuming,

(iii) it fails to start the test from a P_{rs} equivalent to intrinsic PEEP,

(iv) continuing gas exchange during the manoeuvre reduces thoracic volume, causing an over-estimation of the hysteresis loop area,

(v) it usually requires a temporary increase in FiO$_2$, which may affect the curve due to the development of atelectasis,

(vi) measurement depends on the patient making no respiratory effort.

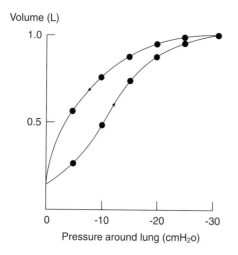

Volume (L)

Pressure around lung (cmH$_2$O)

Figure 1.7 *Pressure–volume curve of the lung during a respiratory cycle, illustrating hysteresis with a greater lung volume achieved for any given pressure during expiration than inspiration. (Reproduced from reference 39.)*

Rapid airway occlusion

Requires no additional equipment, the patient remains connected to the ventilator, it only interrupts ventilation during an inspiratory pause of 3–5 s and has minimal impact on gas exchange, but:

(i) the expiratory limb of the pressure–volume curve is less readily examined,

(ii) measurement depends on the patient making no respiratory effort.

Constant flow inflation or pulse method

Can be used in assist modes of ventilation and disconnection from the ventilator; intermittent airway occlusion or end-inspiratory pause is not necessary, but errors may arise if different time constants within the lung prevent a linear relationship between flow and transthoracic pressure.

Dynamic compliance

Requires an oesophageal balloon to be positioned, cannot be used in patients with airflow limitation because *within*-lung airflow is still present even at end-inspiration and end-expiration and relies on the assumption that respiratory muscles are completely relaxed during end-inspiration and end-expiration.

Intrinsic positive end-expiratory pressure

Intrinsic positive end-expiratory pressure (PEEP$_i$ or autoPEEP) is the presence of a positive alveolar pressure at the end of expiration (Fig. 1.8, (a) and (b)). Under these conditions, expiratory flow has not stopped before the next inspiration occurs, either during spontaneous or positive pressure ventilation. It may arise in three different circumstances:[22]

1. Insufficient Te to allow expiration to the equilibrium (relaxed) volume due to airflow obstruction and/or high ventilatory requirements.
2. Dynamic airway collapse and resulting flow limitation due to emphysema.
3. Continuing expiratory muscle contraction at end-expiration (often contributing to apparent Peep$_i$ although not normally assigned as a cause).

PEEP$_i$ increases inspiratory work during spontaneous breathing and reduces the ability to trigger the ventilator during assisted modes of ventilation as greater inspiratory effort is needed. These aspects may be overcome by applying external PEEP approximately equal to that of the patient's PEEP$_i$. Measurement of PEEP$_i$ may therefore be used to allow better synchrony of the machine with patient demand. It can also be employed to assess the response to bronchodilators. Values of up to 20 cmH$_2$O are not uncommon in asthma or COPD. Recognition of PEEP$_i$ and consideration of its aetiology are helpful. A patient with PEEP$_i$ due to airflow limitation and hyperinflation, for example, would potentially benefit from a prolonged expiratory time and application of extrinsic PEEP, whereas extrinsic PEEP applied to a patient with PEEP$_i$ due to expiratory muscle activation alone would merely increase the patient's work of breathing further.

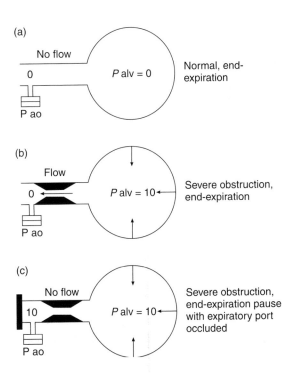

Figure 1.8 *Measurement of static PEEP$_i$. In the absence of airflow obstruction, alveolar pressure (P alv) at the end of expiration equals the pressure at the airway opening (P$_{ao}$) (a). With airflow obstruction, however, P alv is greater than P$_{ao}$ at end-expiration (b). This increase in P alv, static PEEP$_i$, may be measured from the airway pressure during an end-expiratory pause with the expiratory port occluded so P$_{ao}$ then equals P alv (c). (Reproduced from reference 40.)*

MEASUREMENT OF INTRINSIC POSITIVE END-EXPIRATORY PRESSURE

Static PEEP$_i$ can be measured by occluding the airway at the end of expiration, with the resulting plateau pressure representing the average PEEP$_i$ present within the non-homogeneous lung (Fig. 1.8 (c)). This method is automatically available on some commercial ventilators, but requires the absence of expiratory effort otherwise a falsely high value will be recorded. A *dynamic* measurement of PEEP$_i$ can be obtained by recording the airway pressure at which inspiratory flow commences during inspiration (Fig. 1.9). Inspiratory flow commences only after airway pressure has exceeded the value of PEEP$_i$. This dynamic measurement reflects the lowest regional value of PEEP$_i$ and may be considerably less than static PEEP$_i$ in patients with airflow limitation and in those with significant pulmonary inhomogeneity. Measurements of PEEP$_i$ should be made without any external PEEP applied. This method can be applied in the non-intubated patient but, commonly, active expiration, e.g. in patients with airflow limitation, overestimates PEEP$_i$. This may be taken into account by measuring gastric and thus intra-abdominal pressure. The rise in gastric pressure may then be subtracted from the measured value of dynamic PEEP$_i$.

Airways resistance

Several factors apart from the elastic recoil of the lungs and chest wall must be overcome to move air in and out of the lungs, including the inertia of the respiratory system itself, frictional resistance at the lung–chest-wall interface, and chest-wall and pulmonary resistance. In most cases, pulmonary resistance is the only factor of significance, with 80% of this being attributable to airway resistance and the other 20% to resistance of the lung tissue itself. Greatest airflow resistance is present in medium-sized airways, as distal to this the increased resistance of individual airways is offset by their large number. Airway resistance falls with increasing lung volume (Fig. 1.10). This is in part due to increased traction on small airways lacking cartilaginous support pulling them open as lung elastic recoil increases during a large inspiration. Conversely, during a

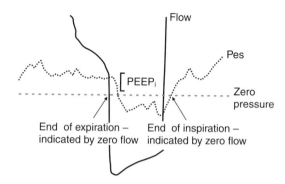

Figure 1.9 *Airflow and oesophageal pressure (Pes) in a patient with obstructive lung disease. Dynamic PEEP$_i$ is given by Pes at end-inspiration, as indicated by the point of zero airflow.*

forced expiration at low lung volumes, the positive pleural pressure is transmitted to the airways, which may be compressed or even collapse. Thus, airways resistance is significantly higher during active expiration due to *dynamic compression* of the airways.

CAUSES OF INCREASED RESPIRATORY SYSTEM RESISTANCE

Airways

- Reduced lung volumes
- Dynamic compression during expiration
- Increased flow rates
- Non-laminar airflow (e.g. in COPD)

Visco-elastic

- Pulmonary fibrosis
- Presence of oedema or areas of consolidation

Determination of airway resistance is useful when assessing the causes of high airway pressures during mechanical ventilation and the response to bronchodilators. Although increased airway resistance usually results from airflow limitation, it is also increased in ARDS or cardiogenic pulmonary oedema; this may reflect oedema in the airway wall and secretions within the airway lumen. An additional factor is a reduction in the number of patent airways due to the marked loss of functional lung volume.

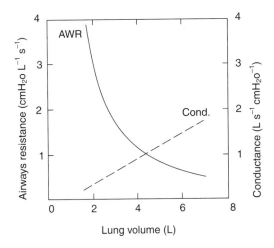

Figure 1.10 *Increase in airways resistance with decreasing lung volume. There is a linear relationship between the reciprocal of airway resistance (conductance) and lung volume. (Reproduced from reference 39.)*

During *laminar* airflow, the relationship between pressure difference (P), flow ($\dot{V}$) and resistance (R) is: $P = \dot{V}R$, so:

$$R = P / \dot{V}$$

and Poiseuille's law applies: resistance being related to viscosity of the air (η), length (l) and radius (r) of the tube:

$$R = 8\eta l/\pi r^4$$

Thus, doubling the length of an endotracheal tube would *double* the resistance to airflow, whereas halving its radius would increase the resistance *16-fold*. The resistance posed by an endotracheal tube is usually not clinically significant, but may be considerable at high levels of minute ventilation or with short inspiratory times.

Increasing flow rates, diameter of the tube and increased gas density all predispose to turbulent flow. During *turbulent* flow a much greater driving pressure is then required to generate the same flow:

$$P \propto / \dot{V}^2 R$$

DETERMINATION OF AIRWAYS RESISTANCE

In the ventilated patient, resistance may be determined with the rapid airway occlusion technique as described for the assessment of static compliance. Before the end of a mechanical inflation with constant inspiratory flow, $\dot{V}$, the airway opening is occluded temporarily until a plateau in airway pressure is achieved (by pressing the expiratory hold knob). The peak airway pressure (P_{max}) falls rapidly to a lower value, $P1$, and then more slowly to a plateau pressure, $P2$, as illustrated in Figure 1.6. Maximum respiratory resistance ($Rtot_{max}$) is then given by $Rtot_{max} = (P_{max} - P2)/\dot{V}$ and minimum respiratory resistance, R_{min} is given by $Rtot_{min} = (P_{max} - P1)/\dot{V}$.

$Rtot_{min}$ represents the instantaneous resistance of the respiratory system, mainly representing the *airway resistance*. $Rtot_{max}$ also reflects the component attributable to time constant inequalities within the respiratory system, and to visco-elastic pressure dissipation within the thoracic tissues. It should be borne in mind that resistance of the respiratory tubing and ETT will contribute towards the values of resistance obtained. Although pre-determined values of *in-vitro* ETT resistance may be subtracted, it has been demonstrated that *in-vivo* values are higher.[23]

Work of breathing

The work of breathing may be increased for a variety of reasons, some of which may co-exist. Lung or abdominal compliance may be reduced, the chest wall may be stiff or airway resistance may be increased. During mechanical ventilation, the work of breathing is more in the assist than control modes, because the patient makes effort in triggering breaths. It will also be increased when there is poor patient–ventilator synchronization. The work of breathing is rarely clinically quantified, but appreciation of workload is useful when excessive or when predicting weaning from ventilation.

A number of methods have been used. For example, the O_2 *consumption* of the respiratory muscles can be measured. In normal subjects, it is less than 5% of total O_2 consumption; with voluntary hyperventilation, it is possible to increase this to 30%. In some patients, the O_2 cost of breathing is a limiting factor on exercise performance. In spontaneously breathing subjects in whom an oesophageal balloon has been positioned, the work of breathing is proportional to the magnitude of negative intrathoracic pressure and the length of time for which it is maintained. Thus, if oesophageal pressure is plotted against time, the area under the curve, termed the **pressure–time product**, is proportional to the work of breathing (Fig. 1.11). Care is required when using this method to pinpoint the beginning of each inspiratory effort with the externally set PEEP as the reference point (rather than zero pressure). This measurement is less meaningful during assisted ventilation because, with positive pressure ventilation, the normal negative pressure swings are reversed during inspiration, whereas with negative pressure support, the normal pressure swings will be augmented as less work is actually performed by the respiratory muscles. An alternative method is to use the **diaphragmatic EMG**, although this requires specialist expertise.

Examination of the **airway pressure contour** in a ventilator-dependent patient can provide useful information on the activity of the patient's respiratory muscles.[24] During mechanical ventilation, the work of breathing is given by the product of pressure across the respiratory system (i.e. from alveolus to atmosphere) and inflating volume. Thus, if Pao is plotted against lung volume, the work of breathing is given by the area under the curve. Computerized bedside monitoring is available for automated determination of the work of breathing using this method.[25] In control mode with the patient fully relaxed, the area under the pressure–volume curve indicates the work carried out by the ventilator to expand the chest. The additional work of breathing carried out by the patient in assist mode is given by the difference between the area under the pressure–volume curve in assist and control modes. A high work of breathing as assessed using this method

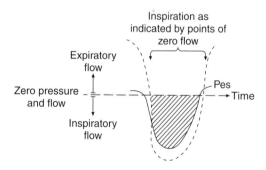

Figure 1.11 *The pressure–time product during inspiration, as indicated by the hatched area, is an indicator of the work of breathing. Points of zero flow are required to define the start and end of inspiration. Pes, oesophageal pressure. (Figure courtesy of Dr N Hart, Muscle Laboratory, The Royal Brompton Hospital, London, UK.)*

may be an indicator of poor patient–ventilator synchronization, and may arise when the inspiratory flow is too low. This typically occurs with high respiratory rates or drive, e.g. in asthma. The phenomenon is called flow deprivation. Some ventilators have the capability of detecting flow deprivation and will automatically increase flow rate to compensate.

RESPIRATORY DRIVE AND CONTROL

Background

In health there is remarkable constancy of arterial CO_2, and ventilation is matched breath by breath to metabolic CO_2 load. Many central and peripheral stimuli influence respiratory drive, which in turn lead to changes in ventilation. One way of evaluating the function of the respiratory control system is to observe the change in output, e.g. minute ventilation in relation to a given input such as an increase in $PaCO_2$. There is, however, considerable redundancy in the system. At the onset of exercise, for example, the sum of the increase in ventilation expected from each of a number of sensory inputs equates to more than is observed in reality. Central integration of these input parameters is complex and in critically ill patients becomes even more so. Increased drive may arise from factors such as sepsis, circulating cytokines or pulmonary afferent stimulation, whereas decreased drive may arise from sedatives/opiates or brain injury. In addition, the normal control mechanisms are disrupted, with time delays between the patient initiating a breath and gas flow from the ventilator, potential poor matching of ventilatory support to the patient's demands and, in heart failure, delay in the circulation time between lung and chemoreceptors. The aim of this section is to highlight a number of ways in which respiratory control may be affected in critically ill patients and the methods of assessment available.

The respiratory centres and CNS input

INTRINSIC RHYTHM GENERATION

Neurons located within the pons and medulla of the brainstem form the respiratory centres. They are responsible for the generation of periodic inspiration and expiration, the nature of which is modified depending upon inputs from elsewhere. Various groups of neurons with discrete functions have been described within the respiratory centre. One view is that, within the medulla, a dorsal or ventral respiratory group is responsible for inspiration and expiration respectively. Cells of the **inspiratory area** have the property of intrinsic periodic firing and are responsible for the basic rhythm of ventilation. Bursts of action potentials result in nervous impulses to the diaphragm and other inspiratory muscles. The intrinsic rhythm pattern of the inspiratory area starts with a latent period of several seconds, during which there is no activity. Action potentials then begin to appear, increasing in a crescendo ramp, over the next few seconds. During this time, inspiratory muscle activity progressively increases. Finally, the inspiratory action potentials cease and inspiratory muscle tone falls.

MODIFICATION OF THE INTRINSIC RHYTHM

This inspiratory ramp can be 'turned off' prematurely by inhibitory impulses from the **pneumotaxic centre**, thereby shortening inspiratory time and increasing respiratory frequency. The **expiratory area** is quiescent during normal quiet breathing as exhalation occurs by **passive** recoil of the lungs and chest wall to their equilibrium position at FRC. On more forceful breathing, for example in a patient with increased airway resistance or during exercise in a normal subject, activity of the expiratory cells results in active expiration.

An **apneustic centre** in the lower pons has an excitatory effect on the inspiratory area of the medulla, tending to prolong the ramp action potentials. In some types of brain injury, an abnormal breathing pattern is seen in which prolonged inspiratory gasps are interrupted by transient expiratory efforts due to damage to the apneustic centre. A **pneumotaxic centre** in the upper pons appears to 'switch off' or inhibit inspiration, thereby fine-tuning inspiratory volume and rate.

During wakefulness, volitional influences are important and the cortex can override the function of the brainstem within limits, e.g. during voluntary hyperventilation or speech. In the ventilated patient, sedatives/opiates are commonly used to reduce cortical drive. Anxiety or pain alters the pattern of breathing via the limbic system and hypothalamus and may make it difficult to match ventilator and patient, particularly if assist modes rather than pressure support are being employed.

Central chemoreceptors

The central chemoreceptors are situated near the ventral surface of the medulla in the vicinity of the exit of cranial nerves IX and X and have been separated into rostral and caudal areas on each side. They stimulate breathing in response to an increase in brain extracellular hydrogen ions. The composition of cerebrospinal fluid (CSF) is governed by the activity of the blood–brain barrier (important in making adjustments over days to weeks), whereas brain ECF is primarily affected by cerebral metabolism and cerebral blood flow, the latter leading to virtually instantaneous adjustments of ECF pH with changes in arterial PCO_2 as molecular CO_2 diffuses readily across the blood-brain barrier. The precise location of the sensors is not known. Thus, the CO_2 level in blood regulates ventilation chiefly by its effect on the pH of brain ECF, and the resulting hyperventilation reduces $PaCO_2$ in the blood and therefore in brain ECF and bulk CSF.

In the presence of CO_2 retention, the expected CSF acidosis is compensated for by homeostatic adjustments, mediated by the blood–brain barrier, and simultaneous renal retention of bicarbonate ions. Thus, in chronic hypercapnia, the CSF pH is normal, with a consequent low minute ventilation for a given $PaCO_2$. This may be advantageous in reducing the work of breathing, but it may slow weaning from a ventilator or increase the risk of nocturnal hypoventilation in the spontaneously breathing patient. An example of this phenomenon is illustrated in Figure 1.12, which shows the hypercapnic ventilatory response breath by breath of a patient with chronic, stable hypercapnic respiratory failure. Before nocturnal non-invasive ventilation (closed circles), there is marked blunting of the ventilatory response. Following a period of nocturnal non-invasive ventilation, there is an increase in the ventilatory response to CO_2. During this period, the patient's daytime arterial blood gases improved ($PaCO_2$ and PaO_2 before ventilation were 6.3 and 9.7 kPa respectively, and after ventilation 5.74 and 10.6 kPa). Much of this increase in ventilatory drive is due to adjustments in bicarbonate and pH (arterial HCO_2^- and H^+ before ventilation = 31.2 and 36.4 mM L^{-1}, and after ventilation = 27.9 and 37.2 mM L^{-1}).

Peripheral chemoreceptors

These are located in the carotid bodies at the bifurcation of the common carotid arteries and in the aortic bodies above and below the aortic arch. The carotid chemoreceptors are the most important in humans. They are stimulated by a decrease in arterial O_2 and pH or an increase in CO_2. There is a relatively small increase in firing rate of the carotid sinus nerve as PaO_2 is decreased from hyperoxia to normoxia and then an exponential increase with the inflection point around 8.0 kPa. The peripheral chemoreceptors are the only receptors to increase ventilation in response to hypoxia and, in their absence, hypoxaemia *depresses* ventilation due to a central inhibitory effect.

In health, $PaCO_2$ is maintained almost constant (±0.4 kPa or 3 mmHg). In other words, the 'error signal' in the control system is so small as to be negligible. This remarkable control is achieved by the rapid response of the peripheral chemoreceptors to oscillations in $PaCO_2$ generated as CO_2 rises within alveoli during expiration, which then falls during inspiration as fresh air is drawn into the lungs. The rate of rise of the $PaCO_2$ oscillation is directly proportional to metabolic CO_2 load, making it a suitable signal for respiratory control.[26] Indeed, modification of the $PaCO_2$ oscillation profile using inspiratory CO_2 pulses delivered either early in inspiration or after a small delay results in a greater increase in ventilation with the early pulses, despite the same mean $PaCO_2$ in both instances.[27] In chronic obstructive airways disease, there is damping of the $PaCO_2$ oscillation, an effect most pronounced in emphysematous patients. Those in whom $PaCO_2$ oscillations are most damped have the highest $PaCO_2$ levels, probably reflecting the severity of their disease and reduced ventilatory drive secondary to damping of $PaCO_2$ oscillations.

In normal subjects given a CO_2 mixture to breathe, only 20% of the increase in ventilation is attributable to the peripheral arterial chemoreceptors. In simple terms, one could regard the central chemoreceptors as providing most of the *drive* to breathe, whereas the peripheral chemoreceptors provide fine precision *control* of breathing.

Cheyne–Stokes respiration

An exception to the rule of tight respiratory control arises in **Cheyne–Stokes respiration**, in which periods of apnoea of 10–20 s alternate with periods of hyperventilation of equal duration. In the critically ill, Cheyne–Stokes respiration is often a poor prognostic indicator. Factors predisposing to Cheyne–Stokes respiration include low end-tidal PCO_2, high chemoreflex sensitivity, increased chemoreflex time and low alveolar lung volume. Thus, a low cardiac output or hypoxia predisposes to periodicity of breathing.

Carbon dioxide retention during oxygen supplementation

Chronically hypercapnic patients may retain CO_2 on delivery of supplementary O_2. Four mechanisms have been proposed to explain this phenomenon.

1. Removal of the hypoxic ventilatory drive by oxygen supplementation in patients who have increased dependence on this respiratory drive due to reduced ventilatory sensitivity to CO_2. Reduced sensitivity to CO_2 may be attributable to a tendency to normalize CSF and arterial pH despite persistent hypercapnia, as described in the section on central chemoreceptors.

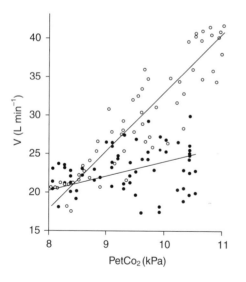

Figure 1.12 *Graph to show a part of the hypercapnic ventilatory response curve during CO_2 re-breathing breath by breath, in a subject with chronic, stable hypercapnic respiratory failure before (closed circles) and several days after (open circles) commencing nocturnal non-invasive ventilation.*

2. Reversal of hypoxic pulmonary vasoconstriction in poorly ventilated areas of the lung leading to increased physiological shunting and so $\dot{V}:\dot{Q}$ mismatching.
3. Increased ratio of dead space to tidal volume ($V_D:V_T$), e.g. due to a change in breathing pattern with an increase in respiratory frequency:V_T, or dilation of proximal airways.
4. Loss of $PaCO_2$ oscillations reducing peripheral chemoreceptor ventilatory drive.

There is no agreement among studies as to which is the predominant mechanism, possibly reflecting genuine differences in patients. In one study of patients with an acute exacerbation of COPD given 100% O_2 to breathe, ventilation was depressed in CO_2 retainers but not in those who did not retain CO_2,[28] giving support to theory (1). Reversal of hypoxic pulmonary vasoconstriction, as indicated by the ventilation:perfusion dispersion ratio, occurred to an equal degree in both CO_2 retainers and non-retainers, suggesting that this was not an important mechanism. In another study of patients during remission, however, supplementary O_2 resulted in a substantial increase in $PaCO_2$ with minimal change in ventilation, suggesting predominance of changes in $\dot{V}Q$ matching or $V_D:V_T$.[29]

Other receptors influencing respiratory control

A number of pulmonary afferents project centrally by way of the cervical vagus nerves, such as **pulmonary stretch receptors** and **lung epithelial irritant receptors,** and these modulate the ventilatory response to CO_2 and hypoxia. Vagal inhibition using cooling of the vagal nerves in anaesthetized rabbits has been shown to stimulate ventilation during modest hypercapnia (shifting to the left and steepening of the hypercapnic ventilatory response curve), but to inhibit ventilation during more intense hypercapnia (flattening of the hypercapnic ventilatory response curve). In humans, pulmonary stretch receptors are likely to be of greater importance in newborn babies than in adults. **Juxta-capillary receptors**, lying in the alveolar walls, result in rapid, shallow breathing during moderate stimulation and in apnoea during intense stimulation. There is evidence that engorgement of pulmonary capillaries and increases in the interstitial fluid volume stimulate these receptors.

They may therefore play a role in the rapid, shallow breathing and dyspnoea associated with heart failure and interstitial infiltration. **Joint and muscle receptors** are likely to be of most importance in increasing ventilation in the early stages of exercise. Many muscles contain **muscle spindles** that sense elongation of the muscle. This information is used to control the strength of contraction. These receptors may be involved in the sensation of dyspnoea that occurs when unusually large respiratory efforts are required to move the lung and chest wall, for example because of airway obstruction. An increase in arterial blood pressure can cause reflex hypoventilation or apnoea through stimulation of the **aortic and carotid sinus baroreceptors**. Conversely, a decrease in blood pressure may result in hyperventilation and a sensation of air hunger. The pathways of these reflexes are largely unknown. Other afferent nerves can bring about changes in ventilation: pain may cause a period of apnoea followed by hyperventilation, and heating of the skin may result in hyperventilation.

Assessment of ventilatory drive

This is of most use when assessing the continued need for ventilatory support. Measurement is made during a period of spontaneous breathing and compared with the value after a period of unsupported breathing.

ARTERIAL BLOOD GASES

The measurement of alveolar or arterial PCO_2 gives a better indication of the normality, or otherwise, of alveolar ventilation than does formal measurement of minute ventilation. In the presence of hypoxia, $PaCO_2$ will be reduced in a predictable fashion.[30]

THE HYPERCAPNIC VENTILATORY RESPONSE

In normal subjects, *minute ventilation* gives an adequate reflection of respiratory drive, but mechanical constraints, e.g. airflow obstruction, may limit ventilation and so other indicators of drive need to be considered. If there is a defect at any stage in the output chain from the ventilatory centres down, transformation into ventilation will be impaired.[31]

Changes in pleural pressure: $P_{0.1}$ and $\delta P_{OesMax}/\delta t$

The oesophageal occlusion pressure, i.e. the oesophageal pressure at 100 ms during an inspiratory attempt against a closed airway at functional residual capacity $P_{0.1}$, has been proposed as a more reliable indicator of drive in airflow obstruction. $P_{0.1}$ has been used within the ICU to:

- assess respiratory centre output while changing the fraction of inspired O_2,[32]
- predict weaning outcome (values of $P_{0.1} \le 6$ cmH$_2$O suggest that discontinuation of mechanical ventilation is likely to be unsuccessful, whereas values of ≤ 4 cmH$_2$O predict success),[33]
- set the appropriate level of assisted ventilation[34] and pressure support.[35]

Technical difficulties determining the true onset of inspiratory muscle activity from pressure data may reduce the reliability of this technique. The maximum rate of change of oesophageal pressure, $\delta P_{OesMax}/\delta t$, has been proposed as an alternative to $P_{0.1}$ and has been shown to have a good correlation with end-tidal pressure ($P_{et}CO_2$) in normal subjects during CO_2 rebreathing and with walk time during an exhaustive exercise test in patients with COPD.[36]

Diaphragmatic EMG

High values of $P_{0.1}$ and $\delta P_{OesMax}/\delta t$ always indicate high ventilatory drive. *Low* values may indicate low drive, a defect of the phrenic nerves or muscle weakness. For instance, in severe COPD, hyperinflation may render the diaphragm so mechanically disadvantaged that there is *functional* weakness and it is no longer capable of generating high inspiratory pressures. $P_{0.1}$ and $\delta P_{OesMax}/\delta t$ will therefore both be reduced for a given central drive. However, drive may be examined by an oesophageal electrode to measure diaphragmatic EMG.

BREATHING PATTERN AND ACCESSORY RESPIRATORY MUSCLE USE

Patients in whom the work of breathing is increased or respiratory muscle strength decreased often compensate by adopting a shallow breathing pattern with increased respiratory frequency. It should be borne in mind that measures that do not take into account respiratory frequency, such as $P_{0.1}$ and $P_{OesMax}/\delta t$ will give a less accurate reflection of drive. Ventilatory drive is particularly difficult to assess in patients with respiratory muscle weakness: output cannot be seen as flow, intrathoracic pressure change or muscle tension as these are all below points on the output chain where the problem is. The diaphragmatic EMG may be distinctly abnormal due to the disease process itself. In these patients, other clues, such as respiratory frequency and detection of activity of respiratory muscles not normally used in quiet breathing (neck accessory muscles, shoulder girdle muscles and abdominal muscles), all assume greater importance.

CONCLUSION

In conclusion, imbalance of the load and capacity of the respiratory muscle pump may result in ventilatory failure. The clinician must be alert to the possibility of respiratory muscle pump overload in patients with a persistent requirement for mechanical ventilation. Strategies to assess the load on the pump and its capacity have been outlined, but further research is needed to determine the prevalence, causes and magnitude of respiratory muscle pump dysfunction. Automated assessment of many aspects of pulmonary mechanics has undoubtedly moved it from a predominant research tool into the clinical field. Intuitively, an appreciation of pulmonary mechanics, with carefully tailored ventilatory strategies, should decrease the work of breathing and so improve outcome. However, further studies are required in this area. It is hoped that future work may lead to the development of 'intelligent ventilators', which assess and respond to the work of breathing undertaken by the patient throughout each breath and are sufficiently specific that they are able to recognize activities such as swallowing or talking.

REFERENCES

1. Polkey, MI, Lyall, RA, Green, M, Leigh, PN, Moxham, J. Expiratory muscle function in amyotrophic lateral sclerosis. *Am J Respir Crit Care Med* 1998; **158**: 734–41.
2. Gibson, G. Diaphragmatic paresis: pathophysiology, clinical features and investigation. *Thorax* 1989; **44**: 960–70.

3. Parthasarathy, S, Jubran, A, Tobin, MJ. Cycling of inspiratory and expiratory muscle groups with the ventilator in airflow limitation. *Am J Respir Crit Care Med* 1998; **158**: 1471–8.

4. Polkey, M, Lyall, R, Moxham, J, Leigh, P. Respiratory aspects of neurological disease. *J Neurol Neurosurg Psychiatry* 1999; **66**: 5–15.

5. Quera-Salva, MA, Guilleminault, C, Chevret, S, *et al.* Breathing disorders during sleep in myasthenia gravis. *Ann Neurol* 1992; **31**: 86–92.

6. Polkey, MI, Kyroussis, D, Hamnegard, CH, *et al.* Diaphragm strength in chronic obstructive pulmonary disease. *Am J Respir Crit Care Med* 1996; **154**(5): 1310–17.

7. Moxham, J, Goldstone, J. Assessment of respiratory muscle strength in the intensive care unit. *Eur Respir J* 1994; **7**: 2057–61.

8. Gabor JY, Cooper, AB, Hanly, PJ. Sleep disruption in the intensive care unit. *Curr Opin Crit Care* 2001; **7**: 21–7.

9. Resta, O, Guido, P, Foschino-Barbaro, MP, *et al.* Sleep-related breathing disorders in acute respiratory failure assisted by non-invasive ventilatory treatment: utility of portable polysomnographic system. *Respir Med* 2000; **94**(2): 128–34.

10. Spitzer, AR, Giancarlo, T., Maher, L, Awerbuch, G. Neuromuscular causes of prolonged ventilator dependency. *Muscle Nerve* 1992; **15**: 682–6.

11. Coakley, JH, Nagendran, K, Honavar, M, Hind, SJ. Preliminary observations on the neuromuscular abnormalities in patients with organ failure and sepsis. *Intensive Care Med* 1993; **19**: 323–8.

12. Deconinck, N, Van Parijs, V, Bleeckers-Bleukx, G, Van den Bergh, P. Critical illness myopathy unrelated to corticosteroids or neuromuscular blocking agents. *Neuromusc Dis* 1998; **8**: 186–92.

13. Leitjen, FSS, de Weerd, AW, Poortvliet, DCJ, *et al.* Critical illness polyneuropathy in multiple organ dysfunction syndrome and weaning from the ventilator. *Intensive Care Med* 1996; **22**: 856–61.

14. DeJonghe, B, Cook, DJ, Outin, H. Risk factors for polyneuropathy of critical illness. In *1999 yearbook of intensive care and emergency medicine,* J-L Vincent, ed. Springer: Berlin, 1999: 322–30.

15. Bolton, CF. Sepsis and the systemic inflammatory response syndrome: neuromuscular manifestations. *Crit Care Med* 1996; **24**: 1408–16.

16. Polkey, MI, Duguet, A, Luo, Y, *et al.* Anterior magnetic phrenic nerve stimulation: laboratory and clinical evaluation. *Intensive Care Med* 2000; **8**: 1065–75.

17. Luo, YM, Lyall, RA, Harris, ML, *et al.* Quantification of the esophageal diaphragm EMG with magnetic phrenic nerve stimulation. *Am J Respir Crit Care Med* 1999; **160**(5 P+ 1): 1629–34.

18. Rieder, P, Louis, M., Jollliet, P, Chevrolet, J. The repeated measurement of vital capacity is a poor indicator of the need for mechanical ventilation in myasthenia gravis. *Intensive Care Med* 1995; **21**: 663–8.

19. Numa, AH, Newth, CJL. Assessment of lung function in the intensive care unit. *Pediatr Pulmonol* 1995; **19**: 118–28.

20. Durbin, C, Kopel, R. A case-control study of patients readmitted to the intensive care unit. *Crit Care Med* 1993; **21**: 1547–53.

21. Suratt, PM, Owens, D. A pulse method for measuring respiratory system compliance in ventilated patients. *Chest* 1981; **80**: 34–8.

22. Marini, JJ. Should PEEP be used in airflow obstruction? *Am Rev Respir Dis* 1989; **140**: 1–3.

23. Conti, G, Blasi, RAD, Lappa, A, *et al.* Evaluation of respiratory system resistance in mechanically ventilated patients: the role of the endotracheal tube. *Intensive Care Med* 1994; **20**: 421–4.

24. Marini, JJ, Capps, JS, Culver, BH. The inspiratory work of breathing during assisted mechanical ventilation. *Chest* 1985; **87**(5): 612–18.

25. Banner, M, Jaeger, M, Kirby, R. Components of the work of breathing and implications for monitoring ventilator-dependent patients. *Crit Care Med* 1994; **22**(3): 515–23.

26. Band, D, Wolff, C, Ward, J, Cochrance, G, Prior, J. Respiratory oscillations in arterial in carbon-dioxide tension as a control signal in exercise. *Nature* 1980; **283**: 84–5.

27. Datta, AK, Nickol, AH. Dynamic chemoreceptiveness studied in man during moderate exercise breath by breath. *Adv Exp Med Biol* (US) 1995; **393**: 235–8.

28. Robinson, TD, Freiberg, DB, Regnis, JA, Young, IH. The role of hypoventilation and ventilation-perfusion redistribution in O_2-induced hypercapnia during acute exacerbations of chronic obstructive pulmonary disease. Am J Respir *Crit Care Med* 2000; **161**: 1524–9.

29. Dick, C, Liu, N, Sassoon, C, Berry, R, Mahutte, C. O_2 induced changes in ventilation and ventilatory drive in COPD. *Am J Respir Crit Care Med* 1997; **155**: 609–14.

30. Wolff, C. The control of ventilation in hypoxia I. *The Newsletter of the International Society for Mountain Medicine* 1997; **8**(1): 3–5.

31. Whitelaw, W. Assessment of output of the respiratory controller. *Semin Respir Crit Care Med* 1998; **19**(4): 361–5.

32. Aubier, M, Murciano, D, Fournier, M, *et al.* Central respiratory drive in acute respiratory failure patients

with chronic obstructive pulmonary disease. *Am Rev Respir Dis* 1980; **122**: 191–9.

33. Murciano, D, Boczkowski, J, Lecocguic, Y, *et al.* Tracheal occlusion pressure: a simple index to monitor respiratory muscle fatigue during acute respiratory failure in patients with chronic obstructive pulmonary disease. *Ann Intern Med* 1988; **108**: 800–5.

34. Sassoon, C, Mahutte, C, Simmons, D, Light, R. Work of breathing and airway occlusion pressure during assist-mode mechanical ventilation. *Chest* 1988; **3** : 571–6.

35. Alberti, A, Gallo, F, Fongaro, A, Valentia, S, Rossi, A. P0.1 is a useful parameter in setting the level of pressure support ventilation. *Intensive Care Med* 1995; **21**: 547–53.

36. Hamnegard, CH, Polkey, MI, Kyroussis, D, *et al.* Maximum rate of change in oesophageal pressure assessed from unoccluded breaths: an option where P0.1 is impractical. *Eur Resp J* 1998; **12**: 693–7.

37. Green, M. Respiratory muscle testing. *Bull Eur Physiopathol* 1984; **20**: 433–6.

38. Polkey, MI, Hamnegard, CH, Hughes, PD, *et al.* Influence of acute lung volume change on contractile properties of the human diaphragm. *J Appl Physiol* 1998; **85**: 1322–8.

39. West, J. *Respiratory physiology* – the essentials, 5th edn, PA Coryell, ed. Baltimore: Williams & Wilkins; 1990.

40. Hughes, J, Pride, N. *Physiological principles and clinical applications*. WB Saunders; 1999.

2

Mechanical ventilation: the basics

JOHN C GOLDSTONE

INTRODUCTION

Mechanical ventilation is used to replace or aid the work usually carried out by the respiratory muscles. As with any technology, several milestones were reached before its general introduction. Anaesthetists were adept at airway control, and intubation of the trachea was required to perform the complex head and neck surgery that resulted from the First World War. Advances in pulmonary physiology improved the understanding of gas exchange, and the introduction of neuromuscular paralysis enabled experience to be gained with positive pressure ventilation to facilitate thoracic surgery.

Surprisingly, the event that precipitated the widespread introduction into clinical practice of devices to ventilate the lungs did not originate in the operating theatre, but was an outbreak of paralytic polio in Scandinavia in the 1950s. It is fortunate that the acute onset of respiratory muscle paralysis presented the simplest scenario for a ventilator to perform, to take the place of the respiratory muscles and push gas into the chest with underlying normal lungs.[1] There was an urgent need for new technology. At the height of the outbreak, medical students were working in 2-hour shifts performing ventilation by hand using simple breathing circuits for many days at a time. New cases overwhelmed the capacity of the acute hospitals. A transfer of technology from industry to medicine occurred with a speed of development that would be unlikely to be possible today. What emerged were devices that were robust and simple. Indeed, for many years these original characteristics applied to most ventilators.

Important events in the 1960s and 1970s changed the potential for ventilation. First, the flow of gas delivered to the patient was controlled directly from a valve that could be opened and shut rapidly. Second, the control of the valve was via a microprocessor. Flow volume and pressure were measured in inspiration and expired gas. The aperture of the valve was controlled by feedback from the flow and volume sensors, and this could be adjusted in milliseconds. The advent of this form of technology enabled the ventilator to be controlled in a myriad of different ways.

Although modern ventilators are capable of generating complex ventilatory modes, they are of a very simple conceptual design (Fig. 2.1). A source of high-pressure air and oxygen (O_2) is connected to a blender by a solenoid valve, the flow from which is controlled by a microprocessor. The operator pre-sets the characteristics of the inspiratory and expiratory phase of the ventilator. By constantly checking measured parameters such as flow, volume and pressure, the ventilator delivers the breath to the patient.

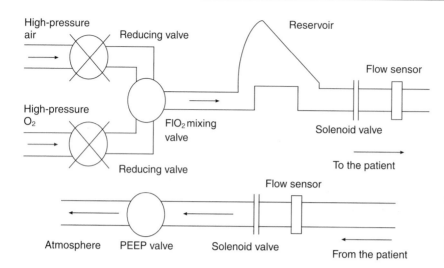

Figure 2.1 *A simplified diagram of a modern ventilator. Sensors that measure flow and pressure control the position of the solenoid valve in the form of a feedback loop.*

The ventilator may be used to perform the normal work of breathing when either the respiratory muscles are weak or the motor nerve function is compromised. Additionally, despite normal respiratory muscles and motor output, when the work involved in breathing is raised, ventilation can be used to perform some of the excessive work.

A simple task for the ventilator would be to provide a constant flow rate over a given time. The valve is therefore adjusted to ensure that the flow is not affected by changes in airway pressure. A more complex task is to provide a constant pressure over a given time period. In this case, the valve may need to be fully open at the beginning of inspiration to produce a constant pressure in the airway. Later on, the flow rate may have to be decreased substantially as soon as the target pressure is achieved, and flow rates may need to be increased or decreased rapidly. The ventilator has the ability to produce a variety of pressure waveforms by rapidly altering flow and sensing pressure. For example, an accelerating or decelerating pattern of inspiratory flow can be used to adjust peak airway pressure, and this feature is used when the lungs are stiff.

INDICATIONS FOR MECHANICAL VENTILATION

Mechanical ventilation is indicated where established or impending respiratory failure exists, which is defined as the inability of the breathing apparatus to maintain normal gas exchange. Mechanical ventilation is used most commonly following major surgery when haemodynamic variables are being normalized. The majority of ventilated patients are postoperative patients (>65% of all patients) who have had major surgery such as cardiac, aortic or neurosurgery and they rarely need mechanical ventilation for more than 24 hours (Table 2.1).[2] The other major groups requiring ventilation are patients with head or chest trauma (<10%), poisoning (<8%) and the critically ill with severe primary respiratory disease (<13%).

Table 2.1 *Main indication for mechanical ventilation in the adult*

Routine anaesthesia and post-operative management of major surgery

Respiratory impairment (parenchymal, airway or chest wall)
- Pneumonia, asthma, lung contusion
- Acute exacerbation in chronic bronchitis or emphysema
- Adult respiratory distress syndrome, cystic fibrosis
- Chest trauma with flail segment, ruptured diaphragm
- Chest wall burns, kyphoscoliosis

Central nervous system or neuro-muscular impairment
- Drug overdose: narcotics, anaesthetics, barbiturates
- Trauma, meningoencephalitis, tumours, infarction
- Brain oedema, raised intracranial pressure
- Intracranial bleed, status epilepticus, tetanus, rabies
- Central hypoventilation
- Polyneuritis, Guillain-Barre, Lambert-Eaton
- Myasthenia gravis, myopathies, paralysing poisons

Circulatory failure
- Cardiac arrest, severe shock (sepsis or other causes)
- Left ventricular failure (pulmonary oedema)

AIRWAY PRESSURE

Airway pressure is dependent on two main factors: how stiff the lungs are and the resistance to airflow.[3] As gas enters the lung, part of the pressure required overcomes flow resistance within the branching airways and part of the pressure is related to the elastic properties of the system (Fig. 2.2). The stiffness of the lungs and chest wall is the compliance of the respiratory system. Pressure is proportional to volume $\times$ 1/total compliance. Airway pressure is also proportional to the flow through the branching airways. Pressure is proportional to flow $\times$ resistance.

$$\text{Airway pressure} = (\text{volume} \times 1/\text{compliance}) + (\text{inspiratory flow} \times \text{resistance})$$

$$Paw = (V \times 1/Crs) + (\dot{V} \times R)$$

The relationship between airway pressure flow and compliance is known as the equation of motion and is expressed as three simultaneous graphs, of pressure, volume and flow, running together with time (Fig. 2.3). Many ventilators have such displays available at the bedside. Most modes of ventilation control one variable of the equation of motion, with the remaining variables being dependent. Compliance and resistance

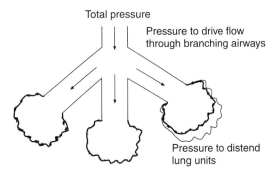

Pressure = (1/compliance × volume) + (resistance × flow)

Figure 2.2 *When gas is pushed into the chest, the airway pressure rises to overcome the elastic recoil of the lung and chest wall and the resistance to airflow through the major branching airways.*

can be measured at the bedside during mechanical ventilation.[4] If no breathing effort is made, the ventilator performs the work to inflate the chest. Much information can be obtained from the pressure waveform generated during constant flow ventilation.

At the beginning of inspiration, very little (if any) volume has entered the chest, yet there is a rapid upstroke of the airway pressure graph. The early rise in airway pressure occurs because the ventilator has to overcome resistance to airflow (Fig. 2.4). An estimate of resistance can be calculated from the initial upstroke

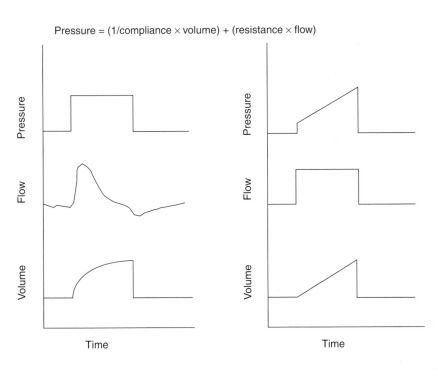

Pressure = (1/compliance × volume) + (resistance × flow)

Figure 2.3 *Simple breath patterns during mechanical ventilation. The left-hand panel shows a constant pressure during inspiration. The right-hand panel shows a constant flow delivered to the patient.*

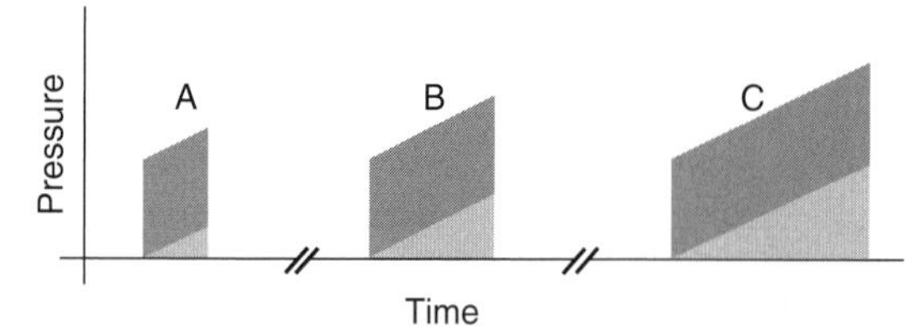

Figure 2.4 *During constant flow ventilation, airway pressure rises as time progresses in inspiration. (A) Early in inspiration, the rise in pressure occurs without a large change in lung volume, and this is due to the resistance of the branching airways. (B) As time continues, airway pressure increases and includes the effect of the recoil of the lung and chest wall. (C) At the end of inspiration, the pressure due to the stiffness of the lung and chest wall (triangular-shaped element) can be calculated from either an inspiratory breath hold or by measuring the height of the triangular part of the diagram.*

of the pressure waveform. If flow is constant, and set by the user, it is therefore easy to obtain from the ventilator display. If the height of the initial upstroke in airway pressure (in cmH$_2$O) is divided by the flow, the resistance (in cmH$_2$O L^{-1} s^{-1}) can be easily calculated.

As time progresses, gas enters the chest and the airway pressure then rises as an upward ramp. The total pressure at this time is the sum of the resistance and elastic forces. From the graphs, it can be seen that the resistance to airflow is a constant increment, and this is represented as equal-sized bars in Figure 2.4. At the end of inspiration, the elastic recoil of the lungs and chest wall is maximal, and the pressure generated peaks.

The effective compliance of the system (lung and chest wall) can be calculated from the volume delivered and the pressure during an inspiratory breath hold, at zero gas flow. When the breath is held in inspiration, pressure drops to equal the static recoil holding the chest open. This can either be measured or estimated as the height of the triangular diagram. Compliance is then calculated as the volume per unit pressure (mL cmH$_2$O^{-1}).[5]

MODES OF VENTILATION

The way in which the ventilator delivers a breath to the patient is described by a confusing nomenclature. As the ventilator is controlled by a microprocessor, numerous possible combinations of breaths are possible, and it is estimated that over 22 different modes of ventilation have been introduced into clinical prac-

Table 2.2 *A descriptive classification of ventilators by the way in which the breath is delivered to the patient*

1 *How is the breath controlled by the ventilator?*
- Pressure control
- Volume control
- Time control

2 *How is the mandatory breath delivered to the patient?*
- All breaths are mandatory
- Mandatory breaths are intermittent
- No mandatory breaths

3 *What type of inspiratory trigger is used?*
- Pressure triggering
- Flow triggering
- No triggered breaths

4 *Are the spontaneous breaths assisted?*
- Pressure support

5 *Is expiration assisted or augmented?*
- CPAP

tice. Although the range of potential breath types delivered to the patient is large, few comparative clinical trials have been performed relating the mode of ventilation with eventual outcome, sometimes making the rational use of such modes difficult.

Often, a mode of ventilation has many synonymous terms. A simple example is the description of full mechanical ventilation. Controlled mandatory ventilation (CMV) is the term used to describe ventilation in which all the breaths delivered to the patient are fixed by the ventilator. In the UK, this is often referred to as intermittent positive pressure ventilation (IPPV). Assist control ventilation is used as a term to describe a mandatory form of ventilation in which all the breaths delivered to the patient are assisted. However, these terms are confusing, as they are vague and ill defined.

Ventilators can be described in terms of the way in which the breath is delivered to the patient. The variable that is controlled could be volume, pressure or time. Each breath from the ventilator can be mandatory or spontaneous, and the breath can be triggered by the machine or the patient, or both (Table 2.2).[6]

Volume control

In this mode, volume is controlled and the other factors from the equation of motion will vary. The ventilator seeks to deliver the pre-set volume to the patient, and this is an advantage in most circumstances in which the patient is not able to make an inspiratory effort and the underlying lung mechanics are normal, as is the case for patients undergoing general anaesthesia. However, pressure at the airway is not controlled and will depend on the dynamics of the system. If the lung and chest wall are stiff, or if airway resistance is high, pressure will rise and, unless this is limited, excessive pressures may result.

Recently, the effect of one form of mechanical ventilation was investigated in patients with acute respiratory distress syndrome (ARDS). In this study, the volume delivered to the patients was controlled and the results were compared with those from a group who received higher tidal volumes. Importantly, mortality when tidal volume was restricted was less than with the standard treatment. With this exception, few other modes of ventilation have had a demonstrable effect on patient outcome.[7,8]

Pressure control

During pressure control ventilation, the airway pressure is pre-set and the volume delivered to the patient is dependent on the mechanics of the system. Tidal volume may vary, and will be high when the system has a low resistance and a high compliance. If resistance and compliance alter, as they may do rapidly in the critically ill, a changing delivered volume to the patient occurs. As pressure is pre-set, high airway pressures are avoided, and this may be advantageous in the presence of stiff lungs with the ever-present danger of barrotrauma.

In the critically ill patient, the lung is not homogeneous in nature; frequently, there are areas of the lung that are stiffer or have a higher resistance to gas flow. Ventilation to the stiffer lung units may require prolonged inspiratory times. Pressure control exerts a constant pressure and may succeed in expanding areas of the lung, particularly if inspiration is prolonged. This may be contrasted to volume control, with which much of the initial volume is delivered to the few remaining lung units whose characteristics are more normal. This may cause over-distension of the normal lung units and may not inflate the stiffer lung units.

PARTIAL ASSISTANCE

In the critically ill, spontaneous breathing is often maintained and ventilatory support is provided as a proportion of the total effort. Another force is acting on the lungs and must be added to our simple diagram, that of the patient's respiratory muscles, Pmus. Pmus is acting to inflate the lungs and, if the ventilator is in total harmony with the patient, Pmus and Paw will work together and are additive (Fig. 2.5).

Triggering the ventilator

The mechanism by which the ventilator senses an inspiratory effort is termed the trigger, and the change in airway pressure during inspiration is the method that is most often used today. Pressure generated by the respiratory muscles within the chest is transmitted into the upper airway and is detected in the mouth. In normal subjects, there is little phase difference between pleural pressure and mouth pressure. Pressure is easily measured using a transducer and most methods used are robust. The transducer measures airway pressure continuously and is programmed to detect the change in pressure that occurs during inspiration. The trigger can be adjusted to react to a smaller change in airway pressure, making it more sensitive. This enables the ventilator to be triggered closer to the beginning of the breath.

All trigger systems have a time delay from the moment inspiration begins to the point when the

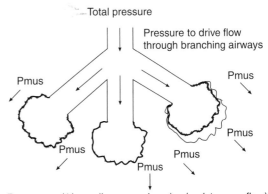

Pressure = (1/compliance × volume) + (resistance × flow)

Figure 2.5 *When the patient is breathing spontaneously, the ventilator assists the breathing effort. If the ventilator and the patient efforts are synchronous, the effects can be seen as additive.*

ventilator delivers a breath. The rate of response of a trigger can be divided generally into two phases. Phase I describes the time during which the pressure builds up to the trigger point and Phase II describes the time from the trigger point to the opening of the inspiratory valve and breath delivery.[9]

If the trigger is insensitive or if the reaction time is delayed, the patient will be breathing against a closed airway, and this ineffective ventilation can amount to a considerable amount of work for the patient. Pressure triggering may occur from other fluctuations of pressure within the airway and it is possible to trigger a ventilator from cardiac oscillations that appear as artefacts.

In lung pathology, e.g. chronic obstructive pulmonary disease (COPD), the rate of transmission of a pressure signal from the pleural space to the airway may be delayed and a phase difference may occur. This slows the response of the ventilator.[10]

Inspiratory flow may also be detected and used as a trigger. Two methods are employed to measure flow. Flow may be measured directly at the mouth or a continuous low flow may be introduced by the ventilator during expiration (bias flow) and the difference between inspiratory and expiratory flow continuously measured. When inspiration begins, some of the bias flow enters the lungs and less of the bias flow is detected at the expiratory sensor of the patient breathing circuit. This inspiratory/expiratory flow difference triggers the breath. Flow triggering tends to increase the sensitivity of ventilators compared with pressure triggering, and the time delay from the start of the breath to delivery to the patient can be reduced considerably.

Intermittent mandatory ventilation

Partial assistance can be delivered to the patient by delivering a pre-set tidal volume at a pre-set flow rate. The number of breaths is also pre-set, and this form of ventilation was originally termed intermittent mandatory ventilation (IMV).

Several problems occur in adults with IMV. The ventilator breath is not timed to spontaneous breathing and the machine breath may coincide with any phase of spontaneous respiration. If the patient is breathing out when the ventilator delivers an inspiratory breath, high airway pressure may be obtained. Furthermore, if the patient receives a number of machine breaths together, there may be insufficient time for adequate exhalation, leading to an increase in functional residual capacity (FRC) and the phenomenon of 'breath stacking'. In order to solve these problems, the ventilator needs to 'know' when the patient is breathing and which phase of breathing is occurring. Synchronized IMV (SIMV) senses inspiration and has the capacity to *trigger* a breath.

In order to make SIMV work effectively, the ventilator must be inhibited from delivering a machine breath during the initial phase of exhalation, and should deliver a breath in synchrony with a spontaneous breath. During SIMV, the ventilator is inhibited at the first part of the expiratory cycle. The amount of inhibition is related to expiratory time. At the start of exhalation, the ventilator is insensitive but, as time progresses, it becomes more responsive. During SIMV, triggering is achieved by monitoring either the pressure generated in the airway or the flow that occurs during a spontaneous breath.

Delivering a volume to the patient from the ventilator does not imply that all work previously performed by the respiratory muscles is now provided by the machine. Inspiratory efforts often occur throughout a mandatory machine breath, especially when the inspiratory flow rate from the ventilator is slow. This is common in COPD, when inspiration is difficult to sense by the ventilator. When machine inspiratory flow is low, the respiratory muscles may contract during the whole of the ventilator breath, at the same level that occurs during spontaneous breathing. The implication is that respiratory muscle rest may not occur, despite the ventilator providing machine breaths that are designed to provide for respiratory muscle work.

Pressure support ventilation

Pressure support ventilation (PSV) has several differences compared with SIMV. During PSV, the only variable that is pre-set is the target airway pressure.[11] The patient determines the respiratory rate and PSV is triggered from airway pressure or from airway flow. When inspiration is sensed, the target pressure is established by delivering maximum flow to the airway, which is then reduced as soon as the target pressure is achieved. As inspiration continues, a constant pressure is maintained. The duration of inspiration is also related to patient effort. Inspiration is most commonly terminated when inspiratory flow is reduced to 25% of the maximum inspiratory flow rate. PSV may also cycle to expiration if the airway pressure exceeds the pre-set level of support, or when inspiratory time is excessive or in response to other parameters designed to prevent excessive inspiratory times.

PSV is controlled by the patient, and the rate and size of tidal volume are not pre-set by the user. Tidal volume is not assured, and this may change beyond that which is clinically acceptable. During sleep, or if centrally acting drugs are administered, PSV will not maintain a minimum level of ventilation.

It is possible either that PSV may be delivering more assistance than is needed or that support is insufficient. The correct amount of pressure support is difficult to judge and, as with SIMV, chronic under-ventilation or over-ventilation is possible.

Proportional assist ventilation

The equation of motion has been used so far to describe how ventilators work when one element (volume, pressure or flow) is controlled. Proportional assist ventilation (PAV) is an attempt to solve the equation of motion rather than just to control one respiratory variable.[12] The pressure required to achieve a tidal volume is, in the partially assisted patient, related to the amount of pressure delivered by the ventilator and the amount of pressure generated by the respiratory muscles. The ventilator may deliver most of the pressure and the respiratory muscles would then be unloaded and the amount of work performed by the muscles would be minimal. The adjustment that is set by the user is the degree of off-loading that the ventilator delivers (expressed either as a ratio or a percentage).[13]

Compliance and resistance can be measured by the ventilator. As the ventilator also measures the tidal volume that is delivered, the pressure that is generated can be calculated. If the patient were breathing spontaneously, the pressure calculated would then represent the pressure developed by the respiratory muscles. The ventilator can be instructed to provide some of this pressure, and this can be varied from all of the pressure (100%) through to none of the pressure. In the simplest version of PAV, values for compliance and resistance can be pre-set, or may be taken from measurements during full mechanical

ventilation. More usefully, measurements of compliance and resistance, measured on-line over millisecond time frames, enable the total amount of pressure required to be measured simultaneously during a breath. If the tidal volume changes, so the amount of pressure changes, reducing for a small breath and increasing for a large breath. What remains constant is the amount the ventilator provides as a fraction of maximum.

RECENT ADVANCES IN MECHANICAL VENTILATION

Greater importance is now placed on maintaining spontaneous ventilation during critical illness. The design of the expiratory valve now enables ventilators to provide cyclical changes in airway pressure and patients can superimpose their own breathing pattern 'on top' of the changing level of background pressure and each spontaneous breath can be additionally assisted.

The advent of the modern ventilator has meant there has been a rapid increase in the number of 'modes' or patterns of mechanical ventilation. Although many studies have investigated intermediate outcome of new ventilator modes, few of these modes have been the subject of prospective trials and there is less evidence to suggest one form of ventilation is superior to another.

Positive end-expiratory pressure

In health, the lungs are held open by the outward recoil of the chest wall. At the end of expiration, the tendency of the lung to collapse is balanced by the outward recoil of the chest wall, such that lung volume is at steady state. The resting end-expiratory volume is termed functional residual capacity. FRC reduces when body posture is changed to the supine position. During anaesthesia and after sedation, FRC falls and the critically ill patient therefore tends towards a FRC which is substantially reduced.[14]

The physiological effect of a low FRC is dependent on the state of the small dependent airways and alveoli. At some stage, airways close and at this point hypoxaemia is common. The application of a positive background pressure throughout the respiratory cycle has the effect of increasing lung volume, splinting the airways open and preventing lung volume falling to low levels at which airway closure is possible. Such pressure is termed continuous positive airway pressure (CPAP) if the patient is breathing spontaneously or positive end-expiratory pressure (PEEP) if this is applied during positive pressure ventilation.

PEEP has been used extensively to treat hypoxaemia and is most effective when lung volume is recruited. This effect is gradual, with improvements in arterial blood gas measurements 1 hour after changing PEEP/CPAP. On the other hand, derecruitment tends to happen promptly.

Periodically, recruitment of lung units may require much higher pressures to be applied to the lungs to open collapsed or partially inflated lung units, and PEEP is important to maintain lung volume once alveoli have been recruited, the so-called open lung strategy.[15] Such forms of lung ventilation may have complex interactions and need to be applied with care.

Increasing the mean pressure in the chest also has an effect on the mediastinum and cardiac chambers. The effect of raising intrathoracic pressure was originally considered to act mainly on the venous system, impeding filling of the ventricles and end-diastolic volume and hence reducing stroke volume and cardiac output. The relationship between the heart and the lungs is now recognized to be more complex and may alter when ventricular function is diminished. Nonetheless, it is important to note that raised intrathoracic pressure may have a deleterious effect on cardiac output, and the net effect may be to depress O_2 delivery to the tissues.

Non-invasive ventilation

Mechanical ventilation does not require endotracheal intubation, and respiratory support is frequently provided with a tightly fitting facemask during resuscitation and by anaesthetists in the operating theatre. This technique has been adapted in order to support patients on the intensive care unit (ICU), using a simple ventilator and accepting that some of the ventilated gas may leak away. Such support is non-invasive and has many advantages. The patients do not need to be intubated, are not sedated and may spontaneously cough and expecto-

rate. Additionally, the facemask may be removed intermittently and the patient may be able to speak and communicate during therapy. This type of treatment is now termed non-invasive ventilation (NIV). NIV is a generic term used to describe any form of positive pressure facemask therapy; it begins with CPAP and includes volume or pressure controlled mechanical ventilation. NIV was initially used for patients with severe chronic hypercapnic respiratory failure as an alternative to mechanical ventilation with an artificial airway. Success in this area is widespread and the treatment is no longer restricted to the ICU, ward-based care now being usual. Frequently, patients require long-term treatment and domicillary NIV is provided with specifically designed ventilators.

NIV is used for acutely ill patients in respiratory failure. It is particularly successful when used at an early stage when the patient can co-operate with treatment effectively. Several studies have demonstrated that NIV decreases morbidity and mortality in acute ventilatory failure due to COPD, possibly due to the decrease in pneumonia associated with endotracheal intubation.[16]

However, not all patients are suitable for this form of therapy. Patients with a decreased level of consciousness, those who are unable to cough and expectorate or to swallow or protect their upper airway are difficult to manage with NIV and may need to be intubated. NIV demands an effective team of nurses, doctors and physiotherapists. In the acutely ill, the first few hours of treatment demand intensive input from the team. The case for NIV in hypoxaemic respiratory failure is more complex, some studies having suggested that treatment may not prevent more invasive therapy involving endotracheal intubation.

PRACTICAL ASPECTS OF MECHANICAL VENTILATION

Some dangers of mechanical ventilation apply to all patients. It is not possible to establish effective, long-term ventilation without securing a sealed connection with the airway via an endotracheal or tracheostomy tube. However, the insertion of this tube requires either general or local anaesthesia, with its attendant risks.

Anaesthesia

The risks of the anaesthesia needed for endotracheal intubation include:

- myocardial depression caused by general or local anaesthetic drugs,
- aspiration of gastric contents,
- a further fall in arterial O_2 tension, especially if intubation is difficult,
- an idiosyncratic reaction to anaesthetic drugs,
- reflex worsening of bronchoconstriction following tracheal intubation or suction of secretions.

These risks are not substantially reduced if topical local, instead of general, anaesthetic is used for the intubation of the trachea.

Sedation and paralysis

IPPV through a nasal or an orotracheal tube is poorly tolerated without some sedation. Often, paralysing drugs are also required initially, especially in neurological disease (status epilepticus, for example) or trauma. In general, the ideal sedative should be very short acting, given by constant intravenous infusion and have minimal side effects, especially affecting the circulation. None of the currently available sedatives is devoid of important side effects. The benzodiazepines often cause tolerance, requiring increasing dosage that leads to a build up of active metabolites and prolonged depressant effects on the central nervous system, which last for days after stopping administration, especially in those patients with renal or hepatic failure. Propofol, an intravenous anaesthetic, and isoflurane, a volatile inhalation anaesthetic, have been used for continuous sedation. They are both short-acting agents with no cumulative effects and their cardiovascular and respiratory effects at sedative doses are minimal in the fit patient. However, the cardiac depressant effects of these two drugs may be important in the patient with poor myocardial function.

There is a wide choice of suitable neuromuscular blocking drugs: vecuronium and atracurium have minimal side effects and are sufficiently short acting to allow rapid regulation of the state of paralysis. All ICU staff should be aware that neuromuscular blocking agents have no sedative effects and that patients may be awake and paralysed if sedation is not prescribed. Another danger of paralysis is the inability of the patient to make spontaneous breathing efforts should there be an accidental ventilator disconnection.

Equipment failure

The risks of equipment failure include accidental disconnection of the ventilator, undetected leaks or malfunction of the endotracheal tube, all leading to alveolar hypoventilation and hypercapnia.

Hyperinflation

Airflow obstruction is defined by the failure of lung emptying and the consequent increase in resting lung volume. At the higher volume, the pressure in the peripheral airway is increased. This pressure is difficult to measure and is termed occult or intrinsic positive end-expiratory pressure or autoPEEP. This effect may be worsened by mechanical ventilation when the mandatory machine breaths may be set in such a way as to allow insufficient time for lung deflation. Subsequent breaths delivered from the ventilator increase lung volume until a new equilibrium is established.

Endotracheal tubes

Mechanical ventilation often requires tracheal intubation and this is a hazardous moment for any critically ill patient. Anaesthetic drugs always depress the circulation and neuromuscular paralysis removes the laryngeal reflexes that may protect against aspiration. Intubation may not be technically straightforward and patients with inadequate lung volume desaturate quickly. A checklist for items needed during intubation is useful.

All artificial airways offer a resistance to airflow. The flow of air through the tube is seldom ideal and never laminar in nature. Turbulent airflow is common, due to the shortness of the tube relative to the internal diameter, the presence of secretions and the possibility of changes in diameter due to kinking.

The work performed by gas flowing through the endotracheal tube depends largely on the diameter of the tube and on the inspiratory flow rate.

The highest work is seen when the internal diameter is 7.0 mm or less, with a minute ventilation greater than 15 L min^{-1}. When inserted, endotracheal tubes in adults are seldom less than 7.00 mm and functional tube diameter changes with use. If secretions are present inside the tube, it is possible for a larger endotracheal tube to function as one of a much smaller diameter. This phenomenon is most prominent after 7 days of use.

As the airway resistance due to the endotracheal tube increases, several effects occur. When the patient initiates a breath, work is performed across the tube. As a result, inspiration occurs before the ventilator can sense a pressure change in the airway, and a time delay occurs such that the respiratory muscles contract before the ventilator senses the beginning of inspiration. Also, when the ventilator does trigger, some of the pressure generated is again dissipated across the endotracheal apparatus and therefore less is available for lung inflation.

It may be possible to remove the effect of the endotracheal tube if airway pressure is sensed closer to the patient. Inspiration is sensed at the earliest possible moment and the work to breath across the tube itself is reduced if the target pressure is also sensed at the distal endotracheal tube. A system of compensation for the resistance of endotracheal tubes is a facility of modern ventilators. Details concerning the type of tube may be entered into the ventilator programme and the resistance of the tube is automatically compensated for.[17]

The position of the endotracheal tube within the airway frequently requires attention. The plastic nature of the tube tends to soften when it reaches body temperature and the tube adopts a configuration that is acutely angled. It is possible for the patient to move the tube to the point where the cuff of the tube lies above the larynx, with only the tip of the tube within the airway. When this happens, air leaks can be heard. A temporary seal can be re-established by further inflation of the cuff. Eventually, the over-inflated cuff sits at the back of the throat, with the endotracheal tube resting above the larynx, and the airway may not in fact be intubated. In this circumstance, it is often necessary to re-intubate the patient.

If humidification of the inspired gases is not adequate, endotracheal tubes may become acutely blocked with secretions, which can completely occlude the airway.

Endotracheal tubes may migrate beyond the carina, entering a major bronchus. This results in partial or complete occlusion, with collapse of the occluded lung and hypoxaemia.

Nosocomial infection

Mechanical ventilation with sedation and the upper airway bypassed with an endotracheal tube carries with it a high risk of infection. Despite immaculate care of the upper airway, secretions collect at the back of the pharynx and can be silently aspirated into the lungs. Additionally, many patients receive some form of sedation during intubation and ventilation, with the result that the cough reflex is impaired. Ciliary clearance is reduced when the airway is intubated. Pathogens that are present in such ventilator-acquired pneumonias (VAPs) may often be of the hospital-acquired type and may be difficult to treat effectively. It has been noted that pneumonias acquired in this manner may be reduced if the pharynx is continuously aspirated with the aid of specially designed endotracheal tubes. If the supine posture is changed to a head-up position, the incidence of VAPs decreases.

Cardiovascular effects of intermittent positive pressure ventilation

Not all the effects of IPPV on the cardiovascular system are adverse. They result from the rise in intrathoracic pressure, especially if PEEP is used, and are mediated through direct mechanical interference with the heart, through indirect reflexes of the autonomic nervous system and through hormone release or changes in blood gases. The predominant direct adverse effects of IPPV upon the right heart are a reduction in venous return (pre-load) and an increase in pulmonary vascular resistance (after-load). The direct effects upon the left heart are less marked and less well established, the widely held view being that both pulmonary venous return (pre-load) and after-load decrease. This effect on left ventricular after-load is due to a fall in ventricular transmural pressure because of the increase in intrathoracic pressure (this also applies to the right ventricle). This mechanism provides a form of 'assistance' to ventricular work that may be beneficial in cardiac failure.[18]

The reflex responses are complex, depending upon multiple neural and chemical feedback loops. The neural reflexes are mediated initially by the vagus nerve, predominantly affecting the heart rate, but stronger reflexes involve the whole sympathetic system, affecting vascular resistances and circulating catecholamines. The reflexes originate from lung and atrial stretch receptors and from the arterial baroreceptors and chemoreceptors (the latter only if arterial CO_2 tension falls or arterial O_2 tension rises in response to IPPV). The humoral reflex response to IPPV includes an increase in antidiuretic hormone (ADH) and reninangiotensin and a decrease in atrial natriuretic peptide, which may be partly responsible for the sodium retention seen in ventilated patients. The changes in catecholamines are partly mediated by $PaCO_2$ changes. The pattern of circulatory changes is variable. The predominant effect is a decrease in both cardiac output (typically by 25%) and arterial blood pressure, an increase in heart rate and a slight increase in systemic vascular resistance; right and left atrial pressures increase relative to atmospheric pressure (transmural pressures *decrease*). This pattern is often modified by blood-gas changes associated with mechanical ventilation because of the powerful stimulant effects of CO_2 upon the sympathetic system.

REFERENCES

1. Snider, GL. Historical perspective on mechanical ventilation: from simple life support system to ethical dilemma. *Am Rev Respir Dis* 1989; **140**: S2–7.

2. Esteban, A, Anzueto, A, Alia, I, *et al*. How is mechanical ventilation employed in the Intensive Care Unit? *Am J Respir Crit Care Med* 2000; **161**: 1450–8.

3. Mead, J, Milic-Emili, J. (1964). Theory and methodology in respiratory mechanics with glossary and symbols. In *Handbook of physiology*. Volume 1, *Respiration*. Washington: American Physiological Society, 1964; 363–6.

4. Gattinoni, L, Mascheroni, D, Basilico, E, Foti, G, Pesenti, A, Avalli, L. Volume/pressure curve of the total respiratory system in paralyzed patients: artefacts and correction factors. *Intensive Care Med* 1987; **13**: 19–25.

5. Tobin, MJ, Van de Graaff, WB. (1994). Monitoring of lung mechanics and work of breathing. In *Principles and practice of mechanical ventilation*. New York: McGraw Hill, 1994; 1300.

6. Branson, RD, Chatburn RL. Technical description and classification of modes of ventilator operation. *Respir Care* 1992; **37**: 1026–44.

7. The Acute Respiratory Distress Syndrome Network. Ventilation with lower tidal volumes as compared to traditional tidal volumes for ALI and ARDS. *N Engl J Med* 2000; **342**: 1301–8.

8. Amato, *et al*. Beneficial effects of the open lung approach with low distending pressures in acute respiratory distress syndrome. A prospective randomized study on mechanical ventilation. *Am J Respir Crit Care Med* 1995; **152**: 1835–46.

9. Sassoon, CSH. Mechanical ventilator design and function: the trigger variable. *Respir Care* 1992; **37**: 1056–69.

10. Murciano, D, Aubier, M, Bussi, S, Derenne, JP, Pariente, R, Milic-Emili, J. Comparison of esophageal, tracheal and occlusion pressure in patients with chronic obstructive pulmonary disease during acute respiratory failure. *Am Rev Respir Dis* 1982; **126**: 837–41.

11. MacIntyre, NR. Respiratory function during pressure support ventilation. *Chest* 1986; **89**: 677–83.

12. Younes, M. Proportional assist ventilation, a new approach to ventilatory support. *Am Rev Respir Dis* 1992; **145**: 114–20.

13. Younes, M, Puddy, A, Roberts, D, et al. Proportional assist ventilation; results of an initial clinical trial. *Am Rev Respir Dis* 1992; **145**: 121–9.

14. Sykes, K. *Respiratory support*. London: BMJ Publishing, 1995.

15. Lachmann, B. Open the lung and keep the lung open. *Intensive Care Med* 1992; **18**: 319–21.

16. Vitacca, M, Rubini, F, Foglio, K, Scalvini, S, Nava, S, Ambrosino, N. Non-invasive modalities of positive pressure ventilation improve the outcome of acute exacerbations in COLD patients. *Intensive Care Med* 1993; **19**: 450–5.

17. Guttman, J, Bernard, H, Mols, G, *et al*. Respiratory comfort of automatic tube compensation and inspiratory pressure support in conscious humans. *Intensive Care Med* 1997; **23**: 1119–24.

18. Lemaire, F, Teboul, JL, Cinotti, L, *et al*. Acute left ventricular dysfunction during unsuccessful weaning from mechanical ventilation. *Anesthesiology* 1988; **69**: 171–9.

3

Mechanical ventilation: ventilatory strategies

HILMAR BURCHARDI

VENTILATORY STRATEGIES FOR ACUTE LUNG INJURY

Pathophysiological conditions

In acute lung injury and early acute respiratory distress syndrome (ARDS), pulmonary membrane permeability is critically increased as a result of an acute systematic inflammatory reaction, either due to direct tissue damage (e.g. aspiration) and/or indirectly (e.g. sepsis). This results in a severe interstitial and intra-alveolar non-cardiogenic oedema.[1] Under the influence of gravity, the fluid-filled lung tissue is compressed, particularly in the dependent parts,[2] and the surface area for gas exchange reduced ('baby lung'), with severe impairment of oxygenation. Surfactant production is impaired so that alveoli tend to collapse. Gas exchange is still maintained in the aerated non-dependent areas of the lungs, although these potentially may be damaged by hyperinflation, and the compressed or fluid-filled alveoli can be re-aerated by lung recruitment as long as interstitial fibrosis has not yet occurred.

The abnormalities in respiratory mechanics depend upon the underlying aetiology.[3] In primary ARDS (i.e. pulmonary, such as pneumonia), lung compliance is decreased but the chest-wall component remains normal. In secondary ARDS (i.e. extra-pulmonary, for example due to surgical causes), chest-wall compliance is decreased (e.g. by abdominal distension), whereas lung compliance may be preserved.

There is also increasing evidence that mechanical ventilation may itself damage the lungs. The mechanisms of this ventilator-associated lung injury (VALI) are various:[4] regional alveolar over-distension, caused by high inspiratory pressure and/or volume, is compounded by the inhomogeneity of lung injury and generates damaging shear forces and, in some areas, repeated opening and closing of collapsed alveoli, which further damages the lung and increases microvascular permeability ('stress failure') and oedema. These potential risks and adverse effects consequently determine the strategy of mechanical ventilation.

Ventilatory principles

The main principles for mechanical ventilation in acute lung injury are:

- 'open up the lungs and keep them open',
- limiting airway pressure and tidal volume,

- permissive hypercapnia,
- variation of the inspiration:expiration (I:E) ratio,
- supplementary spontaneous breathing efforts.

'OPEN UP THE LUNGS AND KEEP THEM OPEN'

To recruit collapsed alveoli requires a higher pressure than is necessary to keep them open. The clinical aim is to 'open up the lungs and keep them open'. The application of external positive end-expiratory pressure (PEEP) increases lung volume and can recruit collapsed alveoli. The distribution of additional gas volume induced by external PEEP will depend on the regional compliance of different lung areas, which may be very variable in inhomogeneous lungs. Thus, it is unlikely that one level of PEEP will be optimal for the whole lung. In ARDS, any increase in lung volume by external PEEP not only reduces intrapulmonary shunt, but also simultaneously hyperinflates non-compressed lung areas, thereby potentially converting well-ventilated alveoli into non-perfused dead space.

Consequently, a compromise is necessary that keeps the lesser compliant alveoli open without over-distending the more compliant areas. Some intensivists recommend applying external PEEP slightly (e.g. 2 cmH$_2$O) above the lower inflection point (Pflex) of the pressure/volume (P/V) curve. However, this is cumbersome and problematic to measure and sometimes no inflection point can be identified. (For a fuller discussion, see Chapter 12.) PEEP induces more recruitment in secondary or extrapulmonary ARDS than in primary or pulmonary causes of ARDS. The increase in intra-abdominal counter-pressure is important in secondary ARDS and it has been proposed that measurement of intra-abdominal pressure (IAP) may better define the optimal level of PEEP than estimating Pflex.

An alternative lung recruitment strategy is to statically distend the lungs with high continuous positive airway pressures (CPAP), e.g. 35–40 cmH$_2$O for 40 s followed by a return to previous PEEP levels.[5] Convincing evidence for this potentially risky manoeuvre is not available.

LIMITING AIRWAY PRESSURE AND TIDAL VOLUME

Transpulmonary pressure should be kept within the normal range that applies at maximum lung capacity. This corresponds to a maximum airway plateau pressure of about 35 cmH$_2$O.[4] In ARDS 'baby lungs', the consequence is a need to reduce tidal volume to avoid high inflation pressures and alveolar over-distension. Tidal volumes of 12–15 mL kg^{-1}, as formerly proposed, cause over-distension. The tidal volume must also be adjusted to the prevailing PEEP level: when using higher PEEP, tidal volumes have to be reduced to avoid some lung areas being in the flatter part of the pressure–volume curve, indicating over-distension. Restriction of the ventilatory excursion may be even more important in inhomogeneous lungs to reduce local tissue stress forces. Consequently, low tidal volumes and a higher level of PEEP are now advised, with tidal volumes as low as 6 mL kg^{-1} being recommended.[10] The consequence might be an increase in PCO_2, although alveolar ventilation can be increased by increasing frequency. There is no benefit in increasing respiratory rate above 25 min^{-1}, however.

PERMISSIVE HYPERCAPNIA

If arterial PCO_2 is allowed to increase from 40 to 80 mmHg, alveolar ventilation can be reduced by 50%. Hickling and co-workers[6] were the first to demonstrate in ARDS that permissive hypercapnia was well tolerated. They showed that mortality was reduced when peak airway pressures were cut by decreasing tidal volumes and limiting peak inspiratory pressures to 40 cmH$_2$O. This concept is now commonly accepted.[7] Acute hypercapnia increases sympathetic activity, cardiac output and pulmonary vascular resistance and dilates both bronchi and cerebral vessels. However, a slow and gradual elevation of PCO_2 is remarkably well tolerated. Contra-indications are co-existing head injury or other risk of cerebral oedema, a recent cerebrovascular accident or significant cardiovascular dysfunction.

VARIATION OF THE I:E RATIO

Once open, the alveoli can be kept open by external applied or intrinsic PEEP (autoPEEP). Intrinsic PEEP occurs when expiration (regional or total) remains incomplete at the end of the available expiratory time. This is a dynamic phenomenon that depends on the actual conditions of ventilation. Thus, intrinsic PEEP can be caused by high tidal volumes, short expiratory time or high ventilatory time constants. Commonly, there is a spectrum of slower and faster alveolar compartments. Fast compartments may be able to expire completely, e.g. 0.5 s. By shortening expiratory time, intrinsic PEEP can deliberately be manipulated: this is the concept of the inverse ratio ventilation or IRV mode, whereby slower alveolar compartments may be kept open by 'individual' intrinsic PEEP, i.e. using regional air trapping to prevent alveolar collapse.

IRV has been advocated in ARDS.[8] The possible advantages are:

- the prolonged inspiration ensures a more homogeneous ventilation,
- during the short expiration, slower compartments will not exhale completely and will remain distended by an intrinsic PEEP.

It has been argued that the pressure-controlled mode (PC-IRV) may be better than the volume-controlled mode (VC-IRV). PC-IRV ensures that alveolar pressures never exceed the set value anywhere within the inhomogeneous lung. Of course, pressure limitation could also be achieved in a volume-controlled mode by setting a pressure limit. A more important argument for the PC-IRV mode may be that inspiratory pressure remains constant, even if lung compliance improves by alveolar recruitment. This will lead to a further increase in tidal volume. In contrast, in VC-IRV, airway pressure decreases when compliance improves, which reduces the chance for further alveolar recruitment unless the pre-set tidal volume is manually re-adjusted.

However, the use of IRV, with the associated increase in mean intrathoracic pressure, will interfere with cardiac output. The benefit from IRV in oxygenation may be lost by reducing O_2 transport, unless these effects are counterbalanced by fluid volume and/or vasoactive drug therapy. Clinical studies do not convincingly demonstrate the superiority of IRV. An important criticism of IRV is that most of the claimed advantages are either unproven or can be achieved more safely with controlled mechanical ventilation (CMV) and an appropriate external PEEP.

SUPPLEMENTARY SPONTANEOUS BREATHING EFFORTS

In modern strategies, there is a general tendency to incorporate spontaneous breathing efforts even if clearly insufficient. Even a small contribution by spontaneous breathing reduces peak airway pressures. This makes mechanical ventilation less 'invasive'. Venous return will also be less affected and O_2 delivery may improve as a consequence of increased cardiac output. Even more importantly, the ventilatory movements of the diaphragm during spontaneous breathing predominantly affect the most dependent, and therefore most collapsed, areas of the lungs. Furthermore, sedation can be kept lower.[9] This may be beneficial for several reasons:

- less disturbance of other organ function, e.g. gastrointestinal motility,
- less accumulation of sedatives,
- easier dosing of analgesics to individual needs,
- improved diagnosis of complications, e.g. cerebral function disturbance,
- enhanced coughing and clearance of bronchial secretions.

Ventilatory strategies

LUNG-PROTECTIVE VENTILATION STRATEGY

Lung-protective strategies have been compared to conventional ventilation in several controlled studies. In one, reduced mortality was shown in the protective ventilation group, but the mortality in the control group was excessive.[5] Another randomized study failed to prove the benefit of limiting tidal volumes. However, a large, multicentre study[10] has provided evidence for this mode of ventilation: volume controlled ventilation (VCV), I:E ratio = 1:1–1:3, peak airway pressures ≤ 30 cmH$_2$O, tidal volumes of 6 mL kg^{-1}, PEEP levels linked to the required FiO$_2$ (ranging from 5 cmH$_2$O for FiO$_2$ = 0.3 up to 24 cmH$_2$O for FiO$_2$ = 1.0). The hospital mortality was reduced from 40% to 31% and the number of ventilator-free days within the first 28 days increased. Furthermore, an index of lung inflammation showed an advantage from the limited tidal volume strategy.

AIRWAY PRESSURE RELEASE VENTILATION

This mode of ventilation allows spontaneous breathing on a pre-set CPAP level interrupted by short (0.5–1.5s) releases from that pressure level for further expiration. The principle of reducing rather than increasing lung volume when applying tidal volume distinguishes this technique from other modes of ventilatory support. It maintains a moderately high airway pressure (about 20–30 cmH$_2$O) for most of the time, thereby keeping the alveoli open. Further, during the short expiratory release, slow compartments remain open by intrinsic PEEP, which therefore resembles the effect of the IRV mode.[11] An essential advantage, however, is the preservation of spontaneous breathing. At any time during the respiratory cycle, the system is open and the patient cannot 'fight against the ventilator'.

Airway pressure release ventilation (APRV; available on the Dräger EVITA ventilator) seems to be particularly effective when ventilating ARDS lungs.[12] It fulfils all the conditions of lung-protective strategies, but additionally (and most importantly) includes the beneficial effects of spontaneous breathing. Even a minimal amount of spontaneous breathing will contribute to an improvement in V/Q mismatch and an increase in systemic blood flow.

APRV would appear to offer several potential advantages in ARDS:

- a short expiratory time, which favours ventilation in the fast compartments,
- continuous airway pressure level to keep the alveoli open,
- spontaneous breathing, which avoids the need for muscle paralysis or deep sedation,
- minimal deviation from an individually adapted 'optimal' lung volume, i.e. level of mean airway pressure, which may reduce the risk of barotrauma or volutrauma.

Although a consensus conference on mechanical ventilation[13] concluded that there are no convincing data to indicate that any ventilatory mode is superior to another in ARDS, studies comparing the different modes in well-defined clinical conditions are still needed. However, it may be difficult to prove superiority of any one mode by measuring outcome if respiratory failure is only one (and not the most common) reason for a fatal outcome. An improvement in physiological parameters may still be a good way to assess new strategies.

Case 1: Polytrauma with ARDS

KTh, a 21-year-old woman, suffered multiple trauma in a traffic accident, with blunt chest injury and bilateral lung contusions. She was intubated at the accident site. On arrival in hospital, thoracic drains were inserted to treat bilateral haemo-pneumothoraces. Because of progressive respiratory deterioration, she was transferred the following day to the university hospital with ARDS. On arrival in the ICU, her arterial $PO_2 = 67$ mmHg and $PCO_2 = 30$ mmHg and her $FiO_2 = 0.6$ (Fig. 3.1; Table 3.1).

(cont.)

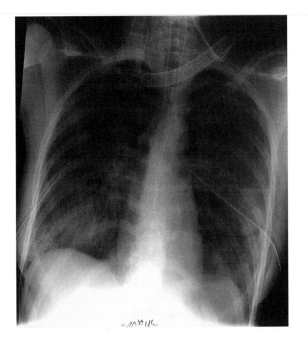

(a)

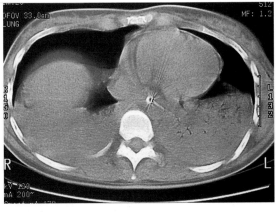

(b)

Figure 3.1 *KTh, a 21-year-old female with polytrauma and ARDS: (a) X-ray and (b) CT scan at arrival in our hospital. In the X-ray, the bilateral lung contusions appear less impressive due to the bilateral pneumothoraces, despite drainage.*

Table 3.1 *KTh, a 21-year-old female with polytrauma and ARDS*

Day	0 arrival	1	2	4	9	16	20
MV	APRV	APRV	APRV	APRV	APRV	APRV	APRV as CPAP
Phigh	30	27	27	25	22	14	6
Plow	8	8	8	8	6	5	5
I:E	3:0.8	3:0.8	3:0.8	3:1.4	4:1	2.5:0.6	2:0.6
RR	18	18	18	19	20	25	25
FiO_2	0.6	0.3	0.4	0.5	0.4	0.3	0.3
$P<->2$	67	63	137	77	84	41[a]	41[a]
PCO_2	30	37	36	44	53	58[a]	52[a]

[a]Venous blood samples.
The patient received no further ventilatory support after day 20. MV, mode of mechanical ventilation; APRV, airway pressure release ventilation; CPAP, continuous positive airway pressure; Phigh, upper APRV pressure (cmH_2O); Plow, lower APRV pressure (analogous to PEEP; cmH_2O); I:E, inspiratory/expiratory duration (s); RR, respiratory rate (per min); FiO_2, inspiratory O_2 fraction; PO_2, PCO_2, O_2 and CO_2 partial pressures (arterial on day 0–9, venous on day 16 and 20; mmHg).

(*cont.*)

Pressure controlled mechanical ventilation was performed using APRV to allow a contribution from spontaneous breathing. Re-positioning of the thoracic drains was necessary. As an extended period of mechanical ventilation was anticipated, a percutaneous tracheostomy (FANTONI method) was performed 3 days after the accident. Intermittent prone/supine positioning was carried out during the next few days. The drains were withdrawn 21 days after the accident, despite a small pneumothorax in the right lung. As the patient was able to breathe with a PS of only 5 cmH_2O, the tracheostoma was allowed to close and she was transferred to a rehabilitation ward at the primary hospital.

VENTILATORY STRATEGIES FOR ACUTE BRONCHIAL ASTHMA AND ACUTE EXACERBATION OF CHRONIC OBSTRUCTIVE PULMONARY DISEASE

Pathophysiological conditions

Many of the basic pathophysiological conditions relevant for mechanical ventilation are similar in acute severe bronchial asthma and in the acute exacerbation of chronic obstructive pulmonary disease (COPD) and therefore these are described together.

The following **basic conditions** determine the strategy of mechanical ventilation.

- Increase in lung volume due to incomplete expiration. Increased airway resistance, decrease in elastic recoil and decrease in expiration time lead to **dynamic hyperinflation**. In COPD, this is aggravated by chronic morphologic changes of emphysema.
- Increase in work of breathing, combined with a high ventilatory demand, results in acute and/or chronic **respiratory muscle fatigue**.
- The consequences are a severe **impairment of pulmonary gas exchange**. In status asthmaticus, acute failure of the ventilatory 'pump' leads to hypercapnia and hypoxaemia. In COPD, oxygenation is impaired and progressive pump failure results in chronic hypercapnia, which may markedly worsen in an acute exacerbation such as acute pulmonary infection.
- The increase in intrathoracic pressure compromises haemodynamics. In COPD, this leads to chronic **cor pulmonale** and episodes of **acute right heart failure**.

The impact of these different factors varies in acute asthma and COPD. In status asthmaticus, airway smooth muscle contraction, wall inflammation and intraluminal mucus cause a marked increase in resistance, which varies within the lungs. In COPD, the loss of elastic recoil and a chronic increase in bronchial secretions prevail, which may critically increase in acute infection.

Increased resistance to flow, high ventilatory demands and short expiratory time, all present to a variable degree, prevent the respiratory system reaching static equilibrium volume at the end of expiration. Inspiration therefore begins at a high lung volume associated with intrinsic or autoPEEP ($PEEP_i$) due to this positive recoil pressure at end-expiration. This phenomenon of dynamic hyperinflation largely dictates the strategy of mechanical ventilation. Dynamic hyperinflation raises intrathoracic pressure, increases the elastic work of breathing and forces the inspiratory muscles to operate at high lung volume, which is a disadvantageous position for pressure generation.[14] Increased intrathoracic pressure and hyperinflation may cause cardiovascular compromise, barotrauma and patient–ventilator dyssynchrony. High alveolar pressure may also increase alveolar dead space and hence ventilatory requirements. The increase in airway resistance results in increased resistive work of breathing and inhomogeneous ventilation distribution with low V/Q ratio regions ('slow compartments'), leading to arterial hypoxaemia (Fig. 3.2). The increased work of breathing may lead to respiratory muscle failure and, as a consequence, to hypercapnia. Furthermore, the interaction of mechanical ventilation and elastic properties of the respiratory system may cause serious complications.[15,16]

In the spontaneous breathing patient, dynamic hyperinflation and the large pleural pressure swings may reduce stroke volume due to changes in pre-load and after-load of both ventricles.[17] The situation is aggravated when initiating mechanical ventilation. The positive intrathoracic pressures throughout the respiratory cycle further decrease venous return and cause hypotension immediately after the institution of mechanical ventilation, a common event in these patients. If the patient is over-ventilated to correct respiratory acidosis, sudden cardiovascular collapse may occur.

Indications for 'invasive' mechanical ventilation

Respiratory function may deteriorate despite conservative treatment in status asthmaticus. In this life-threatening situation, mechanical ventilation is indicated. In patients with COPD, exacerbation is most often caused by acute pulmonary infections and may again necessitate mechanical ventilatory support. Intubation and mechanical ventilation in these circumstances are associated with a higher incidence of complications than in patients ventilated for other causes of respiratory failure. Therefore, the risk:benefit ratio of this decision has to be carefully considered. On the one hand, the risks of mechanical ventilation such as dynamic hyperinflation, barotrauma and nosocomial infection have to be balanced with the risk of acute respiratory or cardiac decompensation and severe arterial hypoxaemia resulting in cardiac or respiratory arrest. Careful observation is necessary in the intensive care unit (ICU) or high dependency unti (HDU), with

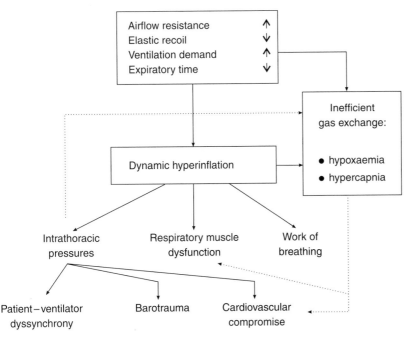

Figure 3.2 *Causes and consequences of dynamic hyperinflation (see text for details).*

readiness for immediate action if there is failure to improve.

GOALS OF MECHANICAL VENTILATION

The goals of mechanical ventilation in asthma are to support pulmonary gas exchange and to unload respiratory muscles whilst allowing time for other therapeutic interventions (such as steroids) to reduce airway inflammation and bronchial reactivity. In asthma, ventilatory support is generally only needed for a short time, e.g. hours to a few days. In COPD, the goals of mechanical ventilation are similar, but ventilatory support may be needed for longer.

COMPLICATIONS OF MECHANICAL VENTILATION

Mechanical ventilation is associated with a number of complications,[15,16] which increase morbidity and mortality:

- mucus plugging, e.g. atelectasis, occlusion of the endotracheal tube,
- ventilation-associated pneumonia (VAP) and nosocomial infection,
- barotrauma, e.g. pneumothorax, subcutaneous emphysema,
- hypotension.

INDICATIONS FOR INVASIVE VENTILATION IN STATUS ASTHMATICUS

The absolute indications for intubation are: coma, apnoea, cardiac arrest and severe arterial hypoxaemia despite high FiO_2. Continued deterioration, despite maximal conservative treatment, often forces the physician to institute mechanical ventilation. Evidence of fatigue, excessive work of breathing and somnolence (cerebral hypoxia) should be looked for carefully: fatal apnoea can occur very suddenly and unexpectedly. Changes in alertness, speech, respiratory rate and extent of accessory muscle use indicate deterioration. In patients with significant bronchial secretions, the decision to proceed to endotracheal intubation should be taken earlier.

Hypercapnia *per se* is not an indication for intubation. Patients who become more comfortable and more able to speak should continue with medical therapy despite a high $PaCO_2$. A progressive increase in $PaCO_2$ with acidaemia (pH < 7.25) may force

matters. Evidence of CVS compromise, arrhythmia or pneumothorax will necessitate ventilatory support. Pneumothorax is best drained before intubation. The indication for intubation and mechanical ventilation is therefore a clinical decision based on an estimate of the risks and benefits.

Intubation

Endotracheal intubation may be extremely difficult in status asthmaticus. Reflex bronchospasm and cardiac arrhythmia, or cardiac arrest, may occur in hypoxaemic patients. Intubation should therefore be performed by the most experienced clinician available. Deep sedation with benzodiazepines is necessary. Ketamine (dosage 3–6 mg kg^{-1}) may be useful as it also causes sympathomimetic stimulation. Some recommend topical anaesthesia, but this may irritate the airways and cause further bronchospasm. In emergency cases, oral intubation is easier to perform. In addition, it allows for placement of a large endotracheal tube (8 mm or greater), which is important for suctioning viscous mucus. A large tube also reduces airflow resistance and facilitates bronchoscopy, which may be necessary for lavage.

INDICATIONS FOR INVASIVE VENTILATION IN ACUTE EXACERBATION OF CHRONIC OBSTRUCTIVE PULMONARY DISEASE

Before initiating invasive mechanical ventilation in COPD patients, it is essential to consider that this may be the starting point of a long process with complications such as nosocomial infection, barotrauma, weaning problems etc.

> In patients with COPD, the use of **non-invasive ventilation** (NIV) should be considered if there is no compelling reason to intubate, such as severe life-threatening hypoxaemia, multiple organ failure or an impending surgical procedure.

The decision to intubate should be based on the clinical situation. Symptoms of life-threatening decompensation are excessive respiratory rate (>35 min^{-1}), severe respiratory inco-ordination, increasing agitation or coma; a pH < 7.25 will not be tolerated for a long period. In contrast to the situation in status asthmaticus, early **percutaneous tracheostomy** may be useful if extubation to NIV is not planned.

The practice of mechanical ventilation

CONTROLLED MECHANICAL VENTILATION

Controlled modes are used initially. It is important to control and limit airway pressure. Pressure controlled ventilatory modes (PCV) prevent excessive airway pressures that might otherwise occur if resistance suddenly increases. There are no controlled studies to support their use, however.

Initiating mechanical ventilation can be difficult and requires continuous adaptation of the ventilatory settings. Patients should initially be deeply sedated to prevent fighting against the ventilator. Muscle paralysis is needed in the acute situation but, if it is used, it should be only for a short period. COPD patients may not adapt to the ventilator easily and a high dose of opiates may be needed to depress respiratory drive. High airway pressure *per se* does not necessarily indicate hyperinflation and may be caused by high airflow resistance in the endotracheal tube or the central airways (e.g. secretions, mucous plugs).

In acute asthma, correction of arterial hypoxaemia is the first priority. In COPD patients, a reasonable target is to keep arterial O_2 saturation about 90% (PaO_2 60–70 mmHg). If this cannot be achieved by $F_IO_2 < 0.4$, a pulmonary shunt, e.g. atelectasis, pneumonia etc. is likely and requires treatment.

> In asthma and COPD, minimizing dynamic hyperinflation is essential.

In controlled modes, there are three strategies that can decrease dynamic hyperinflation:

1. decrease of minute ventilation,
2. increase of expiratory time,
3. decrease of resistance to expiratory flows.

Decrease of minute ventilation

Controlled hypoventilation in mechanically ventilated patients is associated with lower mortality and a reduced number of complications in asthma as well as in COPD patients.[18,19] Large tidal volume and minute volume promote dynamic hyperinflation.[20] Hypoventilation can be performed by decreasing tidal volume or breathing frequency, or both. Tidal volume and breathing frequency as low as 5 mL kg^{-1} and 6 breaths min^{-1}, respectively, have been successfully applied in patients with severe asthma.[18] The degree and duration of hypoventilation depend on the severity of obstruction, which varies greatly between patients. To minimize pulmonary hyperinflation, end-inspiratory airway pressure should be limited to <50 cmH$_2$O (some intensivists even recommend keeping end-inspiratory $Paw \le$ 30 cmH$_2$O).[21]

The risks of permissive hypercapnia are minimal as long as $PaCO_2$ changes do not occur quickly.[22] Provided oxygenation is preserved and conditions of increased susceptibility to a high $PaCO_2$, such as increased intracranial pressure, are not present, values of $PaCO_2$ in excess of 80 mmHg are acceptable. Most authors agree that correction of acidaemia should only be done when it is severe (pH < 7.2). A carefully titrated buffer therapy (TRIS, sodium bicarbonate) or a small increase in alveolar ventilation is then indicated. Attempts to decrease $\dot{V}CO_2$ by manipulation using nutritional support are common, but their value is uncertain. Fever reduction and treatment of infection will also reduce $\dot{V}CO_2$.

Increase of expiratory time

Dynamic hyperinflation can be reduced by increasing expiratory time to allow an almost complete expiration despite airflow limitation. This must be achieved at the expense of shortened inspiration by increasing inspiratory flow (>70 L min^{-1}) and by eliminating the end-inspiratory pause (if volume-controlled modes are used). The strategy of increasing expiratory time, although less powerful than controlled hypoventilation, decreases dynamic hyperinflation and improves cardiovascular function and gas exchange.

Decrease resistance to expiratory flows

Decreasing airway resistance by the use of bronchodilator drugs and corticosteroids is of great importance.[16] External resistances should be minimized by using large endotracheal tubes and optimizing the connecting devices (i.e. PEEP valves, circuit connections etc.). These patients have excessive work of breathing due to multiple factors and it may be important to rest the respiratory muscles by controlled ventilation and sedation. Muscle paralysis should only be used at the initiation of mechanical ventilation. After 24 hours, ventilatory support can be switched to assist modes or mechanically supported spontaneous breathing.

PATIENTS VENTILATED ON ASSISTED MODES

When the patient's status improves, the ventilator is switched to an assist mode (pressure or volume assist) and the process of weaning begins (see below). Assisted modes may be used initially, if NIV is applied. In either case, patient–ventilator interaction needs close attention. By improving patient–ventilator synchrony, weaning may be facilitated. To improve patient–ventilator synchrony the setting of the ventilator must be adapted to the patient and frequently checked.

- Maximize the trigger sensitivity. Decrease the threshold for triggering to a level at which autocycling does not occur; use a ventilator with a short response time; and decrease the resistance of the inspiratory circuit. The settings should be repeatedly reviewed and appropriately adjusted.
- Minimize dynamic hyperinflation. Decrease airway resistance (bronchodilators, corticosteroids) and ventilatory demands (correction of hypoxaemia, sedation and even short-term depression of central respiratory drive by opioids).
- Low levels of external PEEP may increase trigger sensitivity substantially by reducing the elastic threshold load and the work of breathing. This beneficial effect of $PEEP_e$ is most evident in patients exhibiting flow limitation during tidal expiration. On the other hand, if flow limitation does not exist, external PEEP will present a back-pressure to expiratory flow and will cause further hyperinflation. The increase in end-expiratory alveolar pressure counterbalances the beneficial effect on trigger sensitivity. As a rough rule, external PEEP greater than 8 cmH_2O should be avoided. Careful re-evaluation of patient status should be performed after applying external PEEP.
- Initial inspiratory flow must meet the patient's flow demand. Inspiratory flow and machine

inspiratory time must be set high enough to satisfy the needs of the patient, which may alter, necessitating new ventilator adjustments. With pressure support mode (PSV), the patient has the ability to influence the machine breathing pattern as well as tidal volume and this mode might therefore be preferred. In the conventional assist modes, e.g. SIMV, this ability is compromised by the mechanical properties of the respiratory system and the function of the ventilator.

Changes in ventilator settings may modify the patient's respiratory response via modifications in mechanics, chemical reflexes and behavioural feedback systems. For example, by increasing inspiratory flows, an increase in spontaneous breathing frequency may occur due to a reflex excitatory effect of high flows on respiratory output counterbalancing their beneficial effect on dynamic hyperinflation. Thus, in contrast to controlled ventilation, changes in ventilatory settings in patients on assist modes may not always be successful.

Restoring respiratory muscle function by intermittent controlled ventilation

A common cause of delay in weaning COPD patients is an inability of the respiratory pump to meet the ventilatory demand. During assisted ventilation, the respiratory muscle load is difficult to assess and could remain excessive in assisted spontaneous modes. However, recovery can be provided by intermittent controlled ventilation, particularly at night, and other periods of spontaneous T-piece breathing,[23] or after extubation, employing NIV (see Chapter 5).

MECHANICAL VENTILATION IN BRAIN INJURY

Early management

Hypoxia is the second most important cause of mortality and morbidity following traumatic brain injury (see references 24 and 25). In the emergency situation, clearing the airway and providing oxygenation and adequate ventilation must be achieved without delay.

In patients with additional injuries that increase the risk of hypoxia, e.g. chest trauma or massive

EMERGENCY MANAGEMENT FOR OXYGENATION AND VENTILATION

- Secure (or maintain) airway.
- Provide high-flow O_2 to all patients with traumatic brain injury (regardless of severity).
- Provide intubation and ventilation for patients with a Glasgow Coma Score (GCS) of <8 (not eye opening, speaking or obeying commands) or a motor score <5 (withdrawing from pain or worse).
- Avoid and/or treat aspiration.
- Keep arterial O_2 saturation >95%.
- Avoid excessive hyperventilation, e.g. end-tidal CO_2 30–35 mmHg.

bleeding, intubation and mechanical ventilation should be considered at a higher GCS.

INTUBATION

The procedure can considerably increase intracranial pressure and should only be carried out with deep sedation and sufficient pre-oxygenation. Oral intubation is preferred as it is easier and safer if cervical spine injury has not been excluded. On the other hand, experienced physicians sometimes prefer 'blind' nasal intubation, especially for tube replacement in already intubated patients. In suspected or proven cervical spine injury, intubation may provoke further neurological damage and in-line axial stabilization must be ensured manually. A cervical collar should be removed as meticulous manual stabilization is regarded as being safer.

Tracheostomy should be performed at an early stage if a prolonged period of ventilatory support is anticipated. Optimal timing is still a subject of controversy. In a multicentre, randomized, prospective trial, no differences in length of stay, infections, mortality and tracheopharyngeal injury were found between early (3–5 days') and late (10–14 days') tracheostomy.

Further management

Arterial hypoxaemia, hypercapnia and systemic hypotension must be avoided.

These may occur during suctioning, positioning, physiotherapy, especially through lack of analgesia or

In patients with **increased intracerebral pressure**

- hypoxaemia
- hypercapnia
- hypotension

may cause **secondary brain damage**.

sedation, or during the replacement of endotracheal tubes, diagnostic or therapeutic manipulations or transportation for external diagnostic procedures or operations. Close monitoring with pulse oximetry, capnometry, arterial pressure and intracranial pressure monitoring and awareness of the problems are mandatory.

PRINCIPLES FOR MECHANICAL VENTILATION

To avoid hypoxaemia or hypercapnia, mechanical ventilation should be considered early.

Target criteria are arterial O_2 saturation >95%, arterial PCO_2 35–40 mmHg (if hyperventilation is not indicated, see below). A high FiO_2 (0.5–0.6) is often required to give a good margin of safety.

Positive end-expiratory pressure

The easiest way to improve oxygenation is to apply external PEEP. Increasing intrathoracic pressure PEEP may impair venous return and cardiac output and reduce cerebral perfusion. An optimal balance between the respiratory and the cardiovascular effects must be found. The effect of PEEP on cerebral circulation depends on the intracranial compliance, on the absolute level of the intracerebral pressure and on the haemodynamic effects related to the stiffness of the lungs. As long as the intracranial pressure is greater than the venous pressure, PEEP will not increase it. Whenever patients with acute brain injury need PEEP to optimize arterial oxygenation, careful monitoring of changes in intracranial pressure and cerebral perfusion pressure (CPP) is mandatory.

Controlled ventilatory modes

When controlled ventilatory modes are required, pressure or volume control can be used. PCV may be preferred to avoid unexpected airway pressure increases. Under stable conditions, and when peak airway pressure can be kept ≤ 30 cmH$_2$O, the volume controlled mode (VCV) has the advantage of ensuring minute volume and thereby the arterial PCO_2. However, sudden changes, e.g. a pneumothorax, or even coughing, may result in an increase in airway pressure, and a pressure limit control should be set at about 35 cmH$_2$O. PEEP should be set at a moderate level (<8 cmH$_2$O) that has no influence on cerebral perfusion if arterial systemic pressure is maintained (systolic >120 mmHg or mean >90 mmHg). The semi-recumbent position (15° to maximum 30°) of the upper part of the body will compensate for potential effects of PEEP. Fighting against the ventilator must be prevented. In severe brain injury, analgo-sedation will be kept at relatively high levels as a general treatment of the brain damage. The continuous application of muscle relaxants is obsolete, although for acute situations, such as severe coughing attacks, during adaptation to new ventilatory settings or in severe shivering, their short-term application may be useful.

Assisted ventilatory modes

In the later course, and assuming that respiratory drive is intact, assisted modes and supported spontaneous breathing (IMV, PSV, BIPAP) can be chosen. This author prefers the BIPAP modes because the ventilatory system is open at any time. The patient can breathe spontaneously whenever he or she wants to (even during the inspiration phase of the ventilator's cycle) and the pre-set peak airway pressure can never be exceeded (even when the patient is coughing or fighting against the ventilator).

Weaning

The decision as to when the patient can be weaned from mechanical ventilation depends on many factors:

- the severity of the brain damage,
- the clinical situation,
- age,
- complications and concomitant diseases,
- organizational aspects, e.g. the availability of competent personnel.

Weaning is a step-wise process, which must be carefully monitored. It should be started as early as possible because unnecessarily prolonged mechanical ventilation will increase the risk of complications. An unsuccessful weaning trial will not endanger the patient as long as a critical increase in intracranial pressure and a reduction of cerebral perfusion are prevented. If the intracranial pressure is continuously > 30 mmHg, a weaning trial should not be undertaken.

SPECIFIC PROCEDURES

Therapeutic hyperventilation

The prophylactic use of hyperventilation ($PCO_2 \leq 35$ mmHg) during the first 24 hours is not recommended because it may compromise cerebral perfusion. Hyperventilation therapy ($PCO_2 = 30$–35 mmHg) may be necessary for brief periods when there is an acute neurologic deterioration or for a longer period of intracranial hypertension refractory to conventional therapy. In this situation, hyperventilation must be carefully titrated; an arterial $PCO_2 < 30$ mmHg increases the risk of cerebral ischaemia and must be strictly avoided.[24] In the absence of increased intracranial pressure, chronic prolonged hyperventilation ($PCO_2 \leq 25$ mmHg) is not indicated.

COMPLICATIONS

Acute lung injury is a known complication of acute brain injury. The real frequency and cause(s) are controversial. If acute lung injury is not the result of trauma to the chest, the most common causes are:

- aspiration (often during resuscitation phase),
- pneumonia (the second most frequent complication, occurs in 40–50%),
- atelectasis (due to impairment of the normal cough reflex and/or to frequent disconnections from the ventilator for endotracheal suctioning),
- neurogenic pulmonary oedema (due to pulmonary vasoconstriction from increased sympathetic tone, arterial hypertension, or an increase in pulmonary capillary permeability).

These complications aggravate the process and may worsen the secondary brain damage. The therapeutic principles to treat these complications are described elsewhere. However, treatment of the acute lung injury must comply with the special limitations regarding acute brain injury (see above).

Case 2: ARDS plus Traumatic Brain Injury

KO, a 28-year-old male, had a motorcycle accident causing severe traumatic brain injury. He was deeply comatose and was immediately intubated by the emergency team before transportation to the local hospital. Aspiration was considered likely before intubation. A few hours later, he was transferred to another hospital with a neurosurgical department. Scanning revealed right parietal contusion with subarachnoidal bleeding into the ventricle, a subdural haematoma, fracture of the left condylus occipitalis and a pneumo-encephalon. There was also blunt chest trauma with bilateral lung contusion and probable aspiration.

A severe sepsis syndrome with multiple organ failure (severe ARDS, barotrauma, acute renal failure) developed during the next days and the patient was transferred to our ICU 9 days after the accident. On arrival, he was deeply analgo-sedated and under controlled ventilation (Table 3.2). Bilateral pulmonary leakage was treated by thoracic drains. The systemic circulation was supported by 40 μg min^{-1} of nor-epinephrine. X-rays and computerized tomography scans revealed a severe ARDS with some degrees of fibrotic consolidation, barotrauma including a pneumothorax, and emphysema in the mediastinum (Fig. 3.3).

We began mechanical ventilation with the APRV mode. Under this ventilatory setting, intracranial pressure could be kept within a range

(cont.)

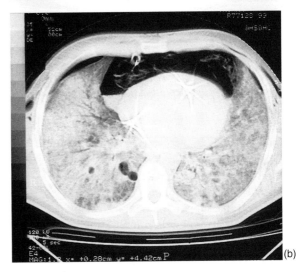

(a)

(b)

Figure 3.3 *KO, a 28-year-old male with polytrauma, sepsis and ARDS: CT scan (a) sagittal and (b) transversal at arrival in our hospital (9 days after trauma) with intrathoracic drains. The patient had severe ARDS and pneumothorax.*

Table 3.2 *KO, a 28-year-old male with polytrauma, sepsis and ARDS*

Day	0 (outside hospital)	0 arrival	1	4	8	9	25	30	49
MV	IRV	APRV	APRV	APRV	APRV	APRV	APRV	ASB-SP	ASB-SP
Phigh	?	29	29	30	26	26	20	ΔP 10	ΔP 10
Plow	?	5	8	10	12	11	8	8	5
I:E	2:1.0	2:0.5	2:1.0	2:0.8	2:0.8	2:1.5	2:2.0	–	–
RR	?	29	29	31	21	26	19	48	27
FiO$_2$	1.0	0.9	0.8	0.5	0.8	0.45	0.35	0.3	0.3
PO$_2$	121	85	87	99	70	84	102	52[a]	50[a]
PCO$_2$	45	53	45	56	56	51	53	47[a]	49[a]
ICP	–	11	11	20	18	19	–	–	–

[a]Venous blood samples.
IRV, inversed ratio ventilation; ASB-SP, assisted spontaneous breathing (ΔP, assist pressure (cmH$_2$O); ICP, intracranial pressure (mmHg). For other abbreviations, see Table 3.1.

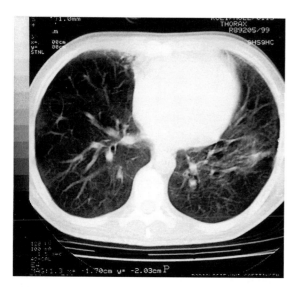

Figure 3.4 *KO, a 28-year-old male with polytrauma, sepsis and ARDS: CT scan at day 26 (35 days after trauma). The ARDS is considerably improved; there is some fibrosis and some bullae.*

(cont.)
of 11–20 mmHg (see Table 3.2). A percutaneous tracheostomy was carried out and intermittent prone/supine positioning performed.

Inotropic support, blood transfusions and continuous veno-venous haemofiltration were necessary. The patient's recovery was slow due to the severely damaged cerebral function (intracerebral hygroma, ventricular drainage, infection). Later, weaning was further delayed by a critical illness polyneuropathy, so that it was 3 months after the accident before the patient was discharged for further rehabilitation (Fig. 3.4).

MECHANICAL VENTILATION IN CARDIAC FAILURE

Ventilatory support in ischaemic heart disease

An increasing in intrathoracic pressure inhibits venous return but decreases left ventricular (LV) transmural pressure, which reduces LV after-load. In the failing heart, which is very sensitive to after-load, the net effect is to improve cardiac output. In contrast, decreasing intrathoracic pressure enhances venous return and may increase LV after-load.[17]

Consequently, CPAP and mechanical ventilation with PEEP have been used to improve cardiac output in LV failure and acute cardiac pulmonary oedema.

When **pulmonary oedema is severe in acute heart failure**, Type 2 respiratory failure occurs[26] because the work of breathing is markedly increased. The excessive intrathoracic pressure swings may also impair diastolic function. Respiratory support is urgently required in this situation and can be achieved by mask CPAP, NIV (bi-level pressure support) or by intubation and mechanical ventilation. CPAP decreases venous return and LV after-load. If LV contractility is markedly impaired, this will result in an increase in cardiac output. If, however, LV contractility is normal, the gain in cardiac output will only be small due to the reduction in venous return. Although CPAP may be sufficient in itself to correct a respiratory acidosis, bi-level NIV is more effective and better tolerated when the PCO_2 is markedly elevated, presumably because NIV provides better unloading of the respiratory muscles. In some patients, perhaps those with predominant systolic dysfunction, intubation and mechanical ventilation will be required, especially if there are contra-indications to NIV (see Chapter 5). Inotropes and LV assist procedures may be needed.

In **chronic congestive heart failure**, the use of CPAP is controversial. In some studies, long-term nocturnal CPAP has been reported to improve daytime cardiac function, but this has not been confirmed by other studies. The mechanisms that could explain a benefit are not fully understood, e.g. decrease in venous return, decrease in LV after-load, vasodilatation by activation of parasympathetic vasodilator mechanisms or reduction in sympathetic tone.[27]

SPECIAL CONSIDERATIONS

Massive obesity increases intra-abdominal pressure, impedes diaphragm function and increases the likelihood of OSA. It may also increase the risk of respiratory failure by impairing sputum clearance and promoting atelectasis and veno-embolism. In acute lung injury, obesity will also increase the risk of complications.

REFERENCES

1. Bernard, G, Artigas, A, Brigham, K, *et al*. Report of the American–European Consensus Conference on ARDS: definitions, mechanisms, relevant outcomes and clinical trial coordination. *Intensive Care Med* 1994; **20**: 225–32.

2. Gattinoni, L, Pelosi, P. Pathophysiologic insights into acute respiratory failure. *Curr Opin Crit Care* 1996; **2**: 8–12.

3. Gattinoni, L, Pelosi, P, Suter, PM, Pedoto, A, Vercesi, P, Lissoni, A. Acute respiratory distress syndrome caused by pulmonary and extrapulmonary disease. Different syndromes? *Am J Respir Crit Care Med* 1998; **158**: 3–11.

4. American Thoracic Society (ATS), European Society of Intensive Care Medicine (ESICM), Société de Réanimation de Langue Française (SRLF). International Consensus Conferences in Intensive Care Medicine: Ventilator-associated lung injury in ARDS. *Am J Respir Crit Care Med* 1999; **160**: 2118–24.

5. Amato, MB, Barbas, CS, Medeiros, DM, *et al*. Effect of a protective-ventilation strategy on mortality in the acute respiratory distress syndrome. *N Engl J Med* 1998; **338**: 347–54.

6. Hickling, KG, Walsh, JSH, Jackson, R. Low mortality rate in adult respiratory distress syndrome using low-volume, pressure limited ventilation with permissive hypercapnia: a prospective study. *Crit Care Med* 1994; **22**: 1568–78.

7. Slutsky, AS. Consensus Conference on Mechanical Ventilation – January 28–30, 1993, at Northbrook, Illinois, USA. Part II. *Intensive Care Med* 1994; **20**: 150–62.

8. Sydow, M., Burchardi, H. Inverse ratio ventilation and airway pressure release ventilation. *Curr Opin Anaesthesiol* 1996; **9**: 523–8.

9. Rathgeber, J, Schorn, B, Falk, V, Kazmaier, S, Spiegel, T, Burchardi, H. The influence of controlled mandatory ventilation (CMV), intermittent mandatory ventilation (IMV) and biphasic intermittent positive airway pressure (BIPAP) on duration of intubation and consumption of analgesics and sedatives. A prospective analysis in 596 patients following adult cardiac surgery. *Eur J Anaesthesiol* 1997; **14**: 576–82.

10. Acute Respiratory Distress Syndrome Network. Ventilation with lower tidal volumes as compared with traditional tidal volumes for acute lung injury and the acute respiratory distress syndrome. *N Engl J Med* 2000; **342**: 1301–8.

11. Hörmann, C, Baum, M, Putensen, C, Mutz, N, Benzer, H. Biphasic positive airway pressure (BIPAP) – a new mode of ventilatory support. *Eur J Anaesthesiol* 1994; **11**: 37–42.

12. Sydow, M, Burchardi, H, Ephraim, E, Zielmann, S, Crozier, TA. Airway pressure release ventilation versus volume controlled inverse ratio ventilation in patients with acute lung injury. *Am J Respir Crit Care Med* 1993; **149**: 1550–6.

13. Slutsky, AS. Consensus Conference on Mechanical Ventilation – January 28–30, 1993, at Northbrook, Illinois, USA. Part I. *Intensive Care Med* 1994; **20**: 64–79.

14. Rossi, A, Polese, G, Brandi, G, Conti, G. Intrinsic positive end-expiratory pressure (PEEPi). *Intensive Care Med* 1995; **21**: 522–36.

15. Georgopoulos, D, Brochard, L. Ventilatory strategies in acute exacerbations of chronic obstructive pulmonary disease. *In Mechanical ventilation from intensive care to home care*. Roussos, C, ed. Sheffield: European Respiratory Society, 1998; 12–44.

16. Georgopoulos, D, Burchardi, H. Ventilatory strategies in adult patients with status asthmaticus. In *Mechanical ventilation from intensive care to home care*. Roussos, C, ed. Sheffield: European Respiratory Society, 1998; 45–83.

17. Pinsky, MR. Mechanical ventilation and the cardio-vascular system. *Curr Opin Crit Care* 1996; **2**: 391–5.

18. Darioli, R, Perret, C. Mechanical controlled hypoventilation in status asthmaticus. *Am Rev Respir Dis* 1984; **129**: 385–7.

19. Tuxen, D. Permissive hypercapnic ventilation. *Am J Respir Crit Care Med* 1994; **150**: 870–4.

20. Tuxen, D. Detrimental effects of positive end-expiratory pressure during controlled mechanical ventilation of patients with severe airflow obstruction. *Am Rev Respir Dis* 1989; **140**: 5–9.

21. Corbridge, T, Hall, J. The assessment and the management of adults with status asthmaticus (state of the art). *Am J Respir Crit Care Med* 1995; **151**: 1296–316.

22. Feihl, F, Perret, C. Permissive hypercapnia. How permissive should we be? *Am J Respir Crit Care Med* 1994; **150**: 1722–37.

23. Esteban, A, Frutos, F, Tobin, M, *et al*. A comparison of four methods of weaning patients from mechanical ventilation. *N Engl J Med* 1995; **332**: 345–50.

24. Maas, A. *Pathophysiology, monitoring and treatment of severe head injury*. New York: Churchill Livingstone, 1993; 565–78.

25. Bullock, R, Chesnut, RM, Clifton, G, *et al.* *Guidelines for the management of severe head injury.* New York: Brain Trauma Foundation, 1995; 1–166.

26. Bersten, AD, Holt, AW. Acute cardiogenic pulmonary edema. *Curr Opin Crit Care* 1995; **1**: 410–19.

27. Scharf, SM. Ventilatory support in cardiac failure. *Curr Opin Crit Care* 1997; **3**: 71–7.

4

Ventilator–patient interaction

JOHN C GOLDSTONE

INTRODUCTION

During mechanical ventilation, the relationship between the ventilator and the patient is not simply a passive one in which the patient's lungs are inflated and the ventilator settings are defined by the user. Rather, many interactions occur and there exists an interface between the patient and the ventilator. For example, ventilation is frequently switched on by the patient inspiration and the ventilator must therefore be able to sense the onset of inspiration. Many other such interactions occur and there may be considerable overlap between them (Fig. 4.1).

TRIGGERING MECHANICAL VENTILATION

Mechanical ventilation is usually delivered so that the patient is able to initiate the breath from the ventilator. Before inspiration occurs, there are several steps that need to be performed and this process is termed triggering (Fig. 4.2).[1,2] In addition, a further set of conditions needs to occur to continue the breath delivered to the patient. The ventilator is constantly checking that inspiration is continuing in order to avoid high airway pressures, which would occur if the patient tried to breathe out during inspiration. The effect of the poorly set ventilator may be harmful.

The trigger can be adjusted to make the ventilator more or less sensitive. In older ventilators, a demand (mechanical) valve was employed as the device that could be opened by the patient at the start of inspiration. Demand valves are difficult to breathe through and, although they are not used in modern mechanical ventilators, they serve to illustrate the problems that a poorly adjusted trigger system imposes on the patient.

The inspiratory trigger

At the start of inspiration, the pressure difference generated in the chest is transmitted to the upper airway, and this is the physiological signal that is sensed by the ventilator to begin inspiration. However, unlike spontaneous breathing, flow does not begin as soon as the pressure at the airway is less than atmospheric. In fact, there is a delay imposed by the breathing system until the pressure in the upper airway equals the opening pressure of the inspiratory valve. This is termed the 'trigger phase'.

As soon as the opening pressure of the demand valve is reached, inspiratory flow begins. If inspiratory flow from the ventilator were unlimited, little further load would be placed on the patient. However, a demand valve imposes a further load because the flow produced by the valve is low, often

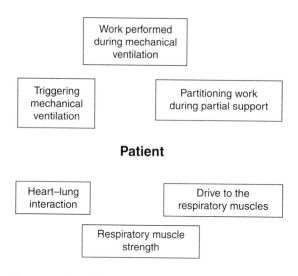

Figure 4.1 *The patient is rarely passively ventilated. There are many interactions that may occur between the patient and the ventilator.*

Clinical effects

The demand valve system had a number of clinical effects on the patient. The ventilator trigger system imposes a considerable absolute delay when no gas can flow to the patient. During this time, all inspiratory effort that is expended is wasted. Furthermore, inspiratory muscle activity is continued and increased, even when the demand valve opens, as flow is insufficient. Such native inspiratory muscle activity, once initiated, does not subside, even when the ventilator begins inspiration.[3] The amount of inspiratory muscle activity can equal or exceed that during spontaneous breathing. This implies that, if the ventilator is adjusted in this manner, no off-loading of muscle activity occurs. The graphic term 'fighting the ventilator' describes, in part, a poorly set inspiratory trigger.

much lower than required. This is particularly the case for patients with high airways resistance, e.g. chronic obstructive pulmonary disease (COPD), who often require high inspiratory flows. When the flow is inadequate for the patient demand, inspiratory effort continues and further negative pressure is generated. The period between the opening of the demand valve and full flow occurring has been termed the 'post-trigger' phase. When insufficient inspiratory flow occurs, the term 'flow starvation' has been used.

Modern triggering systems

A demand valve is nowadays seldom used. In its place, proportional valves are controlled by a microprocessor. A solenoid opens the valve quickly. Additionally, the valve settings can change over small ranges quickly and with minimal time delay, enabling flow to be adjusted precisely and complex pressure waveforms to be created within the airway. The response time to valve opening may be of the order of milliseconds.

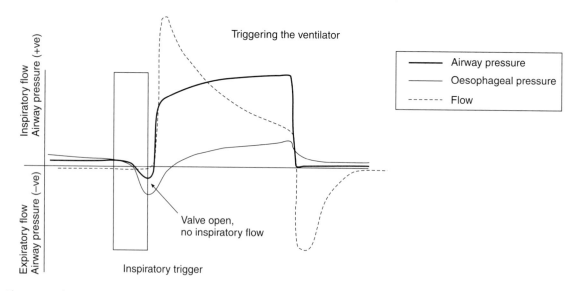

Figure 4.2 *There are two phases that occur before the ventilator allows the patient to breathe freely. The pressure in the airway must reach the set trigger pressure; and, as negative pressure continues, inspiratory flow then occurs.*

Moreover, high inspiratory flow rates can be achieved, such that the time to full flow may be less than 100 ms. The clinical problems of such systems tend now to be related to the way in which the software functions.

Flow triggering

The signal that is used to initiate inspiration may be taken from the inspiratory flow waveform and not the pressure tracing at the mouth. Flow at the mouth will rise when the pressure gradient between mouth and chest is negative. Whereas the pressure changes detected by the ventilator are small, flow signals increase substantially, and may improve the sensitivity of the triggering system.

Although it is possible simply to measure flow within the breathing circuit, this arrangement itself imposes load on the subject. In order to remove this load, flow in the breathing circuit is continuous and is provided at a base level. The flow through the inspiratory limb of the breathing circuit is continuously measured and compared with the flow through the expiratory limb. If no effort is made, the two flows should be equal. During the beginning of inspiration, a small amount of flow enters the patient and the inspiratory flow is greater than expiratory flow. This, then, is the signal to the ventilator to assist the breath.

Clinical problems with triggering

The sequence of events that occur to initiate inspiration is complex and may be described as the inspiratory chain of command (Fig. 4.3). The process involves activation of the inspiratory motoneurons, mainly the phrenic nerve, neuromuscular transmission and then contraction of inspiratory muscles. Movement of the thoracic ribcage then occurs and the volume of the system changes. The pressure within the thorax decreases. At this stage, a pressure difference between the chest and the mouth is established and inspiratory gas flow occurs.

A time delay between the chest and the mouth is a common feature of obstructive lung diseases such as COPD.[4] Initially, inspiratory muscle contraction occurs and pressure in the chest changes prior to any pressure change at the mouth. The time delay between the onset of pressure change in the chest

and that detected at the mouth can be substantial. During this time, the patient will receive no assistance and the term asynchrony has been used. Asynchronous ventilation occurs frequently in mechanical ventilated patients and may go unnoticed unless it is actively looked for.[5]

Other methods of triggering the ventilator

Signals from the brainstem or from the phrenic nerve are difficult to detect and cannot be used to trigger the ventilator. As the muscle is activated, electromyograph (EMG) activity occurs and this can be detected by percutaneous electrodes on the chest wall or over other inspiratory accessory muscles such as the sternocleidomastoid. Electrodes in these positions tend to be helpful when the onset of inspiration needs to be sensed and are useful when substantial contractions of the inspiratory muscles occur. However, they are susceptible to contamination from other adjacent, non-respiratory muscle groups, and the baseline noise sometimes obscures weak inspiratory contractions. Although it is technically possible to trigger ventilation, the system is not robust enough for clinical practice.

Recently, oesophageal EMG has been used to sense inspiration. This technique has been refined to incorporate multi-sensors and is resistant to electrode movement as a source of artefact. Such a system could theoretically move the trigger much closer to the patient and avoid many of the problems associated with triggering.

Improvements in the speed of response can be made if the pressure signal is moved closer to the patient. The pressure waveform may be obtained from the ventilator tubing next to the patient or at the distal part of the endotracheal tube.

RESPIRATORY MUSCLE WORK DURING MECHANICAL VENTILATION

Respiratory muscle activity during controlled ventilation occurs commonly and may be detected clinically or by inspecting airway pressure waveforms. During controlled ventilation, the inspiratory pressure waveform should be the same for each breath.

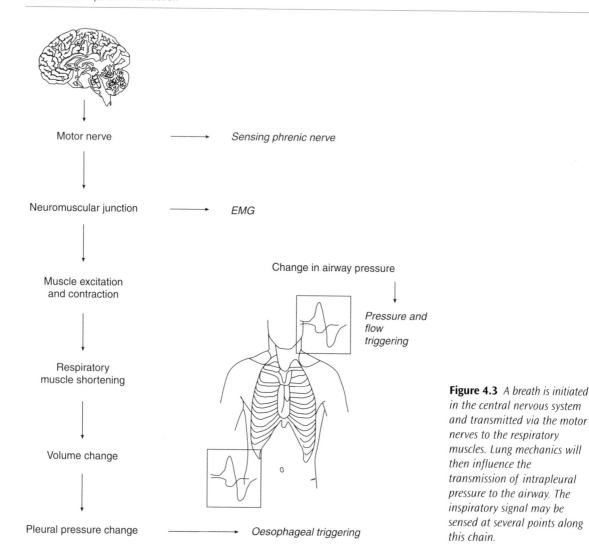

Motor nerve ⟶ *Sensing phrenic nerve*

Neuromuscular junction ⟶ *EMG*

Muscle excitation and contraction

Change in airway pressure

Pressure and flow triggering

Respiratory muscle shortening

Volume change

Pleural pressure change ⟶ *Oesophageal triggering*

Figure 4.3 *A breath is initiated in the central nervous system and transmitted via the motor nerves to the respiratory muscles. Lung mechanics will then influence the transmission of intrapleural pressure to the airway. The inspiratory signal may be sensed at several points along this chain.*

However, this is often not the case, as contraction of inspiratory muscles causes distortion and variation in the pressure waveform from breath to breath.[6,7]

The work of breathing

Mechanical work is defined as a force moving an object over a given distance. This form of work is easy to observe and may be quantified if the force and distance are known. Whereas work commonly occurs during skeletal muscle contraction, not all work may be measured. Internal work occurs when the muscle contracts, for example when holding an object stationary against gravity (Fig. 4.4). As no movement has occurred, no external work is per-

formed, yet the muscle is using energy internally, dissipated as heat and light. Such internal work may be very great indeed. Furthermore, as the muscle tension may be large and is maintained constantly, blood flow is reduced. Failure of force generation from the muscle is rapid and, despite maximal central nervous system drive, fatigue occurs.

EXTERNAL WORK

It is easy to imagine quantifying work when a simple lever and pulley system such as a limb muscle is studied. The respiratory muscles have a complex geometrical arrangement surrounding the ribcage. Moreover, the main inspiratory muscle has a dome-like shape and the force generated by the diaphragm is therefore

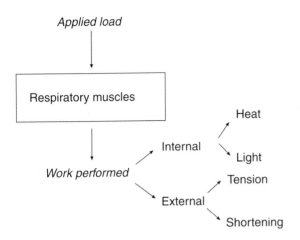

Figure 4.4 *Work is performed during muscle contraction. Internal work may not be easily measured, whereas external work involves movement and can be measured more easily.*

affected by the radii of curvature of the muscle itself. This makes the measurement of work difficult.

External work is performed when gas moves at the mouth. When this happens, pressure within the ribcage decreases and a gradient occurs between the ribcage and the atmosphere. If at this stage no gas flows between the mouth and the lungs, no movement of gas has occurred and no external work is performed. By contrast, internal work is high. When gas flows at the mouth, external work is performed and the work of breathing can be measured. The work of breathing is the integral of pressure and inspiratory volume and is expressed in terms of Joules per minute or Joules per litre of ventilation.

MEASUREMENT

In controlled circumstances, the work of breathing is straightforward to measure.[8] The pressure difference during each breath is recorded. This is the pressure difference that exists between the chest and mouth and is termed transpleural pressure. It is not possible to measure pleural pressure directly. A surrogate is found by measuring pressure elsewhere within the ribcage. Pressure changes in the oesophagus reflect pressure changes within the pleural space. Oesophageal pressure can be measured by passing a balloon catheter transnasally into the stomach and then withdrawing the tube until it is within the mid-point of the oesophagus. The pressure difference between the oesophagus and the mouth is then used for the calculation.

If the subject breathes through a pneumotachograph, inspiratory flow can be calculated and volume measured per breath. On an X–Y plot of volume and pressure, the area of each breath can be clearly seen and overlaid, one breath on top of another, enabling a visual display of work per breath over many iterations. This is typically measured digitally and software-based integration enables the work per breath to be calculated.

OTHER MEASUREMENTS OF WORK DURING BREATHING

Work associated with breathing can be estimated from other techniques. During inspiration, information can be obtained from the oesophageal pressure changes alone and measured as the area under the oesophageal pressure curve during inspiration. The measurement is made from an oesophageal balloon catheter. The pressure changes during inspiration are recorded and the timing of inspiration is made from inspiratory flow measured at the mouth. Oesophageal pressure is integrated from the beginning to the end of inspiratory flow, when flow changes direction. The area under the oesophageal pressure curve is then termed the pressure time product (PTP).[9]

Clearly, PTP is different from the traditional measurement of inspiratory work calculated from volume and pressure measurements. This need not be a problem, providing the two methods are not compared directly. The greatest strength of the PTP measurement may be in establishing trend data. As it is easy to measure and can be performed at the bedside, PTP has been used widely to report how inspiratory work changes during respiration.

The electrical activity of the diaphragm can be used to assess the amount of work performed by the muscle. Diaphragmatic EMG may be detected from electrodes placed adjacent to the diaphragm on the chest wall, or via needle electrodes placed under the skin on the chest wall, or from electrodes mounted on a balloon catheter and swallowed into the oesophagus. The different placements of the detecting electrodes yield different signals and the most robust technique is from oesophageal probes.

During quiet respiration, EMG is phasic and it may not be easy to distinguish it from background noise. As respiratory effort increases, the raw EMG increases in power and is clearly visible. Oesophageal electrodes detect the signal more easily as they are closer to the muscle. Originally, movement of the oesophageal sensors had a great effect on the quality of the EMG signal acquired, limiting the technique to the laboratory. Multiple electrodes have now been developed, straddling the crura of the diaphragm. As the catheter moves, for example during swallowing, one electrode from the array has the maximal signal and this is identified by a computer controlling the array.

A different approach to the problem of measuring inspiratory work is to measure the amount of O_2 used due to respiration.[9,10] In the critical care setting, this is possible because the O_2 consumed during mechanical ventilation can be compared to the amount of O_2 used when respiration is unassisted. The difference between these two states is calculated as the amount of O_2 consumed by the respiratory muscles themselves. Although technically possible, several problems exist at the bedside for critically ill patients. Obtaining steady-state measurements both at rest on the ventilator and then during spontaneous breathing demands little or no other muscle activity, and this is seldom the case in the critically ill. Furthermore, the amount of O_2 consumed may be less than 100 mL min^{-1}. If the total amount of O_2 during breathing is high (the product of minute ventilation and concentration of O_2), the measurement system may be required to detect less than 1% change in the total O_2 presented to the system, a level of fidelity that may not be possible clinically.

CLINICAL APPLICATION

The normal work of breathing is less than 0.6 J min^{-1} at rest. When measured in patients with lung disease such as obstructive lung defects, this may rise by up to fivefold at rest.[11]

In the critically ill, the work of breathing can be used to identify those patients who are breathing against a heavy load. The upper limit of inspiratory work has been identified, above which level breathing cannot be sustained. In small groups of patients studied, this may be at the level of 5 J min^{-1}.

Few large studies have been performed involving critically ill patients and the level of inspiratory work must be judged against the capacity of the inspiratory muscles to perform the work. With normal muscle strength, higher levels of work could be performed and the measurement of work should not be used in isolation to the performance of the whole system.

HEART–LUNG INTERACTIONS

Cardiovascular fluctuations during spontaneous breathing are well recognized and it is not surprising that mechanical ventilation can have profound effects on the circulation.[12] Mechanical ventilation, through its changes in both lung volume and intrathroacic pressure, has an influence on the determinates of stroke volume for both right and left ventricles. It is now appreciated that intermittent positive pressure ventilation (IPPV) has a complex effect on cardiac output rather than merely the decrease in venous blood flow suggested originally.

When lung volume increases, pulmonary vascular resistance (PVR) changes.[13] Pulmonary blood vessels have two major anatomical types. Alveolar blood vessels are closely related to the alveoli and are affected by changes in alveolar pressure. During inflation, alveolar blood vessel resistance increases and the capacity of the vessels decreases. By contrast, extra-alveolar vessels are exposed to intrathoracic pressure changes and volumes. During inflation, the calibre of these vessels increases, resistance falls and their capacitance rises. Clearly, the net effect on PVR during changes in lung volume is a balance, and in health PVR increases with lung inflation. In lung diseases characterized by hyperinflation, PVR is often elevated.

With lung deflation, little change in PVR occurs in the alveolar vessels, whereas the reduced lung volume compresses and reduces the calibre of the extrathoracic vessels and the net effect is to increase PVR at low lung volumes. In the critically ill, diseases that lead to a reduced lung volume, e.g. acute respiratory distress syndrome (ARDS), will tend to increase PVR and this effect will be exacerbated with other changes in the pulmonary vasculature. A goal of ventilatory therapy is to restore lung volume to functional residual capacity (FRC) to normalize PVR in hyperinflated and hypo-inflated lungs.

Lung volume will also impact on the cardiac system through direct mechanical compression of the heart. This may cause a restrictive effect similar to tamponade when pre-existing lung expansion occurs. As inflation pressures are transmitted to the cardiac chambers, so the measurement of cardiac filling pressures becomes inaccurate. Additionally, the cardiac septum may become deviated. This shift in the position of the septum may occur towards or away from the left ventricle, impairing function of either the right or left ventricle.

As the volume of the lungs increases, so intrathoracic pressure changes. During mechanical ventilation, intrathoracic pressure impedes blood flow to the right atrium and decreases right ventricular diastolic filling.

Intrinsic positive end-expiratory pressure

In normal lungs, the pressure in the alveoli reaches atmospheric as the lung empties at the end of each breath and, in the brief moment before the next breath, the pressure in the ribcage is equal to the balancing forces and the system stands still and no gas flows. Thus, the natural tendency of the lungs to deflate further is balanced against the tendency of the ribcage to spring open. This equilibrium point is the FRC.

If too brief a time is allowed for lung deflation, some of the exhaled gas will be trapped inside the lung and this will add volume to the system when the next breath is taken. A new equilibrium point will be established, where FRC is at a higher volume, and the pressure in the alveolus is increased. This can be achieved if the controls of the ventilator are set inappropriately for normal patients who are undergoing mechanical ventilation.

In obstructive lung disease, FRC increases. The resting pressure in the alveolus may be substantially raised.

The effect of intrinsic positive end-expiratory pressure (autoPEEP) was noted in the classic description by Pepe and Marini.[14] They observed the autoPEEP effect in a patient who was admitted to the intensive therapy unit (ITU) with a diagnosis of heart failure and who had a high right-sided filling pressure, a low blood pressure and poor peripheral flow. The patient was receiving inotropic support. The patient was temporarily disconnected from mechanical ventilation to facilitate tracheal suction and physiotherapy, and it was noted that, when disconnected, the filling pressure dropped, the blood pressure increased and the heart rate fell. In this patient, lung over-inflation raised alveolar pressure and this was responsible for the haemodynamic compromise. AutoPEEP acts to raise intrathoracic pressure, impedes venous return and therefore decreases stroke volume and cardiac output.

AutoPEEP was simply measured by Pepe and Marini by using the pressure gauge of the simple ventilator and occluding the expiratory limb of the ventilator tubing (Fig. 4.5). This allows the pressure in the alveolus to equilibrate along the airways and to be transmitted to the inspiratory pressure gauge. At occlusion, the inspiratory pressure jumps up to the level approximate to the level of autoPEEP.

AutoPEEP is now measured automatically on ventilators. The method occludes the inspiratory and expiratory valves and allows the distal airways to equilibrate. It measures the upper airway pressure after a set period of up to 15 s. However, in severe obstruction, this may not be sufficient time for all airways to equilibrate and care should be taken if this technique is employed in these patients.

For many patients, autoPEEP occurs during spontaneous ventilation, with or without some form of ventilator assistance such as pressure support. The occlusion method of measuring autoPEEP is not appropriate in this circumstance, as the patients cannot stop breathing to enable the measurment to take place. The presence of autoPEEP may be suspected in patients who continue to breathe out throughout expiration up to and until the next breath delivered from the ventilator.

Clinical implications

If high, autoPeep prevents venous filling, reduces end-diastolic ventricular volume and therefore reduces stroke volume. When severe, as in the case described by Pepe and Marini, the effect is similar to that seen in cardiac failure, as the pressure within the chest is easy to overlook.

Intrinsic PEEP must be overcome before gas flows into the chest. It acts as an additional load to breathing and ventilators will only cycle to inspiration when autoPEEP is equalled in the upper airway.

The effect of a threshold load induced by autoPEEP can be offset to some extent by the addition of external PEEP. If the pressure in the upper airways is increased by the addition of external PEEP, the effect is to balance the distal and proximal pressures.[15]. As the difference between the two sites of pressure measurement is reduced, so the pressure to begin flow in the upper airway decreases. When they are perfectly matched, the inspiratory effort necessary from the patient to initiate inspiratory gas flow and to make the ventilator 'cycle' to inspiration is

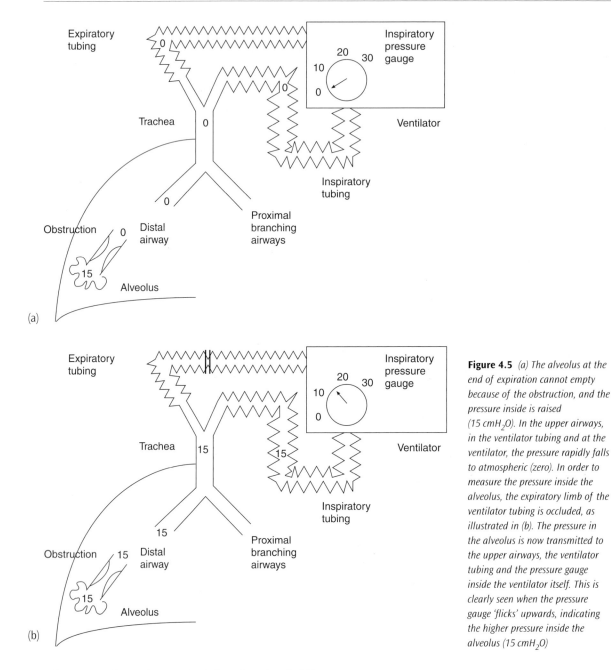

Figure 4.5 *(a) The alveolus at the end of expiration cannot empty because of the obstruction, and the pressure inside is raised (15 cmH$_2$O). In the upper airways, in the ventilator tubing and at the ventilator, the pressure rapidly falls to atmospheric (zero). In order to measure the pressure inside the alveolus, the expiratory limb of the ventilator tubing is occluded, as illustrated in (b). The pressure in the alveolus is now transmitted to the upper airways, the ventilator tubing and the pressure gauge inside the ventilator itself. This is clearly seen when the pressure gauge 'flicks' upwards, indicating the higher pressure inside the alveolus (15 cmH$_2$O)*

minimal. Such a reduction in 'triggering threshold' also ensures that the ventilator provides pressure support for each spontaneous breath made by the patient (Fig. 4.6).

If external PEEP is added to the point in excess of the level of internal PEEP, the effect will be to cause further hyperinflation and the effect of reducing the threshold load is offset. Care should be taken to avoid a further increase in lung volume with the application of distending patterns of ventilation.

RESPIRATORY DRIVE

Breathing during mechanical ventilation is commonplace and respiratory drive may be affected profoundly in the critically ill. At the simplest level, sedative drugs and neuromuscular agents may decrease drive and patients may not trigger mechanical ventilation. The effect of sedative drugs tends to offset the response curve of the central nervous

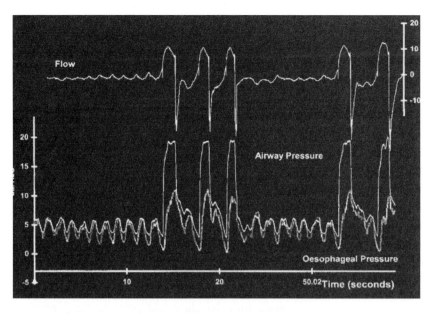

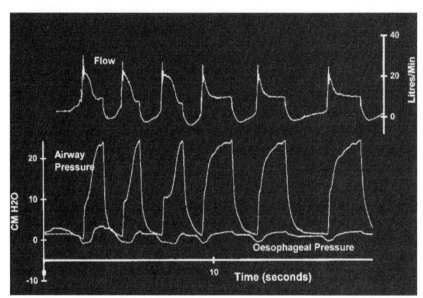

Figure 4.6 *Tracings of flow, airway pressure and oesophageal pressure during mechanical ventilation. The upper panel shows many inspiratory efforts that are not sensed by the ventilator (asynchrony). When external PEEP is added to balance the autoPEEP effect, triggering is successful (bottom panel).*

system to CO_2 and respiratory acidosis, such that higher stimulation levels are needed to begin respiration. Modest over-ventilation may then suppress ventilation and apnoea occurs unless ventilation is adjusted to achieve a higher level of $PaCO_2$ when spontaneous respiration will occur. This may be of little significance in most normal patients recovering after brief periods of ventilation after, for example, elective surgery. For patients who may require high levels of central nervous system drive to breathe, reduction of drive may be significant.

The response of the respiratory muscles to stimulation may be expressed as a frequency–force curve. The relationship between stimulation and response of a skeletal muscle is sigmoid shaped and the curve markedly flattens off as stimulation frequency reaches 40 Hz (Fig. 4.7). Above this frequency, little increase in force is generated.

Normal ventilation occurs at low stimulation frequency and lies on the steep part of the force–frequency curve and consequently large increases in minute ventilation will result from an

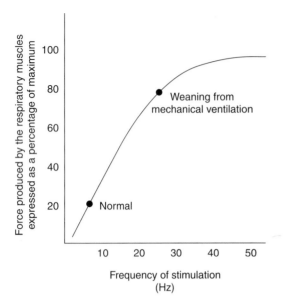

Figure 4.7 *The force generated during respiratory muscle contraction is plotted against the frequency of stimulation. Force rapidly increases as stimulation rises above 5 Hz. There is little increase in force after 40 Hz.*

increase in stimulation frequency. This is well illustrated in patients with a metabolic acidosis who are able to near-normalize their acid–base status by substantial increases in ventilation. Many patients who are critically ill are breathing at the upper range of their frequency–force curve, for example patients with intrinsic respiratory disease such as COPD. In this circumstance, maintenance of respiratory drive is essential. Modest changes in output provoke substantial changes in force generation, precipitating respiratory failure.

The measurement of respiratory drive

It is not possible to measure the output of a motor nerve directly in humans because the amplitude of the electrical potentials cannot be detected percutaneously. Phrenic neurograms may be measured when the nerve can be directly exposed, and this is the case when the phrenic nerve is stimulated to enable native respiration when the spinal cord is damaged at a high level and the patient is ventilator dependent.

An alternative to direct measurement is to assess the result of central drive in terms of the response of the respiratory muscles to the stimulus. For the respiratory muscles, tension within the muscle produces a change in pressure within the chest and thus the response to stimulation is a change in pressure. The pressure is measured at the airway by simple apparatus. Central to the technique is that the airway has to be occluded (often by a rapidly responding solenoid valve) and, if this is done briefly, the respiratory muscles are isometric and the subject cannot detect this brief occlusion and therefore the respiratory pattern is not influenced by the manoeuvre.

In order to standardize the measurement, the pressure generated in the first 100 ms of an occluded breath is measured and this is termed airway occlusion pressure, or $P_{0.1}$. $P_{0.1}$ is raised when respiratory drive is elevated artificially during a hypercapnic challenge and is also high in patients in ventilatory failure. As $P_{0.1}$ is measured before gas flows into the chest and prior to lung inflation, changes in lung mechanics do not affect its measurement. However, as changes in the length of the respiratory muscles will alter the generated pressure for a given stimulus, it is important that lung volume does not alter.

The value of $P_{0.1}$ in assessing patients weaning from mechanical ventilation

It is easy to apply the technique to ventilated patients and, when respiratory drive is elevated, the measured pressure exceeds 5.5 cmH$_2$O. During weaning, when a raised $P_{0.1}$ is found, patients fail to wean. Interestingly, patients who are able to breathe during weaning trials not only have a low $P_{0.1}$ but are also able to increase drive and minute ventilation during a hypercapnic challenge. Patients who are able to breathe spontaneously do so with a lower central drive and also have some ventilatory reserve, contrasting with the fixed capacity of patients who fail.

When airway resistance is high, a considerable time delay may occur between the onset of a negative intrathoracic pressure and pressure changes in the upper airway or mouth. In severe disease, airway occlusion pressure no longer reflects the pressure generated by the muscles and intrathoracic and airway pressures are not related.

Recently, $P_{0.1}$ has been used to assess how much hyperinflation and autoPEEP is present in patients breathing spontaneously. As hyperinflation increases, respiratory drive must accommodate the increased threshold load mentioned previously. The increased drive can be detected as an increase in $P_{0.1}$ and distinguishes hyperinflated patients.[16]

REFERENCES

1. Sassoon, CSH. Mechanical ventilator design and function: the trigger variable. *Respir Care* 1992; **37**: 1056–69.

2. Sassoon, CSH, Gruer, SE. Characteristics of the ventilator pressure and flow-trigger variables. *Intensive Care Med* 1995; **21**: 159–68.

3. Flick, GR, Bellamy, PE, Simmons, DH. Diaphragmatic contraction during assisted mechanical ventilation. *Chest* 1989; **96**: 130–5.

4. Murciano, D, Aubier, M, Bussi, S, Derenne, JP, Pariente, R, Milic-Emili, J. Comparison of esophageal, tracheal and occlusion pressure in patients with chronic obstructive pulmonary disease during acute respiratory failure. *Am Rev Respir Dis* 1982; **126**: 837–41.

5. Fabry, B, Guttman, J, Eberhard, L *et al*. An analysis of desynchronization between the spontaneously breathing patient and ventilator during inspiratory pressure support. *Chest* 1995; **107**: 1387–94.

6. Marini, JJ, Capps, JS, Culver, BH. The inspiratory work of breathing during assisted mechanical ventilation. *Chest* 1985; **87**: 612–18.

7. Marini, JJ, Rodriguez, RM, Lamb, V. The inspiratory workload of patient-initiated mechanical ventilation. *Am Rev Respir Dis* 1986; **134**: 902–9.

8. Marini, JJ, Rodriguez, RM, Lamb, V. Bedside estimation of the inspiratory work of breathing during mechanical ventilation. *Chest* 1986; **89**: 56–63.

9. Collett, PW, Perry, C, Engel, LA. Pressure–time product, flow, and oxygen cost of resistive breathing in humans. *J Appl Physiol* 1985; **58**: 1263–72.

10. Harpin, RP, Baker, JP, Downer, JP, Whitwell, J, Gallacher, WN. Correlation of the oxygen cost of breathing and length of weaning from mechanical ventilation. *Crit Care Med* 1987; **15**: 807–9.

11. Fleury, B, Murciano, D, Talamo, C *et al*. Work of breathing in patients with chronic obstructive pulmonary disease in acute respiratory failure. *Am Rev Respir Dis* 1985; **131**: 822–7.

12. Pinsky, MR. *The effects of mechanical ventilation on the cardiovascular system*. Philadelphia: WB Saunders, 1990.

13. Hakim, TS, Michel RP, Chang HK. Effect of lung inflation on pulmonary vascular resistance by arterial and venous occlusion. *J Appl Physiol* 1982; **53**: 1110–15.

14. Pepe, PE, Marini, JJ. Occult positive end-expiratory pressure in mechanically ventilated patients with airflow obstruction. *Am Rev Respir Dis* 1982; **126**: 166–70.

15. Tobin, MJ, Lodato, RF. PEEP, Auto-PEEP, and waterfalls. *Chest* 1989; **96**: 449–51.

16. Mancebo, J, Albaladejo, P, Touchard, D, *et al*. Airway occlusion pressure to titrate positive end-expiratory pressure in patients with dynamic hyperinflation. *Anesthesiology* 2000; **93**: 81–90.

5

Non-invasive mechanical ventilation in acute respiratory failure

BERND SCHÖNHOFER

INTRODUCTION AND HISTORICAL BACKGROUND

Mechanical ventilation can be provided by either negative or positive pressure ventilation. During the polio epidemics of the 1950s and 1960s, negative pressure ventilation (NPV) was widely used.[1] Ventilation is supported by exposing the chest to subatmospheric pressure to produce inspiration and allowing expiration by returning the pressure around the chest wall to atmospheric pressure. Several devices, such as the Emerson iron lung, cuirass and the Ponchowrap, are available. Although NPV can be successfully employed in acute respiratory failure,[2] because of the size of the devices, the lack of access to the patient and the danger of inducing upper airway obstruction[3] it is not widely used. In the second half of the twentieth century, invasive mechanical ventilation (IMV) was provided through a cuffed endotracheal or tracheostomy tube and became the standard method of providing artificial ventilation as it guarantees control of the airway and the ability to correct acid–base and gas disturbances with security. It also allows close monitoring and control of airway pressures and of tidal volume. Non-invasive mechanical ventilation (NIV), using facial or nasal masks as interfaces, was introduced as an alternative in the late 1970s and early 1980s, usually for domiciliary therapy. According to the underlying pathophysiology of respiratory failure, NIV may be effective in improving alveolar ventilation, reducing dyspnoea, resting the respiratory muscles and reducing dynamic hyperinflation. This chapter focuses on the impact of NIV in acute respiratory failure (ARF), in which it is increasingly applied following a pilot study involving patients with hypercapnic ARF in the early 1990s.[4]

NON-INVASIVE VERSUS INVASIVE MECHANICAL VENTILATION

The main advantage of IMV is the secure access to and protection of the airways. However, a range of adverse effects or complications is associated with IMV (Table

Table 5.1 *Advantages (+) and disadvantages (−) of invasive mechanical ventilation (IMV) and non-invasive mechanical ventilation (NIV)*

Clinical aspect	IMV	NIV
Ventilator-associated penumonia	−	+
Additional resistive work of breathing	−	+
Early and late tracheal injuries	−	+
Deep sedation, paralysis	−	+
Intermittent application of ventilator	−	+
Cough possible	−	+
Eating possible	−	+
Communication possible	−	+
Difficult weaning	−	+
Protection of airways	+	−
Access to airways	+	−
Facial side effects	+	−
Leakage	+	−
Claustrophobia	+	−
Aerophagia	+	−

Table 5.2 *Causes of hypercapnic acute respiratory failure (ARF) in which non-invasive ventilation has been applied*

	RCT	NRCT
Hyercapnic ARF		
Acute exacerbation of COPD	Yes	Yes
Post-extubational	Yes	Yes
Acute exacerbation of asthma	No	Yes
Cystic fibrosis	No	Yes
Hypoxaemic ARF		
Cardiogenic pulmonary oedema	Yes	Yes
Organ transplantation	Yes	Yes
Community-acquired pneumonia	Yes	Yes
Postoperative	Yes	Yes
Trauma	No	Yes
Atelectasis	No	Yes
Opportunistic pneumonia in HIV	No	Yes
Immunocompromised	Yes	Yes
Near-drowning	No	Yes
Lung cancer	No	Yes
Pulmonary embolus	No	Yes

RCT, randomized, controlled trials; NRCT, non-randomized controlled trials; COPD, chronic obstructive pulmonary disease; HIV, human immunodeficiency virus.

5.1). Ventilator-associated pneumonia (VAP) is perhaps the most important,[5,6] the incidence of which is dependent on the duration of IMV as, after 3–5 days, the rate of VAP increases significantly.[7] The rate of nosocomial infection appears to be lower in patients receiving NIV as first-line therapy.[8,9]

SPECTRUM OF ACUTE RESPIRATORY FAILURE TREATED WITH NON-INVASIVE MECHANICAL VENTILATION

Controlled and uncontrolled trials of NIV have been conducted in a broad spectrum of causes of ARF.[10] A limiting factor is that exclusion criteria in many resulted in only a minority of patients being randomized to NIV.[11] As a consequence, the results apply to a restricted patient population and may not be generally applicable. From the pathophysiological point of view, it is useful to differentiate between the hypercapnic and hypoxaemic type of ARF (Table 5.2; see also section 'Non-invasive mechanical ventilation and outcome', below).

TECHNICAL ASPECTS: INTERFACE

One of the most crucial issues is the interface. Several types are commercially available: full facemask, nasal mask, nasal pillows (Fig. 5.1). In some cases, mouthpieces and custom fabricated masks may also be useful. In ARF, the full facemask is usually preferable to nasal masks in our experience. The advantages and disadvantages of mask types are given in Table 5.3.

VENTILATOR MODES FOR NON-INVASIVE MECHANICAL VENTILATION

Both volume-targeted[12] and pressure-targeted ventilation[11,13] can be employed. Critical care ventilators, characterized by high technical quality and elaborate monitoring, and simpler and smaller ventilators, often used for home mechanical ventilation, can be used. In one comparison of the intensive care unit (ICU)-type ventilator and six portable 'home' devices, there were differences between the smaller 'home' devices in terms of re-breathing, the speed to a stable level of pressure support and expiratory resistance.[14] These differences may have clinical impact. Another study investigated the technical performance of nine ventilators used for acute NIV compared to an ICU ventilator.[15] The authors found that most pressure ventilators evaluated were able to respond to high ventilatory demands and even outperformed the ICU device! If the ventilator only supports

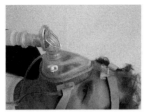
(a)

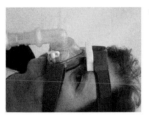
(b)

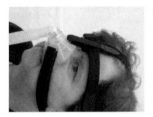
(c)

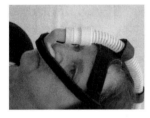
(d)

Figure 5.1 *Interfaces: facemask (a); nasal mask (b); nasal mask with little dead space (c); nasal pillows (d).*

Table 5.3 *Advantages (+) and disadvantages [spectrum from (−) to −] of nasal masks and facemasks*

Clinical aspect	Facemask	Nasal mask
Mouth leak	+	−
Mouth breathing and quality of NIV	+	−
Influence of dental status	+	−
Airway pressure	+	−
Dynamic of improved ABG	+	−
Dead space	(−)	+
Communication	−	+
Eating, drinking	−	+
Expectoration	−	+
Risk of aspiration	−	+
Risk of aerophagia	−	+
Claustrophobia	−	+
Comfort	(−)	+

NIV, non-invasive ventilation; ABG, arterial blood gases.

CO_2-re-breathing may occur with NIV. The risk is greater with a single delivery circuit without a true exhalation valve.[14,17] High respiratory rates and low external PEEP increase the risk of CO_2-re-breathing because of the shorter expiratory time and lower wash-out of the circuit. A minimal expiratory positive airway pressure (EPAP) of 2–4 cmH$_2$O is usually necessary to reduce CO_2-re-breathing in a single tube circuit.

At present, there are no generally accepted recommendations on how to set up NIV. Consideration of gas exchange, muscle load and breathing pattern is appropriate when setting the optimal PSV for each individual patient. Published studies have used a variety of end-points as targets for therapy, such as patient comfort, the level of pressure or volume support, blood gases or breathing pattern.[10–13,18,19] When using bi-level NIV, we start with inspiratory positive airways pressure (IPAP) of 8–10 cmH$_2$O and EPAP of 2–4 cmH$_2$O and quickly increase IPAP as the patient settles. Subsequent adjustment will then depend on the underlying diagnosis, the patient's tolerance and comfort and the physiological parameters such as O$_2$ saturation (SaO$_2$), minute ventilation (aiming for an estimated tidal volume of 10–15 mL kg^{-1}), fall in respiratory rate and disappearance of accessory muscle activity. In ARF due to chronic obstructive pulmonary disease (COPD), an inspiratory pressure support of 15–25 cmH$_2$O and EPAP of 4–6 cmH$_2$O would commonly be used. NIV can be

spontaneous breathing, each breath being triggered, the mode is termed pressure support ventilation (PSV) or assisted spontaneous breathing (ASB). PSV is the most commonly used mode in ARF as it allows the patient more control, which aids tolerance. An important advantage of PSV (over volume support) is the compensation for mild to moderate leak. Patients with ARF are often characterized by agitation, irregular breathing, intrinsic positive end-expiratory pressure (PEEPi) and sleep deprivation. PSV may facilitate patient–ventilator synchrony, whereas the addition of external PEEP will reduce inspiratory muscle work as PEEPi must be overcome before inspiration can begin.[16] In the sleep-deprived patient, however, triggering cannot be guaranteed and a timed mode of ventilation may be better in the patient with more severe respiratory failure.

applied with a mandatory back-up rate, e.g. 12 breaths min^{-1} as patient effort may fall in sleep. Supplemental O_2 (2–10 L min^{-1}) should be administered via the ventilator tubing to maintain the SaO_2 >90%. Some higher-specification machines allow control of inspired O_2.

Triggering is crucial to the success of PSV, i.e. the detection of patient inspiration. Some ventilators have a fixed and others a variable trigger. In the past, ventilators were often pressure triggered. Flow triggering is more sensitive,[20] although so-called auto-cycling may develop due to air leak.[21] This results in rapid switching between IPAP and EPAP, with no real benefit to the patient. Increasing the flow needed to trigger (making it less sensitive) will make this less likely to occur. A new development is a 'moving time' analysis of the pressure contour during a delivered breath (within milliseconds) and these technical advances may improve triggering and comfort. Another technical challenge is how quickly and adequately the ventilator can reach pressure despite variable patient demand. Inspiratory flow depends on the underlying pathophysiology, e.g. resistance and compliance, the given pressure support and inspiratory rise time. The quicker the machine can reach pressure, the lower the work of breathing.[22] Depending on the type of machine, the pressure rise time, or slope, may be adjustable or be manufacturer fixed. A slow rise time is primarily provided for domiciliary use, e.g. for comfort in the non-breathless neuromuscular patient. In ARF, rise time should be short. Indeed, depending on leak, some devices are insufficiently powered to support the short inspiratory time and high pressure support requirements of the dyspnoeic COPD patient. Finally, the detection of end-inspiration may be important for patient comfort. It is adjustable on some ventilators and fixed on others, i.e. switching to expiration when inspiratory flow reaches 70% of the initial flow rate. Again, this is more relevant to domiciliary, long-term ventilation, but may be important when using the spontaneous mode of ventilatory support.

Allowing the patient to maintain control of the breathing pattern may increase compliance. Proportional assist ventilation (PAV) has been proposed as a mode of synchronized partial ventilatory support that unloads both the resistive and elastic burdens and in which support provided is proportional to instantaneous patient effort.[23–25] The majority of studies investigating PAV have been short term. The clinical value of PAV as a NIV mode to treat ARF has not yet been convincingly shown. Controlled ventilation, either as volume assist control (ACV) or pressure-controlled ventilation (PCV), does not require patient effort and cycles automatically if there is no or insufficient ventilatory effort. In contrast to chronic domiciliary ventilation, ACV or PCV is less frequently used when treating ARF, but may be indicated when there is severe overload of the respiratory muscles, profound sleep deprivation or acute O_2-induced narcosis resulting in minimal respiratory effort. These modes should be considered in the failing patient before resorting to endotracheal intubation if to do so is considered safe.

Some NIV studies have compared PSV with volume assist control ventilation in ARF.[18,26,27] No differences were found in outcome, blood-gas changes and degree of muscle rest.[26,27] PSV did, however, have a reduced incidence of side effects and was more comfortable,[18,27] with better leak compensation.[18]

PRACTICAL GUIDELINES TO MANAGE ACUTE RESPIRATORY FAILURE

Based on the literature and clinical experience, a practical algorithm is depicted in Figure 5.2. Compared to conventional treatment with bronchodilators and steroids, NIV is not indicated in patients with a pH >7.35.[28] In other words, patients in whom ARF is not severe enough do not profit from the additional application of NIV. Patients with ARF being considered for NIV should have pH >7.20 and <7.35.[11,29] The use of pH as severity indicator is better than PCO_2 as it distinguishes the acute component of respiratory failure. Using PCO_2 alone would not allow for the chronic component. It is important, when inspecting the pH and other arterial blood-gas results, to take note of any metabolic component that may indicate failure of tissue oxygenation and the development of a lactic acidosis.

IMV and NIV should be seen as complementary treatments in a patient needing ventilatory support. IMV remains the preferred treatment if there are contraindications to NIV (Table 5.4). However, in the early stages, NIV has definite advantages. Treatment strategies should be based on both clinical aspects

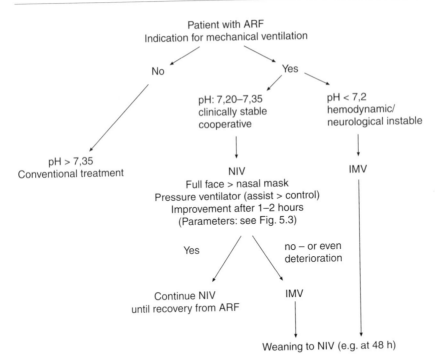

Figure 5.2 *Algorithm for the use of non-invasive ventilation in acute respiratory failure.*

Table 5.4 *Contraindications to non-invasive mechanical ventilation*

Severe acidosis at admission (pH <7.1)
Coma and massive confusion
Massive psychomotor agitation
Significant co-morbidity
Orofacial abnormalities
Irreversible mask intolerance and recent facial surgery
Haemodynamic instability (systolic blood pressure
  <70 mmHg)
Irreversible hypersecretion
Life-threatening, refractory hypoxaemia
Respiratory arrest
Intubation needed to protect upper airways (coma, acute
  abdominal process)
Glottic oedema or closure

(comfort, mental status and mouth and mask leak) and monitoring of physiological parameters (SaO$_2$, pH, breathing frequency and tidal volume) (Fig. 5.3). Success or failure should be judged within the first 1–2 hours (see Fig. 5.2). A lack of improvement in blood gases, a high initial severity of illness score and poor tolerance of NIV are predictors of failure.[30,31] If patients fail to improve, it is important that there is rapid access to intubation as delay increases mortality.[32] In addition to using NIV to prevent intuba-

tion and IMV, it may be employed to accelerate extubation (see Fig. 5.2), thereby reducing the potential for complications, by shortening the period of IMV, and also avoiding the need for re-intubation.[33]

IMPLEMENTATION AND DURATION OF NON-INVASIVE MECHANICAL VENTILATION IN ACUTE RESPIRATORY FAILURE

Despite the evidence for the benefits of NIV, provision is still limited by the lack of resources and, especially, trained personnel. In a survey investigating NIV in acute COPD in the UK, staff and equipment were available in fewer than half of the acute care hospitals.[34] In those hospitals in which NIV was available, it was generally underused. Lack of training, problems with funding and doubts about its value were given as reasons for the failure to provide a comprehensive 'out of hours' NIV service. A meta-analysis of randomized trials[10] may have overestimated its value due to the highly selected study populations included in these studies. Results achieved in enthusiastic departments as part of clinical trials may not be achievable in the real world. In a French multi-centre trial, involving

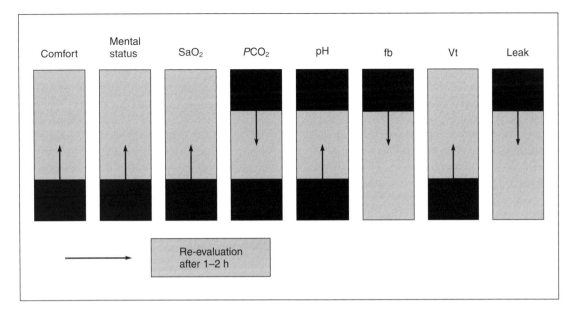

Figure 5.3 *Variables to evaluate non-invasive ventilation. SaO$_2$, O$_2$ saturation; fB, breathing frequency; Vt, tidal volume.*

more than 40 ICUs, poor patient tolerance was a major cause of failure.[35] Success may depend on the quality of NIV provision and yet a complex spectrum of variables influences the implementation phase (Table 5.5). The location for NIV depends on local factors such as equipment, the skills of doctors, nurses and therapists and their 24-hour availability. Patients with a high likelihood of failure (pH <7.25) should be initiated in the ICU or emergency room and, if stabilized, transferred to a high dependency unit (HDU) or specialist ward. In a large, randomized study, the practicality of the early use of NIV in a respiratory ward was examined.[29] For patients with mild to moderate acidosis (pH between 7.25 and 7.35), NIV let to a more rapid improvement in physiological parameters, a reduction in the need for IMV and a significant reduction in hospital mortality. Patients were treated according to a simple protocol using a spontaneous mode bi-level ventilator. Although the providers of the service were not experts, a considerable amount of training was needed, which was required to be on-going. Some practical aspects are illustrated by the following case reports.

Table 5.5 *Factors influencing the success of non-invasive mechanical ventilation*

Location
Interface
Ventilator type, mode and setting
Monitoring
Indication
Motivation of the staff
Training of the staff
Experience of the staff
Size of staff
Time consumption
Organization of team

SUCCESSFUL NON-INVASIVE MECHANICAL VENTILATION IN HYPERCAPNIC ACUTE RESPIRATORY FAILURE (FIG. 5.4)

A patient with end-stage COPD (male, 64 years, FEV$_1$ as an outpatient: 0.70 L, 37% predicted) was admitted with acute exacerbation of respiratory failure. Initial blood gases: PCO$_2$ 8.5, PO$_2$ 4.5 (air) and 6.5 (kPa) with O$_2$ at 2 L min^{-1}, pH 7.28 and respiratory rate 27 min^{-1}. He was co-operative, but agitated, and haemodynamically stable.

The team decided to initiate NIV with a nasal mask. An explanation was given. The head of the bed was maintained at an angle of 45° and a low dose of morphine (5 mg) was given to reduce agitation. Due to mouth breathing, the nasal mask
(cont.)

(*cont.*)

needed to be switched to a full facemask and, to improve the acceptance of NIV, the facemask was initially connected to an Ambu-bag. The patient was ventilated manually in time with his breathing frequency. Thereafter PSV was given with IPAP at 10 cmH$_2$O, progressively increasing to 20 cmH$_2$O. However, excessive respiratory secretions limited acceptability (the patient kept taking the mask off to cough and, after an initial fall in PCO_2, it began to increase again). Fibreoptic bronchoscopy was performed, employing a specially adapted mask, without interrupting NIV.[36] After 4 hours of continuous NIV, PCO_2 was 7.4 and pH 7.33. An NIV-free interval of 15 min allowed the patient to communicate, expectorate and drink. He then continued with NIV. During the first 24 hours on the ICU, NIV was applied for a total of 20 hours. The patient was then transferred to the general respiratory ward, but continued with NIV intermittently and overnight until blood gases normalized.

NON-INVASIVE MECHANICAL VENTILATION FAILURE IN A PATIENT WITH HYPOXIC ACUTE RESPIRATORY FAILURE DUE TO PNEUMONIA (FIG. 5.5)

A patient (male, 42 years) was admitted to hospital. Chest X-ray showed pneumonia involving the right upper and middle lobe. On the ICU, blood gases were: PO_2 4.2 (air) and with 60% O$_2$ 8.8 kPa, PCO_2 3.3 (kPa) and pH 7.45. He was agitated and tachypnoeic (respiratory rate 34 min^{-1}).

NIV was attempted, but the initial period was characterized by several drawbacks: the nasal mask was ineffective and the full facemask leaked and produced claustrophobia. PSV mode was chosen with an inspiratory support of 16 cmH$_2$O. However, patient–ventilator dyssynchrony was apparent. During the first 30 min of NIV, the patient's clinical state deteriorated and he became confused, the blood pressure decreased and the heart rate increased to 130 min^{-1}. Arterial blood gases also failed to improve. NIV failure was obvious and the patient was intubated 2 hours after NIV was initiated. He was ventilated for the following 6 days and required inotropes for the initial 3 days. The pneumonia resolved with broad-spectrum antibiotic treatment. Afterwards, he was successfully weaned without further problems.

Comment This type of patient will often not be successfully managed by NIV and attempting it may expose the patient to risk. In some patients with type 1 respiratory failure, a trial of NIV is appropriate, especially when rapid recovery is likely, for example from pulmonary oedema.

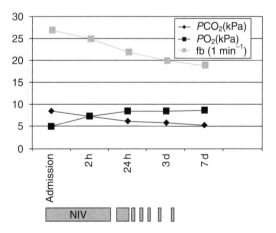

Figure 5.4 *Case report: non-invasive ventilation (NIV) in hypercapnic acute respiratory failure. (fb = breathing frequency.)*

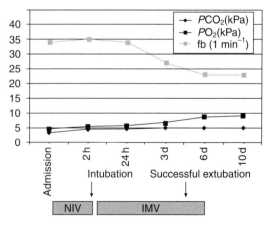

Figure 5.5 *Case report: non-invasive ventilation (NIV) failure in non-hypercapnic acute respiratory failure. (IMV = invasive mechanical ventilation; fb = breathing frequency.)*

DURATION OF NON-INVASIVE MECHANICAL VENTILATION IN ACUTE RESPIRATORY FAILURE

Acute NIV is employed to overcome a life-threatening crisis and the duration of treatment will depend on the precipitating cause. The shortest duration of NIV has been reported in cardiopulmonary oedema (3 hours[37] or 9.3 ± 4.9 hours[38]). In contrast, it takes longer to recover from ARF in COPD. The first 24 hours is the most crucial time whilst awaiting benefit from conventional therapy such as steroids, antibiotics and bronchodilators. We use NIV as much as possible in the first 48 hours. According to the literature, the mean compliance during the first day varies from 4 hours[39] to 6–8 hours.[11,12,29,40] The mean total duration of NIV ranges between 4 and 25 days.[11–13,41]

NON-INVASIVE MECHANICAL VENTILATION AND OUTCOME

Several aspects have been investigated that reflect outcome: intubation and mortality rate, length of stay in ICU and hospital, duration of mechanical ventilation, complication rate (VAP, sinusitis, aspiration, nasal ulceration), cost-effectiveness and time consumption of nursing or medical staff.

Hypercapnic and hypoxaemic acute respiratory failure

The addition of NIV to standard therapy in patients with hypercapnic exacerbations of COPD improves survival and decreases the intubation rate.[10] Two further controlled trials have confirmed these findings.[42,43] COPD patients treated with NIV also have a better survival following discharge compared to conventional treatment,[44,45] although this apparent benefit could be due to selection by survival during the critical illness rather than the effect of NIV versus IMV. Aspects, such as muscle wasting and general nutritional status at discharge could also affect long-term survival. NIV has not been unequivocally shown to be superior to other management strategies in hypercapnic ARF due to causes other than COPD and cardiogenic pulmonary oedema. Table 5.6 summarizes the results of seven randomized, controlled

Table 5.6 *Randomized, controlled trials investigating non-invasive mechanical ventilation in non-hypercapnic acute respiratory failure*

First author	Mortality	ET
Kramer (13)[a]	↘	↘
Wysocki (19)[a]	↘	↘
Antonelli (46)	=	∅
Wood (32)	↗	=
Confalonieri (45)[a]	=	↓
Antonelli (47)	↗	↓
Martin (43)[a]	=	↓

[a]Only a subpopulation of patients with type 1 failure. ET, management by intubation and the provision of mechanical ventilation via an endotracheal tube.

trials. Although in hypoxaemic ARF NIV did not reduce mortality, a significant reduction in intubation rate was found in three trials.[43,45,47]

Cardiogenic pulmonary oedema

The mechanisms by which continuous positive airway pressure (CPAP) or PSV plus CPAP (bi-level PSV) are effective in cardiogenic pulmonary oedema are multifactorial and include lung recruitment, counterbalancing PEEPi, so reducing the work of breathing, decreasing shunt and reducing pre-load and afterload. When compared to conventional treatment, CPAP improves gas exchange and reduces the intubation rate.[37,38,48] Improvement in other outcomes, such as ICU complications, length of stay or mortality, has not been demonstrated. The best modality suited to acute cardiogenic pulmonary oedema has not been investigated. However, adding PSV to CPAP provides greater assistance to inspiration. Therefore, in cardiogenic pulmonary oedema, those with compromised respiratory muscles – indicated by hypercapnia – may benefit most from NIV.[49] PSV may increase the risk of acute myocardial infarction in the presence of symptomatic angina.[50] Whether this is a true causal relationship is unclear, but those at risk may be patients with relative hypovolaemia, from diuretic therapy, or those in atrial fibrillation.

Post-operative patients

Most published evidence for this indication is anecdotal. Both PSV and CPAP have been used. However, some randomized, controlled trials in cardiac, pulmonary, abdominal and transplant surgery have been performed.[47,51–56] It was found that NIV improves physiological parameters without apparent serious side effects. Whether NIV can also modify clinical outcome is unclear.

Patients who are not candidates for invasive mechanical ventilation

The concept of employing NIV when the patient is not a candidate for intubation is an important aspect. Reasons may include advanced physiological age, cachexia or end-stage disease or advance directive. NIV may also provide time for the decision-making process. It aims both to provide effective ventilatory support and to increase patient comfort. Available evidence on comfort is based on retrospective or uncontrolled prospective series. In addition to efficacy, which may be up to 70%,[31,57,58] NIV does appear to be well accepted or tolerated. However, NIV should not be used to prolong the inevitable course towards death. The ethical and economic problems of management in ARF[59] should be better examined in future studies.

Non-invasive mechanical ventilation in weaning, avoiding re-intubation and use at home

In more than 20% of COPD patients receiving IMV, weaning is delayed and sometimes impossible.[60] NIV may be a useful addition to existing weaning strategies. The use of NIV in this way has been reported in uncontrolled studies.[61–63] However, in a multi-centre, randomized study, NIV was performed after short-term IMV.[33] It improved weaning success, survival rate, total time of mechanical ventilation and length of stay in an ICU. Post-extubation failure is also relatively common[64] and the prognosis is poor, with a hospital mortality exceeding 30%. The high mortality of post-extubation failure may relate to clinical deterioration during the period of unsupported ventilation.

A historically controlled study demonstrated the use of NIV to treat post-extubation failure[65] The need for re-intubation, the duration of ventilatory assistance and the length of stay in the ICU were all significantly reduced by NIV. The following is illustrative (Fig. 5.6).

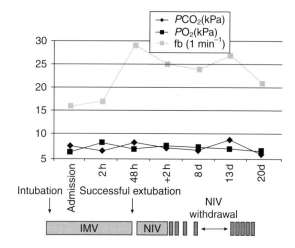

Figure 5.6 *Case report: non-invasive ventilation (NIV) following invasive mechanical ventilation (IMV) in advanced chronic obstructive pulmonary disease. (fb = breathing frequency.)*

CASE HISTORY

A severely dyspnoeic patient with end-stage COPD (female, 67 years, FEV_1 0.58 L, 32% predicted) was intubated by the paramedics at home. Chest radiography (CXR) did not show pneumonia. After 36 hours, sedation was discontinued and, following a successful T-piece trial, the patient was extubated and NIV was initiated. During the next 6 days, her respiratory and clinical state improved, but after discontinuing NIV, she again deteriorated, with progressive hypercapnia. Nocturnal NIV was initiated and led to improved daytime vigilance and a fall in PCO_2 and the patient was discharged to continue this at home.

Comment The role of NIV domiciliary for COPD is contentious, but the practice is increasing. Frequent admissions or significant evidence of sleep-disordered ventilation, with consequent daytime hypersomnolence, are probably the best guides to therapy. Designing properly controlled trials is difficult because of mixed aetiology (OSA, obesity hypoventilation). In currently reported studies, OSA has been specifically excluded, and patients with advanced disease, and predominately advanced emphysema, may explain why, so far, such studies of domiciliary NIV have been negative.

REFERENCES

1. Drinker, P, Shaw, LA. An apparatus for the prolonged administration of artificial respiration. I. A design for adults and children. *J Clin Invest* 1929; **7**: 229–47.

2. Corrado, A, Gorini, M, Villella, G, De Paola, E. Negative pressure ventilation in the treatment of acute respiratory failure: an old noninvasive technique reconsidered. *Eur Respir J* 1996; **9**: 1531–44.

3. Levy, RD, Bradley, TD, Newman, SL, *et al*. Negative pressure ventilation. Effects on ventilation during sleep in normal subjects. *Chest* 1989; **95**: 95–9.

4. Meduri, GU, Abou-Shala, N, Fox, RC, *et al*. Noninvasive face mask mechanical ventilation in patients with acute hypercapnic respiratory failure. *Chest* 1991; **100**: 445–54.

5. Torres, A, Aznar, R, Gatell, JM, *et al*. Incidence, risk, and prognosis factors of nosocomial pneumonia in mechanically ventilated patients. *Am Rev Respir Dis* 1990; **142**: 523–8.

6. Cook, DJ, Walter, SD, Cook, RJ, *et al*. Incidence of and risk factors for ventilator-associated pneumonia in critically ill patients. *Ann Intern Med* 1998; **129**: 433–40.

7. Ruiz-Santana, S, Garcia Jimenez, A, Esteban, A, *et al*. ICU pneumonias: a multi-institutional study. *Crit Care Med* 1987; **15**: 930–2.

8. Guerin, C, Girard, R, Chemorin, C, *et al*. Facial mask noninvasive mechanical ventilation reduces the incidence of nosocomial pneumonia. A prospective epidemiological survey from a single ICU. *Intensive Care Med* 1997; **23**: 1024–32.

9. Nourdine, K, Combes, P, Carton, MJ, *et al*. Does noninvasive ventilation reduce the ICU nosocomial infection risk? A prospective clinical survey. *Intensive Care Med* 1999; **25**: 567–73.

10. Keenan, SP, Kernerman, PD, Cook, DJ, *et al*. Effect of noninvasive positive pressure ventilation on mortality in patients admitted with acute respiratory failure: a meta-analysis. *Crit Care Med* 1997; **25**: 1685–92.

11. Brochard, L, Mancebo, J, Wysocki, M, *et al*. Noninvasive ventilation for acute exacerbations of chronic obstructive pulmonary disease. *N Engl J Med* 1995; **333**: 817–22.

12. Bott, J, Carroll, MP, Conway, JH, *et al*. Randomised controlled trial of nasal ventilation in acute ventilatory failure due to chronic obstructive airways disease. *Lancet* 1993; **341**: 1555–7.

13. Kramer, N, Meyer, TJ, Meharg, J, *et al*. Randomized, prospective trial of noninvasive positive pressure ventilation in acute respiratory failure. *Am J Respir Crit Care Med* 1995; **151**: 1799–806.

14. Lofaso, F, Brochard, L, Hang, T, *et al*. Home versus intensive care pressure support devices. Experimental and clinical comparison. *Am J Respir Crit Care Med* 1996; **153**: 1591–9.

15. Bunburaphong, T, Imanaka, H, Nishimura, M, *et al*. Performance characteristics of bilevel pressure ventilators: a lung model study. *Chest* 1997; **111**: 1050–160.

16. Appendini, L, Patessio, A, Zanaboni, S, *et al*. Physiologic effects of positive end-expiratory pressure and mask pressure support during exacerbations of chronic obstructive pulmonary disease. *Am J Respir Crit Care Med* 1994; **149**: 1069–76.

17. Ferguson, GT, Gilmartin, M. CO_2 rebreathing during BiPAP ventilatory assistance. *Am J Respir Crit Care Med* 1995; **151**: 1126–35.

18. Girault, C, Richard, JC, Chevron, V, *et al*. Comparative physiologic effects of noninvasive assist-control and pressure support ventilation in acute hypercapnic respiratory failure. *Chest* 1997; **111**: 1639–48.

19. Wysocki, M, Tric, L, Wolff, MA, *et al*. Noninvasive pressure support ventilation in patients with acute respiratory failure. A randomized comparison with conventional therapy. *Chest* 1995; **107**: 761–8.

20. Aslanian, P, El Atrous, S, Isabey, D, *et al*. Effects of flow triggering on breathing effort during partial ventilatory support. *Am J Respir Crit Care Med* 1998; **157**: 135–43.

21. Bernstein, G, Heldt, GP, Mannino, FL. Synchronous mechanical ventilation of neonates. *Crit Care Med* 1993; **21**: 1984–5.

22. Bonmarchand, G, Chevron, V, Chopin, C, *et al*. Increased initial flow rate reduces inspiratory work of breathing during pressure support ventilation in patients with exacerbation of chronic obstructive pulmonary disease. *Intensive Care Med* 1996; **22**: 1147–54.

23. Grasso, S, Puntillo, F, Mascia, L, *et al*. Compensation for increase in respiratory workload during mechanical ventilation. Pressure-support versus proportional-assist ventilation. *Am J Respir Crit Care Med* 2000; **161**: 819–26.

24. Younes, M. Proportional assist ventilation, a new approach to ventilatory support. Theory. *Am Rev Respir Dis* 1992; **145**: 114–20.

25. Younes, M, Puddy, A, Roberts, D, *et al*. Proportional assist ventilation. Results of an initial clinical trial. *Am Rev Respir Dis* 1992; **145**: 121–9.

26. Meecham Jones, DJ, Paul, EA, Grahame-Clarke, C, Wedzicha, JA. Nasal ventilation in acute exacerbations of chronic obstructive pulmonary disease: effect of ventilator mode on arterial blood-gas tensions. *Thorax* 1994; **49**: 1222–4.

27. Vitacca, M, Rubini, F, Foglio, K, *et al*. Non-invasive modalities of positive pressure ventilation improve the outcome of acute exacerbations in COLD patients. *Intensive Care Med* 1993; **19**: 450–5.

28. Barbe, F, Togores, B, Rubi, M, *et al*. Noninvasive ventilatory support does not facilitate recovery from acute respiratory failure in chronic obstructive pulmonary disease. *Eur Respir J* 1996; **9**: 1240–5.

29. Plant, PK, Owen, JL, Elliott, MW. Early use of non-invasive ventilation for acute exacerbations of chronic obstructive pulmonary disease on general respiratory wards: a multicentre randomised controlled trial. *Lancet* 2000; **355**: 1931–5.

30. Ambrosino, N, Foglio, K, Rubini, F, *et al*. Non-invasive mechanical ventilation in acute respiratory failure due to chronic obstructive pulmonary disease: correlates for success. *Thorax* 1995; **50**: 755–7.

31. Soo Hoo, GW, Santiago, S, Williams, AJ. Nasal mechanical ventilation for hypercapnic respiratory failure in chronic obstructive pulmonary disease: determinants of success and failure. *Crit Care Med* 1994; **22**: 1253–61.

32. Wood, KA, Lewis, L, Von Harz, B, Kollef, MH. The use of noninvasive positive pressure ventilation in the emergency department: results of a randomized clinical trial. *Chest* 1998; **113**: 1339–46.

33. Nava, S, Ambrosino, N, Clini, E, *et al*. Noninvasive mechanical ventilation in the weaning of patients with respiratory failure due to chronic obstructive pulmonary disease. A randomized, controlled trial. *Ann Intern Med* 1998; **128**: 721–8.

34. Doherty, MJ, Greenstone, MA. Survey of non-invasive ventilation (NIPPV) in patients with acute exacerbations of chronic obstructive pulmonary disease (COPD) in the UK. *Thorax* 1998; **53**: 863–6.

35. Carlucci, A, Richard, JC, Wysocki, M, *et al*. French multicenter survey: non-invasive versus conventional mechanical ventilation. *Am J Respir Crit Care Med* 1999; **159**: A367.

36. Antonelli, M, Conti, G, Riccioni, L, Meduri, GU. Noninvasive positive-pressure ventilation via face mask during bronchoscopy with BAL in high-risk hypoxemic patients. *Chest* 1996; **110**: 724–8.

37. Rasanen, J, Heikkila, J, Downs, J, *et al*. Continuous positive airway pressure by face mask in acute cardiogenic pulmonary edema. *Am J Cardiol* 1985; **55**: 296–300.

38. Bersten, AD, Holt, AW, Vedig, AE, *et al*. Treatment of severe cardiogenic pulmonary edema with continuous positive airway pressure delivered by face mask. *N Engl J Med* 1991; **325**: 1825–30.

39. Foglio, C, Vitacca, M, Quadri, A, *et al*. Acute exacerbations in severe COLD patients. Treatment using positive pressure ventilation by nasal mask. *Chest* 1992; **101**: 1533–8.

40. Hilbert, G, Gruson, D, Gbikpi-Benissan, G, Cardinaud, JP. Sequential use of noninvasive pressure support ventilation for acute exacerbations of COPD. *Intensive Care Med* 1997; **23**: 955–61.

41. Meduri, GU, Turner, RE, Abou-Shala, N, *et al*. Noninvasive positive pressure ventilation via face mask. First-line intervention in patients with acute hypercapnic and hypoxemic respiratory failure. *Chest* 1996; **109**: 179–93.

42. Confalonieri, M, Potena, A, Carbone, G, *et al*. Acute respiratory failure in patients with severe community-acquired pneumonia. A prospective randomized evaluation of noninvasive ventilation. *Am J Respir Crit Care Med* 1999; **160**: 1585–91.

43. Martin, TJ, Hovis, JD, Costantino, JP, *et al*. A randomized, prospective evaluation of noninvasive ventilation for acute respiratory failure. *Am J Respir Crit Care Med* 2000; **161**: 807–13.

44. Bardi, G, Pierotello, R, Desideri, M, *et al*. Nasal ventilation in COPD exacerbations: early and late results of a prospective, controlled study. *Eur Respir J* 2000; **15**: 98–104.

45. Confalonieri, M, Parigi, P, Scartabellati, A, *et al*. Noninvasive mechanical ventilation improves the immediate and long-term outcome of COPD patients with acute respiratory failure. *Eur Respir J* 1996; **9**: 422–30.

46. Antonelli, M, Conti, G, Rocco, M, *et al*. A comparison of noninvasive positive-pressure ventilation and conventional mechanical ventilation in patients with acute respiratory failure. *N Engl J Med* 1998; **339**: 429–35.

47. Antonelli, M, Conti, G, Bufi, M, *et al*. Noninvasive ventilation for treatment of acute respiratory failure in patients undergoing solid organ transplantation: a randomized trial. *JAMA* 2000; **283**: 235–41.

48. Lin, M, Yang, YF, Chiang, HT, *et al*. Reappraisal of continuous positive airway pressure therapy in acute cardiogenic pulmonary edema. Short-term

results and long-term follow-up. *Chest* 1995; **107**: 1379–86.

49. Rusterholtz, T, Kempf, J, Berton, C, *et al.* Noninvasive pressure support ventilation (NIPSV) with face mask in patients with acute cardiogenic pulmonary edema. *Intensive Care Med* 1999; **25**: 21–8.

50. Mehta, S, Jay, GD, Woolard, RH, *et al.* Randomized, prospective trial of bilevel versus continuous positive airway pressure in acute pulmonary edema. *Crit Care Med* 1997; **25**: 620–8.

51. Aguilo, R, Togores, B, Pons, S, *et al.* Noninvasive ventilatory support after lung resectional surgery. *Chest* 1997; **112**: 117–21.

52. Gust, R, Gottschalk, A, Schmidt, H, *et al.* Effects of continuous (CPAP) and bi-level positive airway pressure (BiPAP) on extravascular lung water after extubation of the trachea in patients following coronary artery bypass grafting. *Intensive Care Med* 1996; **22**: 1345–50.

53. Joris, JL, Sottiaux, TM, Chiche, JD, *et al.* Effect of bi-level positive airway pressure (BiPAP) nasal ventilation on the postoperative pulmonary restrictive syndrome in obese patients undergoing gastroplasty. *Chest* 1997; **111**: 665–70.

54. Jousela, I, Rasanen, J, Verkkala, K, *et al.* Continuous positive airway pressure by mask in patients after coronary surgery. Acta *Anaesthesiol Scand* 1994; **38**: 311–16.

55. Matte, P, Jacquet, L, Van Dyck, M, Goenen, M. Effects of conventional physiotherapy, continuous positive airway pressure and non-invasive ventilatory support with bilevel positive airway pressure after coronary artery bypass grafting. *Acta Anaesthesiol Scand* 2000; **44**: 75–81.

56. Pinilla, JC, Oleniuk, FH, Tan, L, *et al.* Use of a nasal continuous positive airway pressure mask in the treatment of postoperative atelectasis in aortocoronary bypass surgery. *Crit Care Med* 1990; **18**: 836–40.

57. Benhamou, D, Girault, C, Faure, C, *et al.* Nasal mask ventilation in acute respiratory failure. Experience in elderly patients. *Chest* 1992; **102**: 912–17.

58. Meduri, GU, Fox, RC, Abou-Shala, N, *et al.* Noninvasive mechanical ventilation via face mask in patients with acute respiratory failure who refused endotracheal intubation. *Crit Care Med* 1994; **22**: 1584–90.

59. Clarke, DE, Vaughan, L, Raffin, TA. Noninvasive positive pressure ventilation for patients with terminal respiratory failure: the ethical and economic costs of delaying the inevitable are too great. *Am J Crit Care* 1994; **3**: 4–5.

60. Esteban, A, Frutos, F, Tobin, MJ, *et al.* A comparison of four methods of weaning patients from mechanical ventilation. Spanish Lung Failure Collaborative Group. *N Engl J Med* 1995; **332**: 345–50.

61. Goodenberger, DM, Couser, JI Jr, May, JJ. Successful discontinuation of ventilation via tracheostomy by substitution of nasal positive pressure ventilation. *Chest* 1992; **102**: 1277–9.

62. Restrick, LJ, Scott, AD, Ward, EM, *et al.* Nasal intermittent positive-pressure ventilation in weaning intubated patients with chronic respiratory disease from assisted intermittent, positive-pressure ventilation. *Respir Med* 1993; **87**: 199–204.

63. Udwadia, ZF, Santis, GK, Steven, MH, Simonds, AK. Nasal ventilation to facilitate weaning in patients with chronic respiratory insufficiency. *Thorax* 1992; **47**: 715–18.

64. Torres, A, Gatell, JM, Aznar, E, *et al.* Re-intubation increases the risk of nosocomial pneumonia in patients needing mechanical ventilation. *Am J Respir Crit Care Med* 1995; **152**: 137–41.

65. Hilbert, G, Gruson, D, Portel, L, *et al.* Noninvasive pressure support ventilation in COPD patients with postextubation hypercapnic respiratory insufficiency. *Eur Respir J* 1998; **11**: 1349–53.

6

Contemporary issues in critical care physiotherapy

MICHAEL BARKER, SHERIC G ELLUM AND SARAH EJ KEILTY

INTRODUCTION

Physiotherapists have a crucial role to play in the treatment of critically ill patients. Over the last 30 years, many innovations have been introduced that have influenced the approach to patient management. At the same time, the case mix of patients seen on the modern intensive care unit (ICU) and high dependency unit (HDU) has changed. Physiotherapy has responded to these changes and has become more evidence based. Traditional physiotherapy practices on the ICU have been challenged[1–4] and this has changed the therapy provided by the critical care physiotherapy services.

This chapter describes the model of physiotherapy practice in our institution. The authors appreciate that structural considerations, e.g. staffing, skill mix, traditional barriers etc., in other hospitals may cause difficulties in the wholesale application of some of the recommendations made. The intention is to focus on the important issues that have lead to a successful implementation of this physiotherapy model.

Implicit in the following discussion is the essential need for holistic assessment to direct the most appropriate treatments. These treatments are grouped together as techniques for preventing intubation, those concerned with tracheostomy management, techniques for secretion clearance and those associated with the rehabilitation needs of the critically ill patient.

TECHNIQUES FOR AVOIDING INTUBATION

Intubation and mechanical ventilation are used to provide ventilatory control and to protect the upper airway during acute severe illness. Positive pressure ventilation via an endotracheal or tracheostomy tube is standard practice. The indications are well documented and the majority of patients wean from ventilation on recovery from the illness prompting ICU admission. However, complications in intubated patients in ICU are relatively common and weaning may be difficult. In some cases, avoidance of intubation by the use of non-invasive ventilatory assistance (NIV) may therefore be appropriate. The physiotherapist will, however, aim to identify reversible factors leading to ventilatory failure in this type of patient and act to prevent deterioration by improving the balance between the respiratory load and capacity of the ventilatory pump. Strategies include improving airway secretion clearance, humidification and patient positioning and techniques of non-invasive respiratory assistance.

Airway clearance techniques

There is a variety of interventions that can be performed to facilitate expectoration of retained pulmonary secretions. The active cycle of breathing techniques (ACBT),[5] used alone or in conjunction with pressure support such as intermittent positive pressure breathing (IPPB), continuous positive airways pressure (CPAP), can be used to aid airway clearance. These techniques may increase tidal volume,[6] improve collateral ventilation,[6] decrease the work of breathing[7] and improve expectoration.

Humidification of the airway is extremely important because the efficiency of mucus transport is dependent on hydrated mucous membrane and correctly functioning cilia. During infection, the viscosity and quantity of mucus are increased. Combined with systemic dehydration and inspiring dry medical gases, this can result in a reduction of mucociliary escalator function, leading to sputum retention, increased airflow resistance and impaired gas exchange.

Positioning to reduce respiratory load

Traditionally, positioning was seen only as a means to facilitate bronchial drainage. Studies show that positioning can reduce the work of breathing by reducing ventilatory demand.[7] The specific position required and the focus of the treatment will depend on the pathology and clinical signs. With unilateral acute lung disease, e.g. consolidation, positioning the patient with the unaffected lung down has been shown to optimize gas exchange by improving ventilation perfusion matching. In the presence of bilateral pulmonary pathology, however, positioning the patient in right-side lying has shown improvements in PaO_2 compared with positioning on the left.[7] This may be attributed to the right lung having a greater volume than the left lung.

Positioning to enhance respiratory muscle function

The forward lean sitting position improves the capacity of the respiratory muscles[8] and reduces the sensation of breathlessness[9] in patients with chronic airflow limitation (CAL). It has been postulated that, in this position, the diaphragm becomes less flattened and longer as it assumes the more usual domed shape, enhancing the length–tension relationship.[9] If the patient is too exhausted to tolerate this position, it can be modified to high side lying, with similar results.

Positive pressure techniques

Non-invasive respiratory assistance has been used since the 1930s. Advances in the technology of ventilators, or flow generators, and interface design have revolutionized the use of non-invasive positive pressure respiratory support. It can be applied to non-intubated patients by a tight-fitting full facemask or nasal mask and by a mouthpiece. It can be applied continuously (CPAP), intermittently with inspiratory assistance alone (PSB) and by combining the two provides both inspiratory positive airways pressure (IPAP) and expiratory positive airways pressure (EPAP) or bi-level positive airways pressure. Patients who do not improve with NIV or who deteriorate may require intubation. A strategic plan in the event of failure of NIV is important at the start of therapy (see Chapter 5).

Continuous positive airways pressure

CPAP was first described in the 1930s for the treatment of extravascular lung fluid. It produces an improvement in oxygenation and in pulmonary compliance and an increase in lung volume.[7] In doing so, CPAP can reduce the work of breathing,[10] has been used successfully to treat acute respiratory distress syndrome (ARDS) in adults[11] and may prevent re-intubation in selected patients.[12]

Intermittent positive pressure breathing

IPPB is patient-triggered inspiratory pressure support and was first described in 1947 . Since then, formal studies have provided conflicting results. Physiological studies have demonstrated that IPPB can bring about a rise in PaO_2 and a reduction in $PaCO_2$,[13] decrease the work of breathing and improve minute ventilation.[14] IPPB, or pressure support breathing, is useful in the treatment of the exhausted patient who has shallow breathing resulting in hypercapnia. It is important that the patient is awake and co-operative. The technique can be applied non-invasively by mouthpiece or mask, but this has to be held in place by the operator and is rarely tolerated by patients for protracted periods of time. This means that IPPB is usually limited to physiotherapy treatment sessions.

Non-invasive ventilation

If patients require longer periods of pressure support, NIV may be effective. Originally, this treatment was used for patients with chronic respiratory failure due to chest-wall disease. There has been considerable improvement in ventilator and interface design and NIV is now used in the treatment of a range of causes of acute respiratory failure (for a full review of NIV in acute respiratory failure, see Chapter 5). The broadening of the application of NIV has moved its use from the ICU to the HDU, postoperative recovery and specialist wards and to the accident and emergency department, creating a requirement for a 24-hour NIV service. Although ideal, this is not always possible because to have suitably trained staff available 24 hours a day requires considerable organization. Significant financial resources are required to fund disposable equipment (masks, circuits etc.) and provide staff and on-going training.

PRACTICAL ASPECTS OF NON-INVASIVE VENTILATION

Many patients tolerate NIV well. Intolerance may relate to mask discomfort, feelings of claustrophobia and asynchrony with the ventilator. It is important that the patient has confidence in the operator and should feel in control of the situation rather than controlled by the situation. A variety of interfaces is available, which have their own advantages and disadvantages. Many manufacturers produce measuring gauges to facilitate fit, but it may be

necessary to try several before the best fit can be achieved. Overall, the nasal mask is preferred as it reduces the feeling of claustrophobia and allows communication with the clinician. The main disadvantage is leak from the mouth, made worse during sleep, and only partially helped by the use of a chinstrap. Full facemasks are usually necessary for extremely dyspnoeic patients. They are, however, claustrophobic and present a risk of aspiration if the patient vomits. Masks may cause skin necrosis, and a strip of foam dressing, placed over the bridge of the nose, may prevent or delay this happening. This is important because NIV will be poorly tolerated if painful. Nasal pillows may maintain ventilatory support while alleviating pressure over the bridge of the nose. They are, however, not a suitable option in severe acute respiratory distress.

Ventilator settings and setting a patient up on non-invasive ventilation

Initially, we set a low pressure, e.g. 10–15 cmH_2O, and demonstrate the flow of air on the back of the hand for reassurance. We then attach the tubing to the mask and hold it to the patient's face for a few breaths, allowing a few triggered breaths. Encouragement should be given to breathe slowly and the spontaneous mode of the ventilator will trigger accordingly. If the respiratory rate is less than 8 breaths/min, or the patient is too tired or weak to trigger breaths, set the ventilator to the spontaneous/timed mode so that machine-initiated breaths will occur in the event of hypoventilation. If supplemental O_2 is required, it may be precautionary to set the spontaneous/timed mode in case of O_2-induced apnoea. Once NIV is established, the head strap can be attached and gently tightened. Over-tightening will exacerbate skin necrosis. Large air leaks should be avoided, especially around the eyes. Once the patient is settled, the operator should watch the chest movement and observe the respiratory pattern. We then slowly increase the pressure to a comfortable level, e.g. 15–25 cmH_2O, and reduce the respiratory rate so that a more efficient breathing pattern is established. It is essential that the operator stays with the patient for the first 30 min so that encouragement and re-assurance can be given.

Monitoring patients on non-invasive ventilation

Monitoring should include clinical assessment combined with physiological variables such as O_2 saturation, blood gases, blood pressure, heart rate and respiratory rate. Arterial blood gases should be measured following 30–40 min of ventilation and ventilator settings should be changed with the aim of increasing pH to more than 7.3. Patients should use NIV for as long as possible on the first day of therapy and especially during sleep. As gas exchange improves, patients can spend increasingly longer periods off the ventilator to allow for airway clearance, mouth care, nutrition and mobility. To assess the need for nocturnal ventilatory support, a trial of overnight oximetry or capnography without ventilatory support may be appropriate before the patient is discharged to the general ward.

NEGATIVE PRESSURE TECHNIQUES

Negative pressure ventilatory support has become less frequently used since the re-emergence of positive pressure ventilation. It may be an option for patients who fail to adapt to positive pressure ventilation. There are two main types of negative pressure devices available: the 'tank' ventilator in which the whole body, except the head and neck, is enclosed; and the cuirass shell, which encloses the anterior thorax and abdomen only. Sub-atmospheric pressure is intermittently applied to the chest wall and abdomen by a pump attached to the chamber and air is drawn into the thorax as the transpulmonary pressure is increased.

The efficiency of negative pressure ventilation is determined by the compliance of the chest wall, airway resistance and the ability to create an airtight seal. It has several limitations. Access is poor with the tank respirator, and synchrony with the patient's breathing pattern can be a problem. The most serious problem with negative pressure ventilation is the tendency to induce upper-airway obstruction, although triggered ventilators are reportedly better in this respect. Alternatively, upper-airway obstruction can be overcome by applying positive pressure by nasal mask and we have employed this approach when intubation was refused or inappropriate for other reasons.

Cuirass ventilation, although of value in domiciliary ventilatory support, is insufficient to assist ventilation in acute CAL respiratory failure. Cuirass ventilation and provision of novel therapy techniques are, however, possible with the Hyeck or RTX (Medivent, UK) machines. These devices have been shown to improve gas exchange in patients with CAL and other causes of respiratory failure, but more clinical trials are needed. A physiotherapy mode using oscillations in pressure up to 600 cycles min^{-1} may facilitate secretion removal. This also warrants further investigation.

SUPPORTING PATIENTS POST-EXTUBATION

Not all patients manage spontaneous breathing in the first few hours post-extubation. Patients at risk of deterioration or who require ventilatory assistance may benefit from NIV. Patients who fail spontaneous breathing trials during assessment for extubation should also be considered for early extubation and NIV as an alternative to tracheostomy.

In the slowly weaning patient, who will usually have a tracheostomy, ambulation can be possible either by bagging or using portable ventilatory assist devices such as the Respironics 'Bi-PAP Harmony ST' (Medicaid, UK) or the 'Voyager' (B&D Medical UK). These can be battery powered and offer triggered and non-triggered ventilatory support modes. They are light and compact devices, which can be carried in a shoulder bag by the therapist or patient. We believe that providing ambulatory respiratory support facilitates rehabilitation.

TRACHEOSTOMY AND DECANNULATION

Tracheostomy is indicated when prolonged ventilatory support is required or the patient is unable to protect his or her airway. There is a variety of tracheostomy tubes available, such as single and double lumen, cuffed and uncuffed, and fenestrated and unfenestrated tubes. Cuffs are most commonly used to provide airway protection from aspiration, which is more likely if the cuff pressure is too low. Too high a pressure, on the other hand, will result in mucosal ischaemia. Cuff pressure should therefore be monitored.[15] A cuff pressure between 15 and 20 cmH_2O is recommended to prevent complications. Single-lumen cuffed tubes are often the initial choice of tracheostomy for economic reasons. The single lumen maximizes the size of the internal diameter for a given external diameter, so reducing resistive load. This resistive load may be of significance during weaning from mechanical ventilation.

Double-lumen tubes have a removable inner tube to prevent the build-up of secretions that may otherwise narrow the internal diameter. In severe situations, this could lead to complete obstruction of the tube. In the extreme example of complete tube obstruction, removal of the inner tube rapidly corrects the emergency, whereas the whole tracheostomy tube would need to be removed in the case of a single-lumen tube. This is perhaps of more relevance in the HDU, where the nurse/patient ratio is lower. A fenestration in the outer double-lumen tube is matched to similar holes in the 'speaking' inner tube to allow air up through the vocal cords. Cuff deflation is often required as well to provide an effective voice. This aspect is important during the weaning process. It is obviously important that the correct, i.e. unfenestrated, inner tube is inserted during periods of controlled ventilation.

A small, cuffless catheter, or mini-tracheostomy, can be inserted when only secretion management is required. It has an internal diameter large enough to pass a size 10-FG suction catheter. Mini-tracheostomy may be favoured as a 'step down' for patients who can breathe spontaneously but require access to aid the clearance of bronchial secretions. A spigot is removed to allow catheter access to clear secretions. Although designed for secretion clearance, its use to provide ventilatory support has been described using inspiratory pressures >50 cmH$_2$O. Intratracheal pressure is, of course, much lower, and surgical emphysema has not been a problem when we have used this approach to avoid formal intubation. Cuffless tubes are rarely used in normal patient care, but have advantages for patients who require long-term tracheostomy and ventilatory support.

Cuff deflation

Once the need for ventilatory support is reduced to a minimum, the primary function of the tracheostomy changes from a means of providing ventilatory support to that of clearance and management of bronchial secretions. Patients breathing spontaneously via a tracheostomy may be managed on the HDU or general ward. When considering removal of the tube, it is important to ensure the patient has an intact swallow. We employ blue dye added to drinking to water. Aspiration can be clearly seen by the appearance of blue dye via the tracheostomy. When demonstrated, further assessment by a speech and language therapist is recommended. However, the significance of minor aspiration is uncertain and swallow often only improves when practised with the cuff deflated.

Speech

Establishing effective communication is important. If the patient can tolerate cuff deflation, a unidirectional speaking valve provides a good voice yet allows continued inspiratory support. Alternatively, fenestrated tracheostomy tubes may be an advantage if a patient finds the addition of a speaking valve increases the work of breathing. It should be noted that, if the leak around the tube within the trachea is minimal, the addition of a speaking valve may lead to distress due to the development of hyperinflation.

Expectoration and cough

It is important when making the decision to decannulate patients that they are able to clear respiratory secretions. Generalized muscle weakness, reduced ventilatory capacity and bypassing of the normal mechanisms of humidification mean the tracheostomized patient is vulnerable to retention of secretions. An assessment of cough effectiveness should be undertaken before decannulation is attempted.

A cough consists of four phases. The **inspiratory phase**, of volumes varying from 200 to 3500 mL above functional residual capacity (FRC), is the first, leading to the **compressive phase**, in which the expiratory muscles contract against a closed glottis, creating an intrathoracic pressure up to 300 cmH$_2$O. During the explosive **expiratory phase**, expiratory flow rates of 6–12 Ls^{-1} are generated in normal adults. A transient supramaximal cough expiratory flow, or cough spike, can be recorded during the initial part of the expiratory phase associated with glottic opening. Although the glottis plays an important role in cough generation, its closure is not essential, as demonstrated by the effective expectoration of sputum by tracheostomized or endotracheal tube-intubated patients. Expiratory flow rates are lower, however, than those generated with a closed glottis and, if combined with respiratory muscle weakness, may reduce cough effectiveness. Laryngeal muscle co-ordination plays an important role because it is essential that the vocal cords are fully abducted to allow rapid expulsion of air. Finally, the **relaxation phase**, with expiratory muscle relaxation and elastic recoil of the lung, allows a return to normal levels of pressures within the thorax.

Evaluation of cough

Normal subjects reach 85–90% of their inspiratory capacity in the inspiratory phase of coughing. Cough may be ineffective when the vital capacity (VC) is <1.5 L and will be so if the VC is <850 mL. A PECF of 160 L min^{-1} may be the minimum value associated with the ability to clear the airways of sputum.[16] This can be measured using a hand-held peak expiratory flow meter or, if available, a pneumotachograph, which is more accurate. Measurement is taken using a mouthpiece with the tracheostomy cuff deflated and the trachesotomy capped off. The testing of respiratory muscle strength on the ICU is fully considered in Chapter 2. Although non-volitional tests may at times be necessary, the invasive nature of these tests makes their use in spontaneously breathing, alert patients difficult. Volitional tests usually provide a reasonable reflection of respiratory muscle strength. Maximal inspiratory muscle strength (MIP), sniff nasal inspiratory pressure (SNIP) and maximal expiratory muscle strength (MEP) have all been shown to be useful when assessing inspiratory or expiratory muscle function. As with all volitional tests, a high value can exclude respiratory muscle weakness, although a low value is more difficult to interpret.

Cough augmentation

A number of techniques can be employed to improve an ineffective cough.

MECHANICAL IN/EXSUFFLATOR (CoughAssist™ MI-E)

The mechanical in/exsufflator (Emerson, MA, USA) assists the clearance of bronchopulmonary secretions. Application of positive pressure, via a facemask, is quickly changed to negative pressure manually or by time cycling to generate a high expiratory flow rate. Positive inflation pressures using 25 cmH$_2$O and subsequent cycling to a negative pressure of -30 cmH$_2$O are suggested starting pressures.[17] Although well established in the USA, the MIE is still largely unused in the UK and Europe. The evidence to support its use has been confined to patients with neuromuscular causes, but these data suggest that MIE can increase PECF rates during unassisted coughing from 1.81 Ls^{-1} to 7.47 Ls^{-1}.[18] Preliminary experience at this centre of improved radio-tracer clearance, compared with standard techniques, suggests that MIE may provide a more effective alternative to cough augmentation in patients with respiratory muscle weakness. It may also be a valuable asset for a broader spectrum of patients across the critical care environment.

MANUALLY ASSISTED COUGH

Manually assisting cough but co-ordinating abdominal pressure by the therapist with patient effort can improve the clearance of respiratory secretions. It is most commonly used for patients with long-term neuromuscular weakness, such as spinal lesions or motoneuron disease. This technique may be beneficial for patients in the critical care environment with underlying restrictive lung disease or respiratory muscle weakness, but requires further study.

REHABILITATION

The negative sequelae associated with immobility are well documented[19] The physiotherapist will aim to improve functional outcomes by the maintenance of joint range and soft-tissue length and increasing strength and endurance by using passive movements, positioning regimens and active therapy. The same exercise principles that apply to training healthy individuals for strength, endurance or power are used in the recovery from critical illness. The concept is of **sport for the sick**. It is useful to consider rehabilitation strategies as those concerned with 'in-bed rehabilitation' and those concerned with 'out-of-bed rehabilitation'.

In-bed rehabilitation strategies

POSITIONING

Positioning is important. Of all the positions used, prone positioning has recently received a lot of attention.[20] It is primarily employed in refractory hypoxaemia in the patient with acute lung injury. Approximately 70% of patients respond with significant improvement in PaO_2:FiO_2 ratio, although, in some, the benefit is not maintained. Since it was first described in 1977, there have been a number of reports and editorials that have mostly explored the mechanisms behind the response. Few have cited complications associated with turning the critically ill patients prone. Some of these complications are relatively minor, such as the loss of central venous access or dependent oedema, and others are more important, such as extubation or cardiovascular instability. Chronic complications such as contractures[21] and myositis ossificans[22] are reported. Guidelines have been published on the management of proned patients,[20] with a focus on the protection of neural structures, such as the brachial plexus and common fibular nerves, in tension-relieving postures. Typical postures to protect the brachial plexus are shown in Figure 6.1. Normally, the illustrated positions should be altered once every 4 hours.

CONTINUOUS LATERAL ROTATION THERAPY

Continuous lateral rotation therapy (CLRT) is considered as an 'in-bed' rehabilitation option, because it is commonly used in severely unstable patients who do not tolerate manual positioning and handling. A continuous rotation of the patient along the longitudinal axis is employed in a specialized bed. These beds can be divided into two categories: those that use rigid table-based rotation units to 'lock' the patient in (mostly used in spinal injury), and those that have air cushion systems (contraindicated in spinal injury). The purpose is to continually change the area of lung dependency to prevent alveolar collapse and to aid the mobilization of secretions. Pressure relief on the skin is also achieved. Studies have shown that changing the area of lung dependency by CLRT improves respiratory function.[23] The mechanisms by which this is achieved are thought to be a combination of increased mobilization of secretions and redistribution of inspired gas to previously collapsed areas of lung.

Controversies surround the use of CLRT and we are not aware of any cost–benefit analyses. Clinical trials of CLRT have suffered from difficulties recruiting sufficient patient numbers to show statistically significant results. A meta-analysis of six trials[24] revealed that CLRT was associated with a decreased incidence of atelectasis and nosocomial pneumonia as well as with a decrease in the ventilation time and intensive care stay. Some patient groups appear to benefit more than others, such as those with sepsis or blunt trauma. All the studies included in the meta-analysis have been carried out in the USA and there are arguments against generalizing these findings. For example, ARDS patients were generally excluded; the practice of respiratory therapy is different in the USA from that in other countries; and the benefit for spinal-injury patients without lung injury may not be transferable to general ICU patients. The optimal rotation settings (depth of rotation, pause time and number of rotations per 24 hours) have also not been established.

ACTIVE MOVEMENTS

If the patient cannot be mobilized out of bed, active movements can still be effectively used when he or she is sufficiently awake to participate. The physiotherapist's primary concern at this stage would be the recruitment and maintenance of anti-gravity muscle groups (quadriceps, gluteal, abdominal and erector spinae muscles), but the triceps, biceps and hand muscles should also be targeted if possible. Active movements should be performed to mimic active **functional** movement patterns, e.g. extension of the lower limb would be performed as a composite movement involving extension at the hip, knee and ankle.

Out-of-bed rehabilitation strategies

The patient should be mobilized out of bed as soon as the opportunity arises. Getting a patient out of bed may seem an easy task, but there are many assessment issues that have to be taken into account to execute the task with minimal risk and optimal efficiency. Even when sitting the patient on the edge of the bed – a commonly used technique to initiate the 'out-of-bed' rehabilitation phase – careful assessment must be conducted. Considerations should be given to the respiratory capacity, haemodynamic stability, muscle strength and

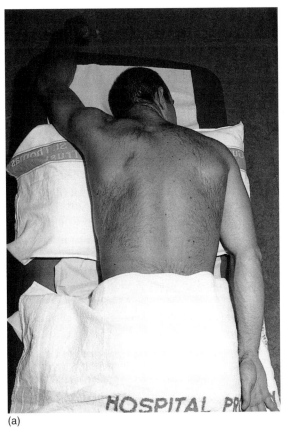 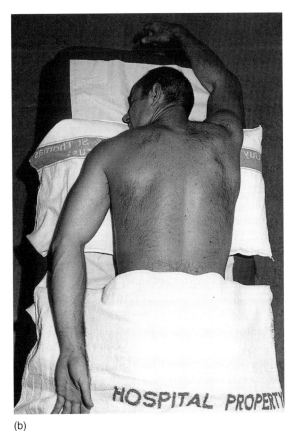

Figure 6.1 *(a) The neck is rotated to the right with the left upper limb in flexion and internal rotation. The right upper limb is placed at the patient's side with the shoulder internally rotated and elbow extended. (b) The mirror image of (a). The neck is rotated to the opposite direction and the upper limbs positioned accordingly.*

neurological co-ordination. The patient's ability to assist in rehabilitation is crucial because this influences the use of moving and handling devices. The methods employed include the following.

- Tilt table. The patient is transferred laterally onto a rigid plinth with footrests and is secured in the anatomical position with straps. The patient is gradually tilted from the horizontal to the vertical/standing position.
- Sitting over the edge of the bed with support, standing from sitting and standing transfers to a chair (via pivoting or stepping around).
- Ambulatory ventilation.

AMBULATORY VENTILATION

Drawing on the use of NIV during exercise in CAL,[25] we have treated similarly deconditioned patients in the ICU. This progressive approach to mobilizing ICU patients is not widely practised and

outcome parameters have not been established. We believe that an exercise regimen positively influences the speed of weaning and decreases ICU stay and cost.

Challenges to 'conventional' chest physiotherapy techniques

PERCUSSION

The use of chest-wall percussion in critical care is waning, due to critiques on its efficacy in acute care.[1] However, percussion may have value in suppurative, chronic lung diseases such as bronchiectasis and cystic fibrosis.[26]

MANUAL HYPERINFLATION

Manual hyperinflation is still commonly used to mobilize retained pulmonary secretions and to recruit collapsed lung. It is effective in treating acute lobar collapse,[27] but its value for patients with lung injury must be questioned. The current ventilation strategy in lung injury is to protect the lung from further trauma by using low-volume ventilation with high positive end-expiratory pressure (PEEP). Disconnecting the patient to manually hyperinflate the lungs thus appears irrational.

HIGH-FREQUENCY OSCILLATION VENTILATION

High-frequency oscillation ventilation (HFOV) is a strategy employed in refractory hypoxaemia using high mean airway pressures with sub-dead-space tidal volumes. A diaphragm that oscillates at 5–6 cycles s^{-1} is used, cycling on top of a maintained CPAP. The physiotherapist is faced with a patient who ought not to be disconnected for chest therapy because de-recruitment and worsening hypoxaemia will ensue. Regular suctioning, even with in-line catheters, can similarly de-recruit the lung. The chest is also visibly oscillating, which precludes manual physiotherapy techniques. Despite this, therapeutic management includes optimal patient positioning and modifying suctioning to only when necessary. (As auscultation is of limited value in HFOV, other parameters are used such as a gradual increase in the proximal operating pressure of the oscillator, known as the 'delta P').

REFERENCES

1. Dean, E. Oxygen transport: a physiologically-based conceptual framework for the practice of cardio-pulmonary physiotherapy. *Physiotherapy* 1994; **80**(6): 347–53.
2. Jenkins, SC, Soutar, S, Loukota, JM, Johnson, LC, Moxham, J. Physiotherapy after coronary artery surgery: are breathing exercises necessary? *Thorax* 1989; **44**: 634–9.
3. Eales, CJ, Barker, M, Cubberley, NJ. Evaluation of a single chest physiotherapy treatment to post-operative, mechanically ventilated cardiac surgery patients. *Physiother Theory Practice* 1995; **11**: 23–8.
4. Barker, M, Eales, CJ. The effects of manual hyperinflation using self-inflating manual resuscitation bags on arterial oxygen tensions and lung compliance – a meta-analysis of the literature. *S Afr J Physiother* 2000; **56**(1): 7–16.
5. Pryor, JA, Webber, BA, Hodson, ME, Batten, JC. Evaluation of the forced expiration technique as an adjunct to postural drainage in the treatment of cystic fibrosis. *BMJ* 1979; **2**: 417–18.
6. Anderson, JB, Qvist, J, Kann, T. Recruiting collapse lung through collateral channels with positive expiratory pressure. *Scand J Respir Dis* 1979; **60**: 260–6.
7. Dean, E. Effect of body positioning on pulmonary function. *Phys Ther* 1985; **65**: 613–18.
8. O'Neil, S, McCarthy, DS. Postural relief of dyspnoea in severe chronic airflow limitation: relationship to respiratory muscle strength. *Thorax* 1983; **38**: 595–600.
9. Sharpe, JT, Drutz, WS, Moisan, T. Postural relief of dyspnoea in severe chronic obstructive pulmonary disease. *Am Rev Respir Dis* 1980; **122**: 201–11.
10. Gherini, S, Peters, RM, Viirgilio, RW. Mechanical work of breathing with positive end expiratory pressure and continuous positive airways pressure. *Chest* 1979; **76**: 251–6.
11. Greenbaum, DM, Millen, JE, Eross, B, Snyder, JV, Grenvic, A, Safar, P. Continuous positive airways pressure without tracheal intubation in spontaneously breathing adults. *Chest* 1976; **69**: 615–20.
12. Dehaven, CB, Hurst, JM, Branson, RD. Post extubation hypoxaemia treated with continuous positive airways pressure mask. *Crit Care Med* 1985; **13**: 46–8.
13. Torres, G, Lyons, HA, Emerson, P. The effects of intermittent positive pressure breathing on intra-pulmonary distribution of inspired air. *Am J Med* 1960; **29**: 946–54.
14. Motley, HL, Werko, L, Cournand, A, Richards, DW. Observations of the clinical use of intermittent positive pressure. *J Aviation Med* 1947; **18**: 417–35.
15. Barry, BN, Bodenham, AR. Airway management in the ICU. *Br J Intensive Care* 2000; **10**: 22–9.
16. Bach, JR, Saporito, LR. Criteria for extubation and tracheostomy tube removal for patients with ventilatory failure. A different approach to weaning. *Chest* 1996: **110**: 1566–71.
17. Whitney, J, Harden, BA, Keilty, SEJ. Assisted cough. A new technique? *Physiotherapy* 2001; **68**: 201–7.
18. Bach, JR. Mechanical insufflation–exsufflation. Comparison of peak expiratory flows with manually assisted and unassisted coughing techniques. *Chest* 1993; **104**: 1553–62.
19. Yasuda, K, Hayashi, K. Changes in biomechanical properties of tendons and ligaments from joint disuse. *Osteoarthritis Cartilage* 1999; **7**(1): 122–9.
20. Barker, M, Beale, R. Optimal positioning for the adult intensive care patient while prone. In *Yearbook of intensive care and emergency medicine*, ed. J-L Vincent. Berlin: Springer-Verlag, 2000; 256–62.

21. Fridich, P, Krafft, P, Hochleuthner, H, Mauritz, W. The effects of long-term prone positioning in patients with trauma induced adult respiratory distress syndrome. *Anesth Analg* 1996; **83**: 1206–11.

22. Willems, MCM, Voets, AJ, Welten, RJTJ. Two unusual complications of prone-dependency in severe ARDS. *Intensive Care Med* 1998; **24**: 276–81.

23. DeBoisblanc, BP, Castro, M, Everret, B, Grender, J, Walker, CD, Summer, WR. Effect of air supported continuous postural oscillation on the risk of early ICU pneumonia in non traumatic critical illness. *Chest* 1993; **103**: 1543–7.

24. Choi, SC, Nelson, LD. Kinetic therapy in critically ill patients: combined results based on meta-analysis. *J Crit Care* 1992; **7**(1): 57–62.

25. Keilty, SEJ, Ponte, J, Fleming, TA, Moxham, J. Effect of inspiratory pressure support on exercise tolerance and breathlessness in patients with severe stable chronic obstructive pulmonary disease. *Thorax* 1994; **49**: 990–4.

26. Gallon, A. Evaluation of chest percussion in the treatment of patients with copious sputum production. *Respir Med* 1990; **85**: 45–51.

27. Stiller, K, Jenkins, S, Grant, R, Geake, T, Taylor, J, Hall, B. Acute lobar atelectasis: a comparison of five physiotherapy regimens. *Physiother Theory Practice* 1996; **12**: 197–209.

7

Diagnostic methods in respiratory intensive care medicine

TORSTEN T BAUER AND ANTONI TORRES

INTRODUCTION

Diagnostic methods in the intensive care unit (ICU) are partly limited by availability. Some methods may be available within the hospital, e.g. computed tomography (CT) of the chest, but transportation of the patient within the hospital may be difficult or even hazardous. However, some techniques are readily available and integrated into the daily routine. The anterior–posterior chest radiograph is routinely performed on a daily basis in most ICUs and longitudinal comparison may facilitate judgement, e.g. new pulmonary infiltrates. Moreover, bronchoscopy can be easily performed in the intubated patient and may even be done while respiratory support is provided using non-invasive ventilation.

The purpose of this chapter is to summarize the potential of the most commonly applied methods for the diagnosis of respiratory disorders and to outline basic practical issues.

PORTABLE CHEST RADIOGRAPHY

Patients usually have multiple medical problems, and portable chest radiography requires careful posi-
tioning of the patient to avoid displacing monitoring devices and indwelling catheters. Anterior–posterior chest radiographs are optimally taken with the patent in the upright position and during deep inspiration. This is usually not possible in the intubated patient, for whom supine films will normally be taken. X-ray exposure timed to the ventilator is difficult, but use of the **inspiratory hold button** ensures deep inspiration. Portable chest radiography remains the cornerstone of imaging techniques in respiratory critical care medicine, despite its disadvantages. The value of routine examinations is debatable.[1]

Monitoring of indwelling patient devices

The correct position of endotracheal tubes should be checked on the chest radiograph. With flexion and extension of the patient's neck, the endotracheal tube moves approximately 3 cm upward or downward. The ideal position is therefore 5 cm above the carina, with the head in a neutral position. Although an endotracheal tube inserted too deeply rarely causes injury, it always extends into the right main bronchus and impairs ventilation of the left lung, despite the fact that modern tubes have side holes to ensure a degree of ventilation to the left lung. One uncommon but serious complication during tube placement is rupture of the posterior membranous portion of the distal trachea or proximal main bronchi. Severe respiratory distress and subcutaneous emphysema, pneumomediastinum or pneumothorax are the symptoms and signs of this complication. Central venous lines and pressure monitors are frequently used to guide fluid therapy and a chest radiograph should be obtained following insertion of a central line catheter to ensue proper positioning. Pressures within the central venous system are measured most reliably when the catheter tip is located between the right atrium and the most proximal venous valves. The catheter tip should therefore be visualized medial to the anterior portion of the first rib, at the junction of the **brachiocephalic** vein and the superior **vena cava** or within the superior vena cava itself. Catheters that are advanced too far increase the risk of cardiac perforation or induction of ventricular arrhythmias.

Pulmonary capillary wedge catheters are helpful for the differentiation of cardiac and non-cardiac pulmonary oedema and optimizing fluid or inotrope therapy. The catheter is introduced via an antecubital, jugular or subclavian vein and advanced through the right side of the heart into the pulmonary artery. Ideally, the tip should not extend beyond the proximal interlobar pulmonary arteries. Complications of pulmonary artery catheters include arrhythmias, pulmonary infarction, pulmonary artery perforation, intracardiac knotting, endocarditis and sepsis. Their routine value has been questioned by the Pulmonary Artery Catheter Consensus Conference.[2] However, this position is not unanimously accepted and a recent meta-analysis found that substituting a non-invasive study for Swan–Ganz catheter placement in the initial evaluation of acutely ill patients may slightly reduce procedure-related events, but may also increase the number of procedures performed.[3]

Thoracostomy tubes are used to drain air and/or pleural effusions, empyemas and haemothoraces. The tubes should be positioned in an anterior–superior location for pneumothorax and in a posterior–inferior location to drain liquids. Chest radiographs may be used to verify the position after the procedure, but ultrasound is more useful in guiding tube placement, especially with loculated collections. Other indwelling devices that may be visualized by the chest radiograph are nasogastric tubes, transvenous pacing wires and intra-aortic counterpulsation devices.

Pulmonary and pleural abnormalities

Atelectasis occurs most often in the left lower lobe, followed by the right lower and right upper lobes. Despite significant intrapulmonary shunting, radiographic appearances may vary from entirely normal to linear, patchy opacities to lobar collapse. Lobar collapse with positive air bronchograms (the positive imaging of the main bronchi) should make the clinician think of consolidation, whereas lobar collapse in the absence of air bronchograms is usually associated with obstruction, e.g. a mucous plug. Both types of lobar collapse may prompt bronchoscopy to obtain microbiological samples or to remove the obstruction. In general, radiograph opacities due to pneumonia appear later and resolve more slowly than do those due to aspiration or atelectasis. Therefore, new pulmonary infiltrates that persist for 48 hours are more suggestive of nosocomial pneumonia. However, the radiographic appearance may be complicated by underlying conditions such as chronic obstructive pulmonary disease or pulmonary oedema.

Because of the effects of gravity in the supine patient, pulmonary vascular redistribution to the upper zones occurs and pulmonary oedema may have an atypical distribution. In addition, the distinction of non-cardiogenic from cardiogenic oedema may be difficult because the usual radiographic signs of pulmonary venous hypertension, cardiomegaly or pleural effusion may not be present and/or are nonspecific. Adult respiratory distress syndrome (ARDS) appears as non-cardiogenic oedema on the chest radiograph. Infiltrates due to ARDS develop rapidly and bilaterally and differentiation from cardiogenic oedema may require determination of the pulmonary capillary wedge pressure with a pulmonary artery catheter, by echocardiography or by other methods (see Chapter 8). Initially, the chest radiograph may be normal. Within 24–36 hours, there may only be little evidence of interstitial perihilar oedema. On days 2–5, the radiographic pattern changes to patchy, ill-defined opacities and then to more confluent, diffuse, bilateral airspace opacities. Massive pulmonary embolism may mimic these appearances and the diagnosis may be difficult to establish. Dynamic spiral contrast-enhanced CT has high sensitivity and specificity for proximal pulmonary embolism (see Chapter 19). Findings on the chest radiograph in lesser pulmonary embolism include peripheral, wedge-shaped pleural-based opacities, atelectasis, elevation of the diaphragm and/or pleural effusion.

Pneumothorax is the most frequently recognized manifestation of extra-alveolar air on the chest X-ray (CXR), but pneumomediastinum may also be present. Mechanical ventilation with positive end-expiratory pressure (PEEP) will exacerbate an air leak once it has developed. In the supine patient, free air within the pleural space rises anteriorly and medially. If there are pre-existing adhesions, the pneumothorax may remain encapsulated, even when the patient is erect. Diagnosis may require CT scanning because differentiation from intrapulmonary air cysts or abscesses may be difficult and significant pneumothorax may not even be apparent on the plain CXR in severe ARDS. Furthermore, scanning may be useful in the evaluation of the later fibroproliferative stage of ARDS.

BRONCHOSCOPY

Flexible bronchoscopy has greatly influenced diagnostic capability in the ICU. It is easy to perform because the airways are readily accessible through the endotracheal or tracheostomy tube. Bronchoscopy may be both diagnostic and therapeutic. For example, in a patient with pulmonary collapse and worsening arterial oxygenation, bronchoscopy may demonstrate mucoid impaction causing lobular collapse, which can be removed at the same time. However, it may sometimes be difficult to identify an obstructed orifice, either because of the variability of bronchial anatomy or because of distal impaction beyond the field of vision. In the USA, pulmonologists with bronchoscopic training are often in charge of ICU patients, but this is not usually the case in Europe. We would therefore encourage training in bronchoscopy to be given to intensive care physicians. Acute respiratory deterioration during bronchoscopy may result from a reduction in alveolar ventilation consequent upon the introduction of airway obstruction. It may also relate to

Table 7.1 *Indications for bronchoscopy in the intensive care unit and high dependency unit*

Emergency interventions
Endoscopic intubation
Malpositioning of the endotracheal tube
Haemoptysis
Chest trauma
Chemical or thermal burns of the tracheobronchial tree
Massive witnessed aspiration
Suspected foreign-body aspiration

Elective interventions
Pulmonary infiltrates associated with clinical signs of infection
Unexplained lung collapse or pleural effusion
Percutaneous tracheostomy
Postoperative evaluation of patents after lung resection or of lung transplant recipients

sedative rugs. If local anaesthesia is employed, only minimal additional sedation is necessary (if any), but coughing may provoke transiently high airway pressure in the intubated patient. In cases of spontaneously breathing patients with respiratory failure who need a bronchoscopic procedure, non-invasive respiratory support can be employed. The bronchoscope is then introduced via the full facemask, but the procedure may be difficult when air leaks cannot be managed.[4]

Table 7.1 summarizes the major indications for bronchoscopy in patients in the ICU or high dependency unit (HDU).

Endotracheal intubation

At intubation, the laryngoscope is usually used to visualize the glottis. The bronchoscope is an alternative if abnormal upper airway anatomy makes intubation difficult, e.g. following trauma or in cervical scoliosis or oropharyngeal disease. The endotracheal tube is slipped over the bronchoscope and used as a guide for intubation when the upper trachea is visualized. Bronchoscopy can also ensure correct endotracheal tube positioning because the distance between the tip of the tube and the carina can be easily assessed. In cervical spine injury, direct laryngoscopic intubation entails the risk of further injury, and fibreoptic nasal intubation is advised in this situation.[5] Although the chest radiograph is usually sufficient to exclude malposition, it is an alternative if profound hypoxaemia calls for urgent assessment.

Haemoptysis

Accurate diagnosis is essential in the management of haemoptysis because massive pulmonary bleeding may rapidly lead to respiratory failure and the need for endotracheal intubation. If severe, elective intubation of the patient prior to bronchoscopy is appropriate. However, massive haemoptysis (between 300 and 1000 mL in 24 hours) is only present in about 5% of cases and not all of these patients need urgent bronchoscopy.[6] Distinction between gastrointestinal, pharyngeal, nasal and pulmonary sources often requires endoscopy. Blood from the lungs is coughed rather than vomited, is partly frothy, alkaline and sometimes mixed with pus. Nausea and vomiting are suggestive of haematemesis, whereas a history of cough, weight loss, fever and night sweats is a clue for haemoptysis. The goals of bronchoscopy are to identify the source of bleeding and prevent blood spilling into unaffected parts of the lung. The options available include endobronchial suctioning, cold saline lavage, use of topical vasoconstrictors (e.g. epinephrine in a dilution of 1:20 000) and/or coagulants, endobronchial balloon tamponade or selective bronchial intubation (see Chapter 9).[7]

Chest trauma, thermal or chemical burns of the tracheobronchial tree

Although car seat belts and the airbag have greatly reduced the incidence of blunt trauma to the thorax in motor vehicle accidents, bronchoscopy is necessary to assess airway damage. Physical and radiographic findings are important determinants of the need for bronchoscopy, e.g. pneumothorax, subcutaneous or mediastinal emphysema, haemothorax, flail chest, atelectasis and haemoptysis. The identification of discontinuation of the tracheobronchial tree ranges from bronchial contusion and laceration to complete tracheal transection.[8]

Thermal inhalation injury to the lungs can be devastating and reliance on the absence of clinical criteria, such as facial or oropharyngeal burns, carbonaceous sputum, wheezing and hoarseness, is insufficient to exclude burn injury. Acute injury produces erythema,

mucosal sloughing and severe airway oedema. Bronchoscopy allows earlier diagnosis and appropriate therapy, including corticosteroids, humidified air, antibiotics and assistance in clearing airway plugs. The role of bronchoscopy after chemical injury is to determine the extent of the chemical burn and to assess or remove secondary complications such as necrotic debris, stenosis or other life-threatening sequelae.[9]

Massive aspiration and suspected foreign-body aspiration

Massive aspiration of gastric contents almost inevitably leads to pneumonia, the severity of which depends on the amount and type of aspirate. Radiographically, aspiration pneumonia most commonly involves the posterior segments of the upper lobes and the superior segments of the lower lobes. Rapid diagnosis and therapeutic intervention decrease morbidity and mortality, although there is no consensus on the role of bronchoscopy after aspiration. The suction channel of the flexible bronchoscope is too small to recover solid material, and the introduction of saline to dilute the aspirate and remove it from the tracheobronchial tree may be harmful if it allows spread into more distal parts of the lung. Therefore, bronchoscopy is probably limited to those patients who develop signs of acute airway obstruction due to the aspiration of larger food particles.

Respiratory compromise due to foreign-body aspiration is rarely severe enough to cause respiratory failure, although acute distress may result if the obstructing object is large or localized centrally. Foreign-body aspiration typically occurs in children or the elderly and manifests as obstructive lobar or segmental over-inflation or atelectasis. If a definite history of aspiration is given or a foreign body is seen radiographically, rigid bronchoscopy is preferable to effect removal. Flexible bronchoscopy is more readily available, however, and may be more appropriate for initial inspection, particularly of the distal parts of the tracheobronchial tree.

Pulmonary infiltrates associated with clinical signs of infection

New pulmonary infiltrates in mechanically ventilated patients suggest nosocomial pneumonia,

Table 7.2 *Diagnostic tools for nosocomial pneumonia in the intensive care unit and high dependency unit*

Non-invasive	Invasive
Sputum	Percutaneous needle aspiration
Culture	Lung needle[a]
Gram stain	Pleural effusion
Blood culture	Protected specimen brush
Serology	Bronchoalveolar lavage
Legionella pneumophila	Conventional
Atypical bacteria	Protected
Viruses	Blind
Endotracheal aspirate[b]	
Urinary antigen	
Legionella pneumophila	
Streptococcus pneumoniae	
Molecular technique	
Polymerase chain reaction	

[a]Not recommended in mechanically ventilated patients.
[b]In intubated patients.

especially when associated with other signs of infection. Quantitative bacterial cultures may be helpful to differentiate between colonization and infection (see Chapter 15) and various diagnostic tools are available (Table 7.2). The best approach is currently contentious, but bronchoscopy may reduce mortality in ventilator-associated pneumonia.[10] A consensus statement[11] provides a clinical algorithm to guide management (Fig. 7.1). As this issue is discussed in detail in Chapter 15, only the basic aspects of diagnostic techniques are provided here.

NON-INVASIVE METHODS

The sensitivity of blood culture in nosocomial pneumonia is low and lacks specificity in the critically ill. Micro-organisms isolated in blood cultures should only be considered to be the definitive cause when also isolated from respiratory samples. The quantitative culture of samples from the lower respiratory tract may assist in differentiation from colonization. For endotracheal aspirates, a cut-off of 10^5 colony-forming units mL^{-1} (cfu) gives an acceptable sensitivity and specificity in diagnosis in the presence of clinical signs.[12] Detection of bacterial antigen in urine is useful for *Legionella* or *Streptococcus pneumoniae*.[13,14] whereas molecular methods currently lack specificity.

BRONCHOSCOPIC METHODS

Bronchoscopic specimens may be contaminated by material from the upper airway or the endotracheal tube. To avoid this, one approach is the use of the protected specimen brush (PSB), positioned via the bronchoscope at the orifice of a radiographically identified segmental bronchus. The catheter is advanced approximately 3 cm out of the fibreoptic bronchoscope and the inner cannula is then protruded to eject a distal carbon wax plug. After suctioning material, the brush is retracted back inside the inner cannula, which is then pulled back into the outer cannula and removed from the bronchoscope. The threshold for quantitative bacterial cultures from a PSB is 10^3 cfu mL^{-1}.

Bronchoalveolar lavage (BAL) samples a larger portion of lung parenchyma, has good sensitivity and is especially useful in immunocompromised patients. The specificity of BAL is limited by contamination with upper-airway bacteria found in up to one-third of specimens. There are several ways of performing BAL, such as directed and non-directed non-bronchoscopic and directed bronchoscopic methods. Growth above 10^4 cfu mL^{-1} in quantitative bacterial cultures is usually significant, no matter which BAL technique is employed.[11]

Unexplained lung collapse or pleural effusion

Atelectasis is often encountered in the ICU/HDU setting because of relative hypoventilation in non-intubated patients, e.g. post-laparotomy or in association with pressure-limited ventilation strategies. In the ventilated patient, a recruitment manoeuvre may be successful in re-expanding the lung. Persistent lobar collapse may be caused by an endobronchial lesion or a mucous plug. Endoscopy may therefore be both diagnostic and therapeutic. Pleural effusions have many causes but, in the critically ill, they are commonly related to congestive cardiac failure, pulmonary infection, neoplasm, excessive fluid replacement during resuscitation or hypoproteinaemia. Pleural effusion due to heart failure is usually bilateral and evidence for this may be provided by echocardiography or a pulmonary artery catheter. In unilateral effusion, diagnostic

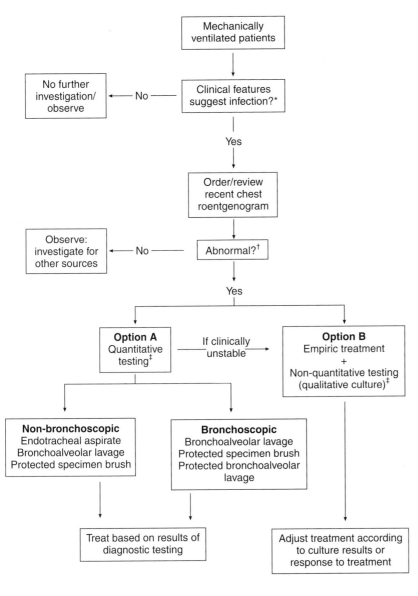

Figure 7.1 *Clinical algorithm for the diagnosis of nosocomial pneumonia. *Two or more of the following criteria: body temperature >38 °C or <36 °C, leucocytosis or leucopenia, purulent tracheal secretion, decreased PaO_2. †Radiographic evidence of alveolar infiltrates, air bronchograms, new or worsened infiltrates. ‡There is no definitive evidence to support either option A or B. Therefore, the clinician should choose the appropriate test based on its sensitivity and specificity, potential adverse effects, availability and cost. (Adapted, with permission, from reference 11.)*

aspiration is indicated, with care being taken to minimize the risk of pneumothorax in mechanically ventilated patients.

Percutaneous dilatation tracheostomy

Tracheostomy prevents complications associated with prolonged translaryngeal intubation and eases weaning from mechanical ventilation.[15] Percutaneous dilatation tracheostomy is a safe alternative to surgical placement. Bronchoscopy may be helpful during this procedure to verify a midline insertion of the guide wire. Although experienced personnel may not need to employ bronchoscopy, it is mandatory to have a bronchoscope available in case complications develop.

Postoperative evaluation of patients after lung resection or of lung transplant recipients

Patients with lung resection or transplantation may develop a number of complications, such as suture granuloma or anastomotic air leak. Bronchoscopy is of critical importance in the diagnosis of anastomotic dehiscence. In addition, pulmonary infiltrates may indicate infection or rejection in lung transplant recipients.

Bronchoscopy allows the identification of pulmonary infections with BAL or pulmonary rejection by transbronchial biopsy. Bronchiolitis obliterans syndrome remains a major late complication and may be an immediate problem in the lung transplant patient.[16] Bronchoscopy is again needed for tissue sampling.

BEDSIDE DIAGNOSTIC ULTRASOUND

Ultrasound is important in the diagnosis of various conditions in the ICU or HDU.[17] It has considerable value in the assessment of the pleura or pleural space. For the aspiration of fluid, simple marking of the overlying skin is adequate, without the need for real-time imaging. The method of drainage depends on the fluid aspirated. If it is clear and odourless, a non-infectious aetiology is usual and simple aspiration is often adequate. Bacterial culture and other laboratory parameters will be employed to identify the cause, e.g. haemoglobin, glucose, lactate dehydrogenase and cholesterol (see Chapter 17). When the ultrasound shows loculations, or the aspirate is bloody or purulent, a chest tube should be considered. The application of ultrasound in the respiratory ICU is not limited to the diagnosis of pleural collections or the placing of drains.[18]

Transoesophageal echocardiography is a Doppler technique that uses the oesophagus as an acoustic window. In ventilated patients, it may be used to assess left ventricular function, valvular disease, endocarditis and prosthetic valve dysfunction. Transoesophageal echocardiography has been increasingly used for the diagnosis of pulmonary embolism and is superior to transthoracic echocardiography in evaluating a cardiac source of embolism. In comparison with radiological procedures, it had limited accuracy for detecting pulmonary embolism with acute cor pulmonale in one study.[19] Only when the pulmonary embolism was located in the main or right pulmonary artery could transoesophageal echocardiography be reliable in confirming the diagnosis. Its performance was better in the presence of shock due to massive pulmonary embolism. In comparison with pulmonary scintigraphy or autopsy, the sensitivity of transoesophageal echocardiography for the diagnosis of

massive pulmomonary embolism was 99%, with a specificity of 100%.[20]

OTHER BEDSIDE PROCEDURES IN THE INTENSIVE CARE UNIT

Portable CT of the chest is now available in some centres and is of value for critically ill patients who cannot be moved from the ICU.[21] It is especially useful in the evaluation of ARDS, differentiating intrapulmonary from pleural abscess, assessing the mediastinum and in tracheo-oesophageal or tracheopulmonary fistula. CT is the modality of choice for establishing the diagnosis of exogenous lipoid pneumonia resulting from the aspiration of hydrocarbons and mineral oil. The measurement of lung permeability employing nuclear isotopes in acute lung injury may be useful, although other indirect techniques such as PICCO are more likely to be useful in monitoring (see Chapter 8).

ACKNOWLEDGEMENT

Dr Torsten Bauer has been in part supported by the Bochumer Arbeitskreis für Pneumologie und Allergologie, Bochum, Germany (BAPA).

REFERENCES

1. Tocino, I. Chest imaging in the intensive care unit. *Eur J Radiol* 1996; **23**: 46–57.
2. Pulmonary Artery Catheter Consensus Conference: consensus statement. *Crit Care Med* 1997; **25**: 910–25.
3. Duane, PG, Colice, GL. Impact of noninvasive studies to distinguish volume overload from ARDS in acutely ill patients with pulmonary edema: analysis of the medical literature from 1966 to 1998. *Chest* 2000; **118**: 1709–17.
4. Vitacca, M, Nava, S, Confalonieri, M, *et al.* The appropriate setting of noninvasive pressure support ventilation in stable CQPD patients. *Chest* 2000; **118**: 1286–93.
5. Fuchs, G, Schwarz, G, Baumgartner, A, Kaltenbock, F, Voit-Augustin, H, Planinz, W. Fiberoptic intubation in 327 neurosurgical patients with lesions of the cervical spine. *J Neurosurg Anesthesiol* 1999; **11**: 11–16.

6. Dweik, RA, Stoller, JK. Role of bronchoscopy in massive hemoptysis. *Clin Chest Med* 1999; **20**: 89–105.

7. Jean-Baptiste, E. Clinical assessment and management of massive hemoptysis. *Crit Care Med* 2000; **28**: 1642–7.

8. Hara, KS, Prakash, UB. Fiberoptic bronchoscopy in the evaluation of acute chest and upper airway trauma. *Chest* 1989; **96**: 627–30.

9. Freitag, L, Firusian, N, Stamatis, G, Greschuchna, D. The role of bronchoscopy in pulmonary complications due to mustard gas inhalation. *Chest* 1991; **100**: 1436–41.

10. Fagon, JY, Chastre, J, Wolff, M, *et al.* Invasive and noninvasive strategies for management of suspected ventilator-associated pneumonia. A randomized trial. *Ann Intern Med* 2000; **132**: 621–30.

11. Grossman, RF, Fein, AM. Evidence-based assessment of diagnostic tests for ventilator-associated pneumonia. Executive summary. *Chest* 2000; **117**: 177s–81s.

12. El-Ebiary, M, Torres, A, Gonzalez, J, Puig de la Bellacasa, J, Garcia, C, Jimenez de Anta, MT. Quantitative cultures of endotracheal aspirates for the diagnosis of ventilator-associated pneumonia. *Am J Respir Crit Care Med* 1993; **147**: 1552–7.

13. Dominguez, J, Gali, N, Blanco, S, *et al.* Detection of *Streptococcus pneumoniae* antigen by a rapid immunochromatographic assay in urine samples. *Chest* 2001; **119**: 243–9.

14. Benson, RF, Tang, PW, Fields, BS. Evaluation of the Binax and Biotest urinary antigen kits for detection of Legionnaires' disease due to multiple serogroups and species of *Legionella*. *J Clin Microbiol* 2000; **38**: 2763–5.

15. Kearney, PA, Griffen, MM, Ochoa, JB, Boulanger, BR, Tseui, BJ, Mentzer, RMJ. A single-center 8-year experience with percutaneous dilational tracheostomy. *Ann Surg* 2000; **231**: 701–9.

16. Meyers, BF, Lynch, J, Trulock, EP, Guthrie, TJ, Cooper, JD, Patterson, GA. 1999. Lung transplantation: a decade of experience. *Ann Surg* 1999; **230**: 362–71.

17. Beagle, GL. Bedside diagnostic ultrasound and therapeutic ultrasound-guided procedures in the intensive care setting. *Crit Care Clin* 2000; **16**: 59–81.

18. Lichtenstein, D, Meziere, G, Biderman, P, Gepner, A. The comet-tail artifact: an ultrasound sign ruling out pneumothorax. *Intensive Care Med* 1999; **25**: 383–8.

19. Vieillard-Baron, A, Qanadli, SD, Antakly, Y, *et al.* Transesophageal echocardiography for the diagnosis of pulmonary embolism with acute cor pulmonale: a comparison with radiological procedures. *Intensive Care Med* 1998; **24**: 429–33.

20. Krivec, B, Voga, G, Zuran, I, *et al.* Diagnosis and treatment of shock due to massive pulmonary embolism: approach with transesophageal echocardiography and intrapulmonary thrombolysis. *Chest* 1997; **112**: 1310–16.

21. White, CS, Meyer, CA, Wu, J, Mirvis, SE. Portable CT: assessing thoracic disease in the intensive care unit. *Am J Roentgenol* 1999; **173**: 1351–6.

Monitoring

RICHARD BEALE

INTRODUCTION

Respiratory critical care involves much more than a narrow consideration of the respiratory system. Most patients who require respiratory critical care also have involvement of other organ systems. Lung injury and the requirement for respiratory support may be either the primary problem, often leading to secondary systemic consequences, or the secondary consequence of another primary disease process. Nevertheless, optimum management of the respiratory system is crucial if the patient is to recover, because very few critically ill patients avoid respiratory problems altogether. Effective respiratory system monitoring is therefore vital, and this chapter aims to provide an overview of the more commonly used techniques.

Monitoring constitutes such a routine part of the care of critically ill patients that it is often taken for granted. In a modern intensive care unit (ICU), increasingly complex equipment is employed to measure and display various aspects of patient physiology. Indeed, as computer technology advances, measurements and variables that were once solely the preserve of the research laboratory are now readily available at the bedside. These advances challenge our ability to understand and use this extra information to benefit our patients. In some cases, there are several different technologies that will provide a particular piece of information, and the decision about which choice is made can have far-reaching organizational consequences.

In order to make such choices appropriately, it is important to consider the purpose and process of monitoring as it applies to a critically ill patient. Monitoring is much more than making a single measurement, because it implies the ability to take a measurement repeatedly, even continuously, in order to follow over time the physiological process that the measurement represents. Usually, this is with the aim of detecting deterioration or improvement, often in relation to therapeutic interventions. Frequently, the ability to track a physiological process by scientific measurement may be limited by the technology available. Although this seems an obvious statement, its implications are more subtle. Necessarily, processes and problems can become defined by the methods used to measure them, even if these methods are far from ideal. In turn, this can mislead the clinician if the limitations and surrogate nature of a measurement are forgotten or ignored. Arguably, much of the current controversy over the use of the pulmonary artery catheter arises from precisely this phenomenon. An understanding of the strengths and weaknesses of alternative monitoring approaches is therefore essential in order to avoid these pitfalls.

The first major area of respiratory critical care monitoring involves the adequacy of gas exchange, which is most frequently assessed using arterial blood-gas analysis, oximetry and capnography. The second involves monitoring of the most frequently used supportive therapy, mechanical ventilation, and involves increasingly sophisticated bedside measurements of respiratory mechanics. The third is the closely related area of haemodynamic monitoring, especially as it relates to heart–lung interaction and the effects of fluid resuscitation upon the injured lung. It is only possible to touch the surface of these areas in this chapter, but specialist texts are available to provide extra detail.

ARTERIAL BLOOD-GAS ANALYSIS

Monitoring arterial blood gases through repeated intermittent measurement of withdrawn blood is a mainstay of respiratory monitoring in any ICU. Standard blood-gas analysers provide measurement of the O_2 (PO_2) and CO_2 (PCO_2) tensions and the pH of the blood sample being analysed. Although arterial blood is used most frequently, the same principles can also be applied to venous samples, and arterio-venous differences in these variables can provide useful information. It is crucial to remember that the measured PO_2 and PCO_2 tensions derive from gas *dissolved* in the plasma rather than the total amount of O_2 or CO_2 present in the sample.

Principles of measurement

Most blood-gas analysers use an O_2 electrode of the Clark[1] or polarographic type to measure the PO_2. In this system, electrons are provided from a cathode and react with dissolved O_2:

$$O_2 + 2H_2O + 2e^- \rightarrow H_2O_2 + 2OH^-$$

$$H_2O_2 + 2e^- \rightarrow 2OH^-$$

Four electrons are used to reduce each molecule of O_2, so the overall current generated is proportional to the amount of dissolved O_2, i.e. the PO_2. In the Clark electrode, the cathode and anode are within an electrolyte solution separated from the blood (or other fluid being measured) by a membrane permeable to O_2.

Measurements of pH and PCO_2 share the same basic principle. In a pH electrode, blood is drawn into a capillary tube of pH-sensitive glass bathed in a buffer solution that maintains the pH outside the glass at a constant value. A potential is thus generated across the glass that is proportional to the pH of the blood sample within the capillary.

In the CO_2 electrode, a pH-sensitive glass electrode is bathed in bicarbonate solution and covered by a CO_2-permeable membrane. When blood is passed across the other side of the membrane, CO_2 diffuses into the bicarbonate solution and reacts with the water present:

$$CO_2 + H_2O \rightarrow H_2CO_3 \rightarrow H^+ + HCO_3^-$$

The hydrogen ion concentration (pH) is then measured in the same way as before, and the system can be calibrated for PCO_2 because the pH change is linearly related to the logarithm of the PCO_2.

Temperature correction of blood-gas measurement

Most blood-gas analysers maintain the electrode temperature at 37°C, but few patients have blood at precisely that temperature. If the patient is relatively hypothermic, the blood sample will therefore be heated in the electrode, resulting in decreased gas solubility and decreased O_2 affinity for haemoglobin, and therefore an artificially raised blood-gas tension. The reverse is true if the blood sample is cooled in the analyser (i.e. the patient is hyperthermic). Most analysers include formulae to correct for this effect on PO_2, PCO_2 and pH in their software, if the true patient temperature is entered into the machine.

During cardiac surgery, there are two different approaches to the effect of temperature upon pH that are commonly utilized. The first is to correct for the effect of temperature during patient cooling on cardiopulmonary bypass and aim at a normal pH for the temperature (the pH increases approximately

0.015 pH unit per degree centigrade of cooling), and is known as the pH-stat approach. The second is to keep the pH normal at 37°C regardless of the patient's actual temperature, and is known as the alpha-stat approach. It remains unclear as to which approach is more beneficial.

CONTINUOUS BLOOD-GAS ANALYSIS

The major drawbacks of the conventional approach to blood-gas analysis are the intermittent nature of the measurement and the requirement to draw blood. In an attempt to overcome these disadvantages, continuous on-line blood-gas sensors have been developed.

Principles

Most critically ill patients, especially those who are unstable, have indwelling arterial lines in place to facilitate frequent arterial blood sampling and continuous arterial blood pressure measurement. One approach that overcomes the problems of traditional blood-gas sampling is to place small sensors within a cassette that can be placed in the arterial line circuit close to the cannula in such a manner as to allow blood withdrawal, measurement and return in a closed fashion. A more sophisticated solution is to utilize miniaturized sensors for the measurement of PO_2, PCO_2 and pH that are sufficiently small to fit on a probe that can be passed through a 20-G arterial line. Technically, it is possible to miniaturize a Clark electrode sufficiently for this purpose,[2] but attempts to do the same for pH and PCO_2 electrochemical electrodes have been more troublesome.

An alternative approach is to use optical sensor technology, sometimes called optodes. Such sensors may utilize the principles of absorbance, fluorescence, phosphorescence or chemiluminescence, the details of which are described elsewhere. The best known and most widely used of the available commercial devices is probably the Paratrend 7® device from Diametrics. This device previously used a combination of an electrochemical (Clark-type) PO_2 sensor and absorbance PCO_2 and pH sensors, but the latest probes rely entirely upon optical technology and are similarly sized to a standard arterial line.

Although continuous pulse oximetry and capnography had initially appeared to make the use of continuous indwelling (and therefore invasive) blood-gas analysis largely unnecessary, developments in intensive care have demonstrated some of the limitations of these techniques. Pulse oximetry is critically dependent upon the quality of the perfusion signal in the tissue within the probe area, and peripheral perfusion is often severely limited in very sick patients. Moreover, due to the flat shape of the upper part of the haemoglobin O_2 dissociation curve, there is very little change in O_2 saturation (SO_2) for dramatic changes in PO_2. This has become of greater importance with the increasing use of lung recruitment manoeuvres, where it is often not feasible to measure changes in absolute lung volume, and where changes in PO_2 may be the best and most important bedside surrogate for judging clinical response (Fig. 8.1). This is greatly facilitated by the use of continuous, online measurement.

OXIMETRY

Under normal circumstances, nearly all the O_2 carried in the blood is attached to haemoglobin, yet traditional blood-gas analysis only provides information about that very small proportion dissolved in the plasma. Oximeters are devices designed to measure the degree to which haemoglobin is saturated

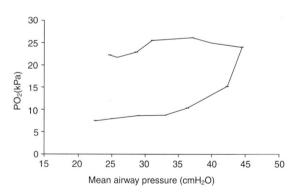

Figure 8.1 A high-pressure recruitment manoeuvre in a patient with acute respiratory distress syndrome performed using a high-frequency oscillator (Sensormedics 3100B). Changes in PO_2 act as a surrogate for changes in lung volume, and demonstrate recruitment and hysteresis. SpO_2 measurements would not illustrate this effect because this patient is on the flat, upper portion of the O_2-dissociation curve.

with O_2, and fall into two major categories. Both use the principles of light absorption, but serve different purposes. The first group comprises the bench-top oximeters, often called co-oximeters. These machines utilize light at several wavelengths to separate the quantities of oxyhaemoglobin (HbO_2), reduced haemoglobin (Hb), methaemoglobin (MetHb) and carboxyhaemoglobin (COHb) in a heparinized blood sample, and express the arterial O_2 saturation (SaO_2) as:

$$SaO_2 = \frac{HbO_2}{HbO_2 + Hb + MetHb + COHb} \times 100$$

Originally, co-oximeters were freestanding devices, but now many modern blood-gas machines can be supplied with in-built oximeters, providing both blood-gas and oximetry profiles.

Unlike co-oximeters, pulse oximeters are true monitoring devices, providing continuous measurement of *in-vivo* HbO_2, usually referred to as SpO_2. The introduction of pulse oximetry constituted a major advance in respiratory monitoring, and today these devices are ubiquitous in modern respiratory, critical care and anaesthetic practice.

Principles of pulse oximetry

Pulse oximeters use the principles of spectrophotometry to provide a value for the arterial haemoglobin O_2 saturation. Light at two wavelengths, usually 660 nm (red) and 940 nm (infrared), is shone from two light-emitting diodes (LEDs) situated in a finger or ear probe. Oxyhaemoglobin (HBO_2) absorbs more infrared light than reduced haemoglobin, whilst reduced haemoglobin absorbs more red light than oxyhaemoglobin. The two diodes are switched on and off rapidly (approximately 600 times s^{-1}), and each sequence allows the detector within the probe to measure the transmission of red light and infrared light, and to control for ambient light. There is a pulsatile (alternating current, AC) component to the absorption signal due to the pulse of arterial blood flowing within the detection area, and a non-pulsatile (direct current, DC) component due to absorption of light by non-pulsatile arterial blood, venous and capillary blood and other tissues. The device relates the pulsatile component to the non-pulsatile component at each wavelength, so calculating a ratio:

$$\text{Ratio } R = \frac{AC_{660}/DC_{660}}{AC_{940}/DC_{940}}$$

Using an algorithm that describes the relationship between R and measurements of haemoglobin O_2 saturation made *in vivo* using a bench-top oximeter, the pulse oximeter saturation (SpO_2) is then calculated. In terms of accuracy, most manufacturers claim that the 95% confidence limit for measurements is $\pm 4\%$ at SaO_2 levels above 70%. Accuracy deteriorates when SaO_2 falls below this level, partly because of the difficulty in obtaining reliable human calibration data in conditions of extreme hypoxaemia. Different probe types can also alter device performance, with ear probes tending to have a faster response time than finger probes. Clearly, the averaging and sampling algorithms employed by different manufacturers are also of importance, and these are constantly being improved.

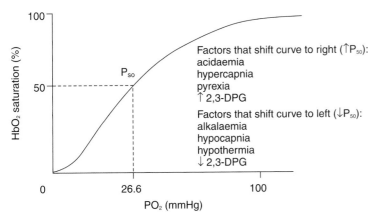

Figure 8.2 O_2-dissociation curve for haemoglobin. 2,3-DPG, 2,3-diphosphoglycerate.

Although pulse oximeters are widely used, they have a number of significant shortcomings that may mislead the clinician. These include:

- lack of responsiveness at high PO_2 values,
- dependence upon adequate tissue perfusion,
- inability to discriminate between abnormal haemoglobin species,
- interference from dyes,
- susceptibility to ambient light,
- false alarms and susceptibility to motion artefacts.

LACK OF RESPONSIVENESS AT HIGH PO_2 VALUES

Because pulse oximeters measure haemoglobin O_2 saturation, they provide very little information about changes in arterial PO_2 once the flat portion of the O_2 dissociation curve has been reached (Fig. 8.2). This means that the dramatic changes in PO_2 seen during recruitment manoeuvres in responsive mechanically ventilated patients cannot readily be tracked with a pulse oximeter.

DEPENDENCE UPON ADEQUATE TISSUE PERFUSION

Under circumstances in which cardiac output and tissue perfusion fall, the ability of the device to detect a pulsatile signal becomes impaired. Many manufacturers also provide a plethysmograph trace, which gives some information as to the adequacy of perfusion. Some devices increase the amplification of the displayed trace as the signal decreases, whereas others provide the ability to alter the amplification manually, or display a perfusion index. The latter approach is more useful if the plethysmograph trace is being used to assess perfusion. Eventually, perfusion may become too poor for an analysable signal to be detected, and an error message will be displayed. Unfortunately, in some situations, inaccurate SpO_2 values may be displayed first, especially if perfusion is sufficiently poor to become gradually impaired by the contact pressure from the probe itself. Under these circumstances, the values obtained should be checked by arterial blood-gas analysis and bench-top co-oximetry.

INABILITY TO DISCRIMINATE BETWEEN ABNORMAL HAEMOGLOBIN SPECIES

The two most commonly encountered abnormal haemoglobin species are COHb and MetHb. Both interfere with pulse oximeter measurements if present in significant amounts. COHb has a very similar absorption spectrum to HbO_2, and pulse oximeters provide readings for SpO_2 that are actually the sum of the HbO_2 and COHb present. Therefore, in situations of severe carbon monoxide poisoning, pulse oximetry may lead the user to believe that the patient is well saturated when the opposite is actually true.

MetHb absorbs similar amounts of light at both 660 nm and 940 nm, giving an absorption ratio of 1. This equates to a SpO_2 value of about 85% on the oximeter calibration curve, so the more MetHb present, the more the SpO_2 reading will tend towards 85%. If methylene blue is used to treat the methamoglobinaemia, although it is highly effective, it will also result in falsely low SpO_2 readings because of its blue colour.

INTERFERENCE FROM DYES

Both methylene blue and indocyanine green may be given intravenously to critically ill patients for a variety of purposes, and both interfere with the signal detected by the pulse oximeter.

AMBIENT LIGHT

Although the LED activation sequence within the oximeter probe is designed to correct for ambient light levels, bright sunlight and some forms of high-intensity artificial light may still interfere with signal detection.

FALSE ALARMS AND SUSCEPTIBILITY TO MOTION ARTEFACTS

A persistent problem with the use of pulse oximeters is the number of false alarms generated. Some authors have suggested that only one in five alarms is genuine. Movement artefact is usually the cause, due either to interference from motion or the probe becoming detached. Poor perfusion may also have this effect, when the local SpO_2 falls as a consequence. Although staff using these devices have largely become inured to this phenomenon, it can be problematic when attempting to analyse trends retrospectively. It can also lead to genuine alarms being ignored. Certainly, no other routinely used monitoring device provides quite so many false alarms.

Oxygen content

Because most of the O_2 present within a blood sample is bound to haemoglobin, calculation of the O_2 content requires knowledge of the PO_2, SaO_2 and Hb:

$$CaO_2 \text{ (per 100 mL blood)} = [Hb \text{ (g dL}^{-1}) \times 1.34 \times SaO_2] + [0.0031 \times PaO_2 \text{ (mmHg)}]$$

For a patient with normal results, i.e. a Hb concentration of 15 g dL^{-1}, SaO_2 of 97% and arterial PO_2 of 100 mmHg, this equates to:

$$CaO_2 \text{ (per 100 mL blood)} = [15 \text{ (g dL}^{-1}) \times 1.34 \times 0.97] + [0.0031 \times 100 \text{ (mmHg)}]$$

$$CaO_2 \text{ (per 100 mL blood)} = 19.8 + 0.3 \sim 20 \text{ mL dL}^{-1}$$

This calculation clearly illustrates how little of the O_2 present in an arterial blood sample is reflected in the PO_2 measurement.

The systemic O_2 delivery (DO_2I) can be calculated by multiplying the arterial O_2 content by the cardiac index as follows:

$$DO_2I = Hb \text{ (gdL}^{-1}) \times 1.34 \times SaO_2 \times 10 \times CI$$

where CI represents cardiac index, the content is multiplied by 10 to convert it to 'per litre' and the dissolved O_2 content is ignored because it is largely insignificant.

MIXED VENOUS OXYGENATION

The principles of oximetry can also be applied to the venous circulation, to facilitate the assessment of systemic O_2 consumption. There are two approaches to this and both require the presence of a pulmonary artery catheter. Aspiration of blood from the distal lumen of a pulmonary artery catheter provides a true 'mixed venous' sample, the saturation of which can then be measured in the normal fashion with a bench-top oximeter.

The mixed venous O_2 content can then be calculated:

$$CvO_2 \text{ (per 100 mL blood)} = [Hb \text{ (g dL}^{-1})] \times 1.34 \times SvO_2 + [0.0031 \times PvO_2 \text{ (mmHg)}]$$

From this, systemic O_2 consumption (VO_2I) can be calculated:

$$VO_2I = Hb \text{ (gdL}^{-1}) \times 1.34 \times (SaO_2 - SvO^2) \times 10 \times CI$$

where CI represents cardiac index, and the dissolved O_2 content is ignored.

With the development of fibreoptic pulmonary artery catheters, continuous measurement of SvO_2 *in vivo* using the principles of reflectance photometry has become possible. Light at two or three wavelengths (usually including 660 nm and 805 nm) is shone through the pulmonary artery catheter fibreoptic bundle and the reflectance signal analysed. Proprietary empirical formulae are used that allow blood to be regarded as a particulate suspension. Correction for the haematocrit is required, and this may be done manually or by analysis within the device of the reflectance data.

SvO_2 changes as the relationship between O_2 delivery and O_2 consumption changes. If O_2 delivery falls but O_2 consumption remains constant, it follows that O_2 extraction must increase. This will be manifest by a fall in SvO_2.

$$O_2 \text{ extraction ratio (OER)} = \frac{VO_2I}{DO_2I} \approx \frac{SaO_2 - SvO_2}{SaO_2}$$

Changes in SvO_2 occur almost immediately in response to changes in O_2 delivery, i.e. changes in cardiac output, Hb concentration or SaO_2, and in response to changes in O_2 consumption. Continuous monitoring of this variable therefore provides a rapid and sensitive monitor of the condition of a critically ill patient, although interpretation of the precise cause for the change can be more difficult.

Continuous monitoring of SaO_2 and SvO_2 can also be used to calculate shunt fraction as follows:

$$\frac{Qs}{Qt} = \frac{1 - SaO_2}{1 - SvO_2}$$

This provides a convenient approximation for the standard equation that can be readily performed at the bedside.

CAPNOGRAPHY

Various techniques have been used to provide similar information for CO_2. These have taken two major forms; expired gas CO_2 analysis (capnometry and capnography) and transcutaneous CO_2 analysis.

Principles of expired carbon dioxide analysis

CO_2 is produced as the product of aerobic metabolism and diffuses passively into the circulation. About 5–10% is dissolved in plasma and a similar amount binds to terminal amine groups on haemoglobin and other proteins within the blood, with the remainder being buffered to HCO_3^-. CO_2 is eliminated through the lungs by alveolar ventilation (V_A), but there is also a proportion of dead-space ventilation (V_D) that does not contribute to CO_2 clearance, with the sum of these being the total expired minute ventilation (V_E). The alveolar $PaCO_2$ varies according to the ventilation–perfusion (V/Q) relationships within the lung. In areas without perfusion (true dead space), $V/Q = \infty$ and the $PaCO_2$ equals the inspired PCO_2 and is zero. At the other extreme, where ventilation falls and so V/Q also falls, the $PaCO_2$ becomes very close to the venous $PvCO_2$ (45 mmHg under normal circumstances).

The alveolar dead-space fraction can be calculated from a modification of the Bohr equation and provides an indication of the V/Q relationship:

$$\frac{VD}{VT(alv)} = \frac{PaCO_2 - PACO_2}{PaCO_2}$$

where VD/VT is the dead-space fraction, $PaCO_2$ is the arterial PCO_2 and $PACO_2$ is the alveolar PCO_2, which can be represented by the end-tidal CO_2 measured with a capnograph.

Techniques for measuring expired carbon dioxide

Measurement of CO_2 in expired gases is now routinely used in many situations in critically ill patients and has become an obligatory safety requirement during general anaesthesia, especially in the intubated patient. In addition to providing a numeric display of the CO_2 concentration (capnometry), virtually all modern devices provide a graphical display of the CO_2 waveform (capnography), which provides important extra information. There are several techniques available for making the CO_2 measurement: mass spectrometry, Raman spectroscopy, colorimetry and infrared spectroscopy – which is by far the most widely used. The infrared absorption peak for CO_2 is at 4.26 μm, but this is close to that of N_2O, and between those of H_2O, leading to potential interference. The presence of other gases (helium, O_2, nitrogen and nitrous oxide) may also cause broadening of the CO_2 absorption spectrum. Nevertheless, these problems have been overcome in modern devices through the use of specific filters, reference cells and known correction factors. To be reliable in clinical use, capnographs require regular calibration using appropriate calibration gas mixtures.

Mainstream and sidestream capnographs

In mainstream capnographs, a measuring cell is positioned directly in the breathing circuit, usually mounted on a specially designed catheter mount in close proximity to the endotracheal tube. The cell is usually heated to around 40°C to prevent condensation on the cell window interfering with the measurement. The cell, which may be quite heavy and cumbersome, must be supported in such a manner that the patient's skin is protected and the endotracheal tube is not kinked or pulled out. In sidestream capnographs, gas is aspirated from the breathing system at a constant rate through a fine-bore sampling tube and passed through the measuring chamber. Such systems are often more convenient to use, but there is a slower response time compared with mainstream systems due to the delay while the aspirated gas sample reaches the cell. The sampling rate also has to be appropriate to the overall ventilatory pattern, and is usually of the order of 50–500 mL min^{-1}, which may have a significant impact upon the volume measurements recorded by the ventilator. If the sampling rate is higher than the expiratory gas flow, contamination of the sample with fresh gas may occur. Some systems return the sampled gas to the breathing system, but most vent it to air, which may have implications for scavenging. Another problem with these systems is that of condensation from the warm expired gases being sampled, particularly if artificial humidification is being used. There is nearly always a water trap in the system to prevent the sensing chamber becoming wet, but the sampling tube may still become blocked with water or secretions. The multiple connectors required with these systems also provide potential sites for leaks from the breathing circuit.

Clinical use of capnography

Although the end-tidal PCO_2 ($P_{ET}CO_2$) is clearly very closely related to the $PaCO_2$, it is not possible to predict one from the other, especially if there is a degree of lung disease. For that reason, the $P_{ET}CO_2$ is best considered as a monitored variable in its own right, rather than as a surrogate for $PaCO_2$.

The most common and probably most important application is to detect oesophageal intubation or endotracheal tube displacement.[3] Sometimes, there may be some CO_2 present in the stomach, initially providing potentially misleading information about tube position. Because any CO_2 is not replenished, the presence or otherwise of a normal capnograph waveform still allows rapid confirmation of correct tube placement (Fig. 8.3). The consequences of undetected tube misplacement are catastrophic and it is now generally considered mandatory to use capnography during anaesthesia in intubated patients for safety reasons. Capnographs are not routinely employed in all ICU patients, although they should certainly be available for acute situations and have been built into some ICU ventilators. Capnograph use is also increasingly regarded as mandatory for safety reasons during the transport of critically ill patients.

TRANSCUTANEOUS CARBON DIOXIDE TENSION MEASUREMENT

Transcutaneous CO_2 measurement provides an alternative to capnography for the non-invasive monitoring of CO_2.[4] Unfortunately, the technology is relatively cumbersome and expensive, and transcutaneous PCO_2 may not be a very good reflection of $PaCO_2$ in critically ill patients. Although there are a number of technical approaches to measuring transcutaneous PCO_2, most commercially available systems use a solid-state CO_2 electrode, often combined with an O_2 electrode. The major advantage of the approach is that it can be applied to patients who have not been intubated and do not have an arterial catheter in place.

Transcutaneous PCO_2 measurement detects the CO_2 that escapes through the skin surface. This comes mainly from capillary blood in the *dermis* and cells in the *epidermis*. Due to the countercurrent arrangement of the capillaries, the PCO_2 is highest here rather than in the arterioles or venules. This CO_2, together with the epidermal production, means that the skin PCO_2 is higher than the $PaCO_2$. If skin perfusion falls, the removal of CO_2 away from the skin is impaired, and the skin PCO_2 becomes progressively higher compared with the $PaCO_2$. This can be overcome by heating the skin area where the PCO_2 electrode is attached, but this has effects on local skin metabolism, on

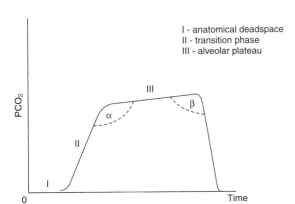

I - anatomical deadspace
II - transition phase
III - alveolar plateau

Figure 8.3 *A typical capnograph waveform. The slope of phase III is increased (as is the α angle) in patients with reduced V/Q matching, e.g. chronic obstructive pulmonary disease. The β angle increases as rebreathing increases.*

the solubility of CO_2 and on the dissociation of CO_2 from haemoglobin. For these reasons, the transcutaneous PCO_2 will still be higher than the $PaCO_2$ but, because the effects of temperature are largely predictable, appropriate correction factors can be employed during the calibration process. Burning of the skin at the electrode site occasionally occurs.

These practical limitations mean that transcutaneous CO_2 monitoring is rarely used in adult ICU practice. It is still occasionally seen in some paediatric ICUs, but it has largely been supplanted by capnography and intermittent or continuous blood-gas analysis. One area where it is still useful is that of sleep studies for obstructive sleep apnoea.

VENTILATORY MONITORING DURING MECHANICAL VENTILATION

Monitoring respiratory system mechanics and patient–ventilator interaction is a crucial aspect of respiratory critical care. At one time, gaining information of this kind was complex and relied upon apparatus and techniques usually only available in the respiratory physiology laboratory. Today, with modern computerised ventilators, an increasing amount of information is available at the bedside, and can both guide adjustment of ventilator settings and allow assessment of patient progress.

Basic principles

In order to ventilate the lungs, it is necessary to overcome the elastic forces generated by both the lungs and the chest wall. Although estimating pleural pressure through the use of an oesophageal balloon can separate these, this is not often done in routine clinical practice. Therefore, it is usually the mechanics of the total respiratory system that is being considered. There are also resistive forces that arise as a consequence of the flow of gas through the tubes of the ventilatory circuit and the airways.

Elastance (E) is described by the equation:

$$E = \frac{\Delta P}{\Delta V}$$

where P is pressure and V is volume. More commonly, the term compliance (C) is used, which is the reciprocal of elastance:

$$C = \frac{\Delta V}{\Delta P}$$

These measurements may be either static or dynamic, depending on whether they are made at zero gas flow. Static compliance uses the plateau pressure or end-inspiratory pressure as the upper pressure for the calculation of change in pressure. Dynamic compliance uses the peak inflation pressure, which includes that component of the airway pressure generated as a result of airways resistance.

If the lung and the chest wall are considered separately, they can be regarded as being in series, so that:

$$\frac{1}{C_{RS}} = \frac{1}{C_L} + \frac{1}{C_{CW}}$$

where C_{RS} is the compliance of the total respiratory system, C_L is lung compliance and C_{CW} is chest-wall compliance. Separation of the lung and chest-wall components requires knowledge of the pleural pressure, usually represented clinically by the oesophageal pressure measured with an oesophageal balloon or catheter.

Resistance can be described as:

$$R = \frac{\Delta P}{\Delta \dot{V}}$$

i.e. the change in pressure for the rate of change of volume.

The product of compliance and resistance is the time constant of the system. In diseased lungs, there will be a number of different time constants related to the degree of heterogeneity of the injury. This is particularly so in the case of severe acute lung injury (acute respiratory distress syndrome, ARDS).

Commonly measured pressures

Nearly all ICU ventilators provide information about a number of different 'airway' pressures, although, in reality, these are usually measured at the ventilator end of the patient–ventilator circuit. These pressures are listed below and each has a specific importance.

PEAK AIRWAY OR INFLFATION PRESSURE

This is the highest airway pressure recorded during the respiratory cycle and comprises a component required to overcome the elastance of the lung and a component to overcome airways resistance. Therefore, peak inflation pressure (PIP) is not the pressure to which the alveolus is exposed directly and is not the best pressure against which to judge the likelihood of barotrauma.

PLATEAU PRESSURE

This is the pressure that is recorded once inspiratory flow has ceased and there is a pause with zero gas flow. It is the pressure used to calculate static compliance. Although it is commonly provided on many ventilators, a true plateau pressure will not be reached unless the duration of the inspiratory pause is sufficient for full equilibration to take place.

END-INSPIRATORY PRESSURE

This pressure is measured using either a manual or programmed end-inspiratory pause of sufficient duration to ensure that a true plateau has been reached. This may be between 2 and 5 s. End-inspiratory pressure is therefore the 'real' plateau pressure and represents the alveolar pressure at the end of inflation. It is a better marker of the likelihood of barotrauma than PAP.

In controlled ventilation, the difference between PIP and plateau pressure, divided by the preceding flow rate, is used as one approach to calculating resistance.

MEAN AIRWAY PRESSURE

This is the inflation pressure averaged over the whole respiratory cycle and appears to relate most closely to both the haemodynamic disturbance associated with mechanical ventilation and changes in oxygenation, particularly when inverse ratio ventilation (IRV) is used. This is often explained on the basis that mean airway pressure (MAP) represents mean alveolar pressure and therefore represents 'how much lung is

open for how long'. Because it is usually measured by a pressure transducer in the ventilator, and also includes the PIP, MAP clearly includes a resistive component. Nevertheless, in clinical practice the concept seems to be useful. One of the fundamental principles of mechanical ventilation in patients with acute lung injury is to improve oxygenation by optimizing lung recruitment, thereby achieving better matching of ventilation and perfusion. MAP is therefore a useful measurement when altering ventilator settings to improve oxygenation.

END-EXPIRATORY PRESSURE AND POSITIVE END-EXPIRATORY PRESSURE

Positive end-expiratory pressure (PEEP) is routinely employed in mechanically ventilated patients in order to improve oxygenation. It improves lung recruitment, prevents lung collapse and may thereby improve ventilation–perfusion matching. Changes in PEEP also alter MAP. PEEP is set on the ventilator and is usually measured in the ventilator circuit. During the expiratory phase, gas is released from the circuit until the pressure has fallen to the set level of PEEP; this is usually the pressure displayed on the ventilator. If there is a delay in lung emptying, the pressure may fall more rapidly in the ventilator circuit than in the lung itself, so that the intra-alveolar pressure is higher than the displayed pressure. This happens when the absolute duration of the expiratory phase is too short to permit full emptying of the lung, resulting in gas trapping. It typically occurs with global obstruction to expiratory flow, as in asthma, or with more localized delay in lung emptying, as may occur in acute lung injury. This is termed intrinsic PEEP (PEEPi) or autoPEEP and may contribute very significantly to the total PEEP. Indeed, ventilatory strategies that employ inverse ratios may have some of their effect on oxygenation via this mechanism. PEEPi is measured by instituting an end-expiratory hold of sufficient duration to allow gas equilibration to occur with the ventilator circuit closed. This is usually of the order of 2–5 s, but up to 20 s may sometimes be required.

PEEPi may also exist as a dynamic phenomenon in patients being ventilated with spontaneous modes when the patient attempts to trigger a new breath before lung emptying is complete. The quantification of dynamic PEEPi requires the use of an oesophageal balloon to provide an approximation of pleural pressure. Dynamic PEEPi is then measured as the negative pressure change in oesophageal pressure required in order to initiate inspiratory flow. If the amount of dynamic PEEPi is significant, it may make ventilator triggering and patient weaning much more difficult. The presence of such dynamic air trapping can also usually be detected from visual inspection of flow–time or flow–volume curves, where expiratory flow has not ceased before the next breath starts in a spontaneously breathing subject.

Pressure, flow and volume diagrams

Modern, computerized ventilators frequently display information about pressure, flow and volume graphically, providing extra information compared with pressure measurements alone. The curves most frequently displayed are either pressure–time and flow–time curves, or the pressure–volume and the flow–volume relationships.

PRESSURE–TIME AND FLOW–TIME DIAGRAMS

Although easier to obtain than pressure and flow–volume loops, these simple displays of pressure and flow over time provide much important information about the patient–ventilator interaction that is readily accessible from simple visual inspection. A number of common phenomena are illustrated in Figures 8.4 to 8.9. Figure 8.4 illustrates the airway and alveolar pressure changes during volume-controlled (constant flow) ventilation. Note the difference between PAP and plateau pressure, representing alveolar pressure that occurs as a consequence of airway resistance. Figure 8.5 shows the same phenomena during pressure-controlled ventilation (decelerating flow). Note that alveolar pressure takes time to reach the set level of inflation pressure and, if an end-inspiratory hold manoeuvre demonstrates that this has not occurred, this suggests that the absolute duration of the inspiratory phase is insufficient. Figures 8.6 and 8.7 illustrate the presence of PEEPi during volume and pressure-controlled ventilation. Note particularly the failure of expiratory flow to reach zero before the next breath commences. This phenomenon is still seen in spontaneous ventilation modes where dynamic PEEPi is present (so-called dynamic hyperinflation). Figures 8.8 and 8.9 demonstrate how the pressure–time diagram can be used as a surrogate for a pressure–volume curve during volume-controlled ventilation. Because flow is constant, so is the rate of change in volume, and time can therefore be regarded as a surrogate for volume. Thus, the graph becomes

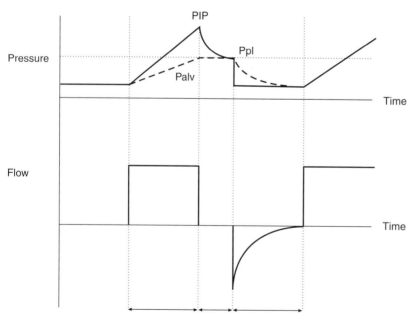

Figure 8.4 *Pressure and flow waveforms during volume-controlled ventilation. PIP, peak inflation pressure; Ppl, pleural pressure; Palv, alveolar pressure.*

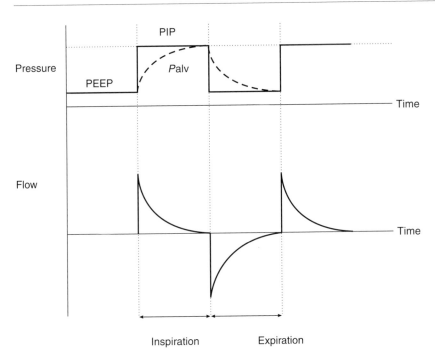

Figure 8.5 *Pressure and flow waveforms during pressure-controlled ventilation. PIP, peak inflation pressure; PEEP, positive end-expiratory pressure; Palv, alveolar pressure.*

an inverted version of a pressure–volume trace, demonstrating the same changes in shape associated with improving or worsening compliance. The slower the flow, the closer to a static curve this will become.

PRESSURE–VOLUME CURVES

The pressure–volume curve has become an important measurement for adjusting the ventilator settings in patients with severe lung injury. Although it

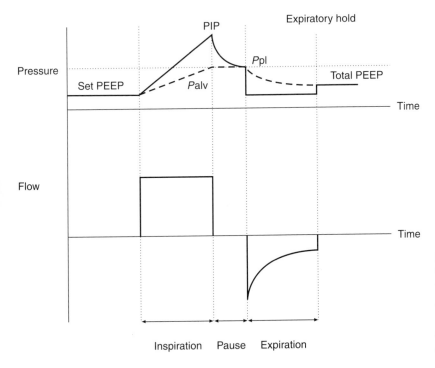

Figure 8.6 *Pressure and flow waveforms during volume-controlled ventilation with static intrinsic PEEP. Set PEEP, level of PEEP set on the ventilator ('external' PEEP); PIP, peak inflation pressure; Ppl pleural pressure; Palv, alveolar pressure.*

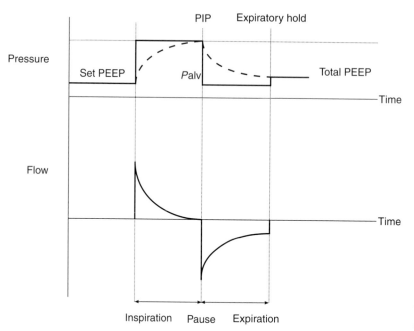

Figure 8.7 *Pressure and flow waveforms during pressure-controlled ventilation with static intrinsic PEEP. For abbreviations, see Fig. 8.6.*

is still predominantly a research tool, the lessons learnt from its use have become part of standard clinical strategies, and modern ventilators allow approximation of the curve at the bedside. The realization that ventilator-induced lung injury is an important component of the syndrome of acute lung injury and that strategies designed to mini-

mize this can result in a reduction in mortality in patients with ARDS has led to more attention being devoted to ensuring that the lung is ventilated at optimum volume. If lung recruitment is inadequate or not maintained, there is cyclical opening and collapse of alveoli, resulting in progressive lung damage, inflammation and cytokine release, which

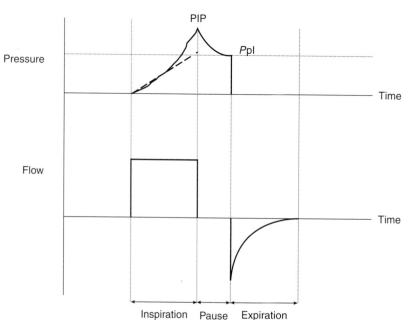

Figure 8.8 *Pressure and flow waveforms during volume-controlled ventilation demonstrating worsening compliance (e.g. over-distension). PIP, peak inflation pressure; Ppl, pleural pressure.*

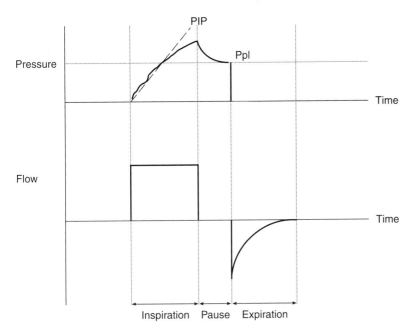

Figure 8.9 *Pressure and flow waveforms during volume-controlled ventilation demonstrating improving compliance (e.g. recruitment). PIP, peak inflation pressure; Ppl, pleural pressure.*

produces secondary systemic damage. If the lung is over-distended, there will be progressive 'volu-trauma' and 'barotrauma'. Modern strategies are there-fore designed to ensure that the lung is recruited and kept open, but that tidal ventilation does not lead to over-distension. The static pressure–volume curve provides a tool with which to do this (Fig. 8.10). Typically, the curve is sigmoid in shape in mechanically ventilated patients with lung injury. The lower portion represents the area of collapse, where static compliance is poor. The linear centre portion represents that lung volume at which lung segments are open and compliance is good. The

flattened upper portion represents the zone of over-distension, where compliance once again deterio-rates. Lower and upper inflection points separate these different portions of the curve. Broadly speaking, modern ventilator strategy is based upon determining where the lower inflection point is and setting the PEEP level slightly above this to ensure that tidal ventilation occurs within the region of maximum compliance. Similarly, the tidal volume is set to ensure that the area of over-distension is avoided. Typically, this means a tidal volume of the order of 6 mL kg^{-1}.

Unfortunately, measurement of the pressure–volume curve is not always straightforward. There are a number of approaches, of which the best known is probably the 'super-syringe' technique.[5] Originally described using a 2-L syringe, with the inflation volume being measured by an electrical signal proportional to the administered volume, this approach utilizes stepwise inflation of the lung. Volumes of between 50 mL and 200 mL are used and static pressure measurements are taken at each step. The procedure should start from the relaxation volume of the lung (functional residual capacity, FRC), especially if the lower inflection point is to be established accurately. This requires the removal of PEEP and disconnection from the ventilator, and the procedure may take several minutes, all of which may result in considerable

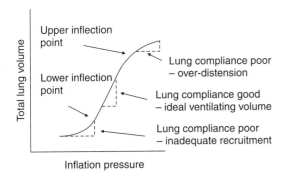

Figure 8.10 *Pressure–volume curve of the lung demonstrating potential for lung damage with inadequate recruitment or over-distension.*

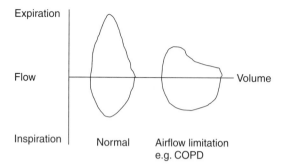

Figure 8.11 *Flow–volume loops demonstrating a normal pattern (left) and the typical pattern seen with airflow limitation and dynamic hyperinflation (right). COPD, chronic obstructive pulmonary disease. The display seen on mechanical ventilators shows inspiration as the upward deflection and the shape of this part of the flow–volume loop will be influenced by the ventilatory mode employed.*

instability and desaturation in patients with severe lung injuries. This has resulted in other approaches also being used. These include using different known-volume ventilator breaths and recording the static end-inspiratory pressure after each, allowing a curve to be constructed from the results of a number of breaths together. Another approach is to use the ventilator to inflate the lung with a known volume at a constant but very low flow. This minimizes the resistive (dynamic) component of the inspiratory phase and provides a good approximation of a static inspiratory curve. The expiratory curve obtained after such a manoeuvre does not reflect static conditions, although a variety of occlusion techniques applied during expiration have been developed to provide a complete loop. This then provides information about the degree of hysteresis (if any) that is present.

FLOW–VOLUME CURVES

In mechanically ventilated patients, the ventilator generates inspiratory flow and expiratory flow is largely passive. Consequently, it is virtually impossible to obtain reproducible forced expiratory flow measurements, but useful information can still be obtained from the shape of the flow–volume curve, especially about the presence of airflow limitation (Fig. 8.11). For patients with significant expiratory flow limitation, the expiratory phase of the curve has a characteristic concave shape. When there are secretions in the airways (or water in the ventilator tubing), the curve has a typical spiky nature to it, as opposed to flow being smooth.

HAEMODYNAMICS AND THE MEASUREMENT OF LUNG WATER

Optimum haemodynamic management is a crucial component of the treatment of critically ill patients with respiratory impairment, especially those who require mechanical ventilation. Although it is beyond the scope of this chapter to provide a detailed appraisal of haemodynamic monitoring techniques, some aspects deserve comment. A major challenge in all critically ill patients is to achieve the correct balance between giving enough fluid resuscitation to allow adequate cardiac performance and avoiding fluid overload. This applies especially to patients with acute lung injury, because this condition is characterized by the development of non-cardiogenic pulmonary oedema.

Use of cardiac filling pressures

Traditionally, central venous pressure (CVP) and pulmonary artery occlusion pressure (PAOP) have been used to assist clinicians with the assessment of vascular filling. Unfortunately, there is often a significant degree of confusion about the true value of these measurements. The first is whether they are being employed to assess overall volume status (as surrogates for total blood volume) or to assess cardiac filling. More usually, it is the latter that is required, but both CVP and PAOP are prone to considerable measurement error (zeroing and levelling the transducer, correct waveform analysis etc.), as well as being significantly altered by mechanical ventilation and the

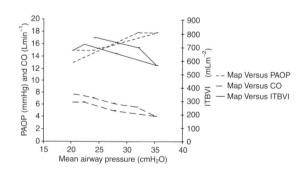

Figure 8.12 *During a high-pressure recruitment manoeuvre, cardiac output and intrathoracic blood volume (ITBV) fall, while pulmonary artery occlusion pressure (PAOP) rises, reflecting the rise in intrathoracic pressure. MAP, mean airway pressure.*

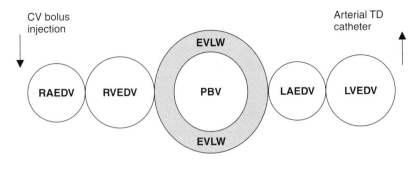

CV bolus
injection

Arterial TD
catheter

ITBV = RAEDV + RVEDV + PBV + LAEDV + LVEDV
EVLW = ITTV − ITBV

Figure 8.13 *Principles of extravascular lung water (EVLW) measurement by indicator dilution. CV = central venous, TD = thermodilution, RAEDV = right atrial end-diastolic volume, RVEDV = right ventricular end-diastolic volume, PBV = pulmonary blood volume, LAEDV = left atrial end-diastolic volume, LVEDV = left ventricular end-diastolic volume, ITBV = intrathoracic blood volume, ITTV = intrathoracic thermal volume*

presence of significant cardiac or pulmonary disease. In a study of patients with ARDS, Lichtwarck-Aschoff and colleagues[6] demonstrated the lack of agreement between changes in conventional filling pressures and changes in cardiac index, demonstrating the unreliability of this approach. Figure 8.12 shows the effect of a high-pressure recruitment manoeuvre on PAOP, cardiac output and intrathoracic blood volume (see below), demonstrating how misleading filling pressures can be.

Nevertheless, as measurements in their own right, CVP and pulmonary artery pressures can provide very valuable information about the performance of the right heart under the extra stresses imposed by severe lung injury (where acute pulmonary hypertension is common), and mechanical ventilation results in high intrathoracic pressures.

Measurement of lung water

Because severe acute lung injury is characterized by increased oedema formation, some authorities have proposed that measurement of lung water should be incorporated into the definitions of acute lung injury and ARDS in order to improve their robustness. In addition, quantification of the abnormal increase in lung water (i.e. the degree of oedema) would have considerable potential advantages for clinicians when judging the balance of good versus harm during the volume resuscitation of critically ill patients. Unfortunately, chest radiography, which is still the most common approach to judging the degree of pulmonary oedema, is neither specific nor quantitative. Developments in indicator dilution techniques have now made it possible to measure lung water at

the bedside, and this has been demonstrated to be of considerable potential value in the monitoring of patients with acute lung injury.

Initially, the technique relied upon double indicator dilution, using chilled indocyanine green solution, which provided an intravascular dye indicator and a thermal indicator that also distributed into the extravascular space. The indicator was injected into the right atrium via a central venous line and was detected via a femoral artery catheter. Cardiac output was calculated in the standard fashion from the thermodilution wash-out curve, and then used in combination with the transit times of the two indicators to calculate their relative distribution volumes. The distribution volume of the intravascular dye represents the blood volume between the injection and detection points (known as the intrathoracic blood volume, ITBV). The distribution of the thermal indicator (known as the intrathoracic thermal volume, ITTV) contains the intrathoracic blood volume, but also includes other structures. Although there is negligible distribution into vessel walls and cardiac muscle, the only major extravascular distribution volume is in the lungs, because this is the only major capillary bed between the injection and detection points. The difference between the ITTV and the ITBV is the extravascular thermal volume, which is a good approximation to lung water and is therefore known as the extravascular lung water (EVLW; Fig. 8.13). A further derivation of this technique has made it possible to obtain bedside measurements of lung water from thermodilution alone.[7] Although not quite as reliable as when the double indicator approach is used, the thermodilution method is sufficiently reliable in most clinical situations and is considerably more convenient and less expensive.

A further benefit of this monitoring approach has been the recognition that ITBV, being a central blood volume closely related to cardiac filling and therefore pre-load, allows a volumetric approach to fluid resuscitation that is more robust than that using filling pressures. Together, knowledge of cardiac output, ITBV and EVLW greatly facilitates the management of haemodynamic instability in the context of severe acute lung injury, although only one study currently exists that demonstrates that management based on the lung water approach translates into a beneficial outcome for patients.[8]

CONCLUSION

This chapter provides only a brief overview of the principles behind a number of the standard monitoring techniques applied during respiratory critical care. Nevertheless, as monitoring devices become more advanced and more ubiquitous, it is crucial to have some understanding of how they work in order to take full advantage of the benefits they can provide, as well as to avoid errors of misinterpretation. All monitoring devices and techniques have limitations that can mislead the unwary user. Another important consideration is that there are often several different ways of obtaining the same information and some devices are more robust and have lower running costs than others. Considerable training is required if modern monitoring devices are to be used to their full potential. Decisions about which devices to purchase must therefore be broadly based and should balance absolute capability and the ability to harness that capability within the complex infrastructure that

is a modern ICU. Respiratory critical care is dependent to a large degree on technological support of the critically ill patient, and keeping abreast of that technology is a major challenge for the clinician.

REFERENCES

1 Clark, LC. Monitoring and control of blood and tissue oxygen. *Trans Am Soc Artif Inten Organs* 1956; **2**: 41–8.
2. Rithalia, SV, Bennett, PJ, Tinker, J. The performance characteristics of an intra-arterial oxygen electrode. *Intensive Care Med* 1981; **7**: 305–7.
3. Sayah, AJ, Peacock, WF, Overton, DT. End-tidal CO_2 measurement in the detection of esophageal intubation during cardiac arrest. *Ann Emerg Med* 1990; **19**: 857–60.
4. Rithalia, SVS. Developments in transcutaneous blood gas monitoring: a review. *J Med Technol* 1991; **15**: 143–53.
5. Matamis, D, Lemaire, F, Harf, A, *et al*. Total respiratory pressure–volume curves in the adult respiratory distress syndrome. *Chest* 1984; **86**: 58–66.
6. Lightwarck-Aschoff, M, Zeravik, J, Pfeiffer, UJ. Intrathoracic blood volume accurately reflects circulatory volume status in critically ill patients with mechanical ventilation. *Intensive Care Med* 1992; **18**: 142–7.
7. Pfeiffer, UJ, Lichtwarck-Aschoff, M, Beale, RJ. Single thermodilution monitoring of global end-diastolic volume, intrathoracic blood volume and extravascular lung water. *Clin Intensive Care* 1994; **3** (Suppl.): 38–9.
8. Mitchell, JP, Schuller, D, Calandrino, FS, Schuster, DP. Improved outcome based on fluid management in critically ill patients requiring pulmonary artery catheterization. *Am Rev Respir Dis* 1992; **145**: 990–8.

9

Respiratory emergencies I: medical

RICHARD M LEACH

INTRODUCTION

Respiratory emergencies are a common cause of cardiorespiratory collapse in the intensive care unit (ICU) patient. The management of haemodynamic instability associated with sudden hypoxaemia is often a greater challenge than that associated with primary circulatory disturbances. Prompt identification of the cause and appropriate therapy are essential. This chapter discusses those respiratory emergencies not discussed elsewhere in this book, specifically massive haemoptysis, aspiration syndromes, acute large airways obstructions and infective emergencies.

MASSIVE HAEMOPTYSIS

Massive haemoptysis is a dramatic, life-threatening clinical emergency. Delayed or inappropriate treatment is common and, as a consequence, patients with potentially treatable conditions die.[1,2] It is usually defined as the expectoration of 500–1000 mL of blood in 24 hours or any life-threatening haemoptysis in a patient with co-existing respiratory compromise.[3,4] Massive haemoptysis accounts for less than 20% of all episodes of haemoptysis. In a recent review from a tertiary referral centre, 38% of cases were classified as trivial (flecks of blood in sputum),

48% as moderate (<500 mL or 1–2 cups daily) and only 14% as massive (>500 mL or more than 2 cups of blood daily).[5] Most cases of haemoptysis are due to infective causes (approximately 80%), including tuberculosis, pneumonia, lung abscess and bronchiectasis, and only a minority are due to malignancy (approximately 20%).[1–6] The bronchial circulation is usually the source of bleeding. Death results from asphyxia, caused by flooding of the alveoli, and only rarely from circulatory collapse.[6] Mortality is directly related to the rate and volume of blood loss and the underlying pathology. In patients expectorating >600 mL of blood within a 4-hour period, the mortality is reported to be 71%, compared to 45% in patients expectorating the same quantity over 4–16 hours and 5% during 16–48 hours.[7]

Clinical evaluation

A good history is essential and may provide valuable information regarding the cause of haemoptysis. The characteristic clinical picture of diseases such as tuberculosis, bronchiectasis and bronchogenic carcinoma may direct subsequent investigation and management. However, few patients are able to localize the site of bleeding in the thorax. Chest examination may reveal localized crepitations or consolidation, but widespread soiling of the tracheobronchial tree, due to coughing, often results in diffuse clinical signs. The examination of expectorated blood may provide clues. Food particles suggest the possibility of haematemesis, but blood in the nasogastric aspirate does not differentiate between haematemesis and haemoptysis as coughed-up blood is often swallowed. Purulent material in the sputum may indicate bronchiectasis or a lung abscess (Fig. 9.1) and microbiology may isolate tubercle bacilli. Associated haematuria raises the possibility of an alveolar haemorrhage syndrome.

Chest radiography (CXR) should be obtained in all patients (Fig. 9.2). It may provide important diagnostic information, including evidence of a mass, cavity or abscess. However, the CXR may be unhelpful[6] and potentially misleading as lesions seen on CXR do not always correlate with the site of bleeding. Soiling (with diffuse alveolar shadowing) due to the widespread distribution of the tracheobronchial blood during coughing and aspiration may further obscure the site and cause of bleeding.

Management of massive haemoptysis

Successful management requires a team approach, involving the intensivist, chest physician, radiologist, anaesthetist and surgeon. Management decisions are often difficult and there is little evidence to direct appropriate therapy, even in specific diseases such as bronchiectasis. The key aspects of management are as follows.

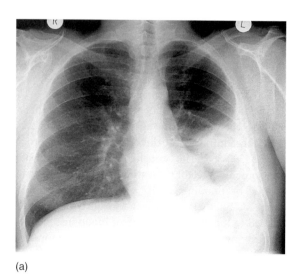

(a)

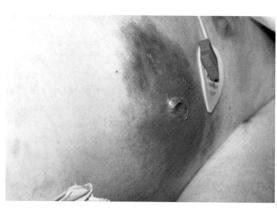

(b)

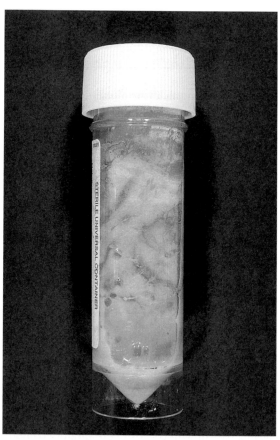

(c)

Figure 9.1 *A 41-year-old man with lung abscess presenting with haemoptysis. (a) Lung abscess on chest radiography. (b) Subsequent development of empyema necessitans over left chest wall (see also Plate 1). (c) Subsequent discharge of pus from abscess (see also Plate 2).*

(a)

(b)

(c)

(d)

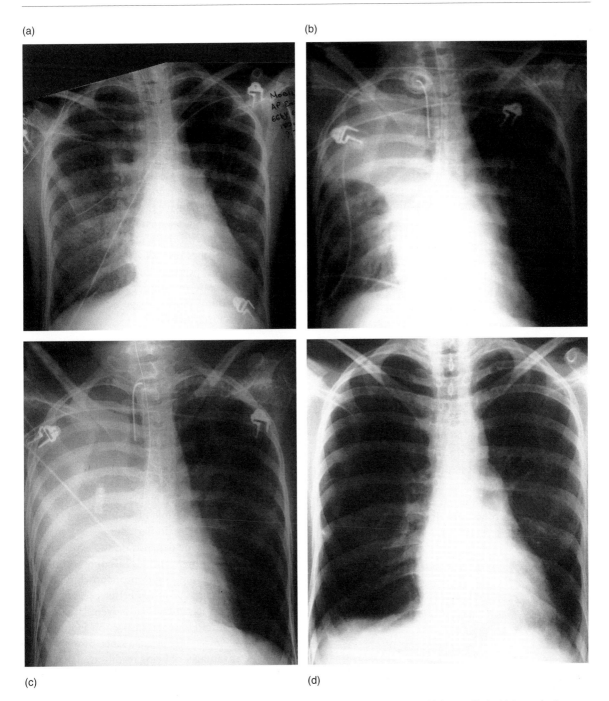

Figure 9.2 *Sequence of four chest radiographs following massive haemoptysis due to tracheobronchial aspergillosis. (a) Onset of minor bleeding in the right upper lobe with some minor 'soiling' of the right lower lobe. (b) Subsequent massive haemoptysis with collapse/consolidation of right upper lobe at 12 hours. (c) 'White out' right lung at 24 hours, with the patient lying right side down to prevent soiling of the 'good' (left) lung. (d) Resolution at 14 days.*

1. Maintain a patent airway and ensure adequate oxygenation by providing supplemental oxygen, if necessary by endotracheal intubation and mechanical ventilation: asphyxia is the greatest immediate risk to the patient.

2. Promote drainage and prevent further alveolar 'soiling', particularly of the unaffected lung, by positioning the patient slightly head down in the lateral decubitus position with the 'presumed' bleeding side down.

3. Determine the cause, site and severity of the bleeding: haematemesis and upper airways bleeding from the nose, pharynx or larynx may be confused with haemoptysis.
4. Excessive chest manipulation, including physiotherapy and spirometry, should be avoided as this may increase or restart bleeding. Cough suppression with codeine 30–60 mg every 6 hours may be helpful.
5. Institute appropriate therapeutic measures, including antibiotics and bronchodilators, depending on the underlying pathology and clinical circumstances.

Bronchoscopy is the most useful initial investigation for identifying the source of bleeding and also allows bronchial toilet to be performed (Fig. 9.3). It is, however, easy to be misled when there is widespread soiling of the bronchial tree, and over-zealous suctioning of blood clots may encourage further bleeding. CXR, computer tomography (CT) and arteriography also have important roles in establishing the diagnosis and assessing progress.

The unaffected lung may have to be ventilated independently until bleeding can be controlled. To achieve this, the endotracheal tube should be positioned in the right or left main bronchus. In the emergency situation, the endotracheal tube is advanced into the right main bronchus (which is in the same axis as the trachea) until breath sounds can no longer be heard in the left side of the chest. If the patient is not bleeding from the right side, the endo-

tracheal cuff can be inflated and the right lung selectively ventilated. If bleeding is originating from the right lung, a Foley or Fogarty catheter should be positioned in the right main bronchus and inflated. The endotracheal tube is then withdrawn until the left lung is ventilated. Urgent bronchoscopy should be arranged to establish the site and cause of bleeding and reposition the endobronchial tube as required. Double-lumen tubes (Carlens or Robertshaw) will also isolate the affected lung, but are difficult to maintain in position, require experienced personnel and have the serious limitation that the small lumens hinder suctioning and prevent flexible bronchoscopy. In the acute situation, the use of double-lumen tubes provides little additional benefit. The use of positive end-expiratory pressure (PEEP) to increase intrathoracic pressure and tamponade the site of haemorrhage during mechanical ventilation is rarely helpful.

Determining the site and cause of haemoptysis

Once the patient has been adequately stabilized, the site and cause of bleeding must be established.

- Early bronchoscopy is essential and is generally accepted to be superior to other diagnostic techniques, including bronchial arteriograms and CT.[6,8] Rigid and flexible fibreoptic bronchoscopy has been used with similar diagnostic yields and the choice of scope depends on the experience of the admitting physician.[2,9] If bleeding is considerable and ongoing, rigid bronchoscopy in the operating theatre provides better access for suctioning and the patient can be ventilated during the procedure. However, inspection is limited to the large, lower airways. Flexible bronchoscopy has the advantages of being readily available, it can be passed through an endotracheal tube (8.0 mm diameter or larger) and allows examination of subsegmental and upper lobe bronchi, which account for 80% of bleeding sites. The disadvantage is limited suctioning capability compared to rigid bronchoscopy. The flexible scope may be passed through the rigid bronchoscope to provide the benefit of both methods.
- If bronchoscopy is unsuccessful, spiral CT with contrast may detect the site of bleeding, tumours,

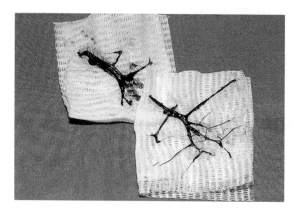

Figure 9.3 *Blood cast of the left bronchial tree removed at fibreoptic bronchoscopy in a 16-year-old girl with haemoptysis due to meningococcal meningitis and disseminated intravascular coagulation.*

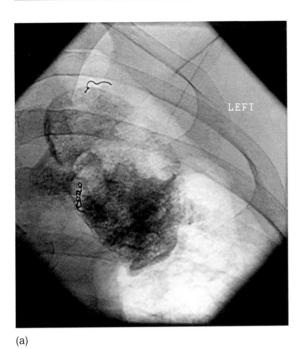

(a)

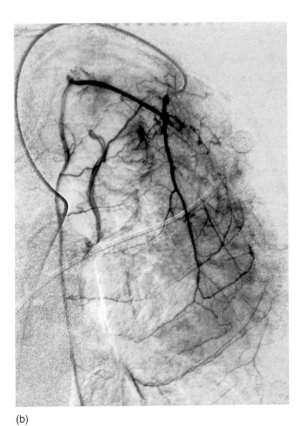

(b)

vascular malformations and other structural abnormalities. A combination of bronchoscopy and CT scanning has the highest diagnostic yeild.[1,2,6] Occasionally, radionucleotide scans may define the site of bleeding and the underlying pathology. Transfer to the radiology or nuclear medicine department requires that the patient is relatively stable, and this may limit their use.

• If bleeding continues, bronchial arteriography and occasionally pulmonary angiography are indicated (Fig. 9.4).

Control of haemoptysis

Establishing the best practice for the treatment of massive haemoptysis is limited by the paucity of comparative trials. In general, control of bleeding is usually required during on-going investigation and includes immediate temporizing measures or bronchial embolization. This is followed by definitive surgery, if feasible, when the patient's condition has been stabilized.

IMMEDIATE

Initial control of haemoptysis is achieved by directing boluses of iced saline with adrenaline (10 mL; 1:10 000 dilution) at the bleeding site through the bronchoscope.[10] This simple technique is successful in 95% of cases for the temporary control of bleeding.[4] The application of topical thrombin to the bleeding

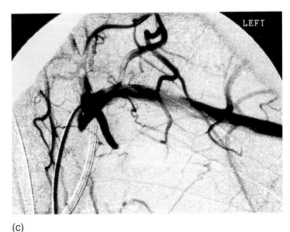

(c)

Figure 9.4 *A 40-year-old man with haemoptysis from an old tuberculous cavity. (a) Bleeding into the cavity on radiography. (b) Angiogram demonstrating multiple sites of bleeding within the cavity. (c) Angiogram after embolization and control of bleeding.*

lesion is also effective in > 70% of patients.[11] Alternatively, tamponade of the affected segmental or subsegmental bronchus with a Fogarty or Foley catheter is successful in > 80% of cases.[12] Occasionally, intravenous vasoconstrictors (vasopressin, terlipressin) may be useful to reduce heavy bleeding.

BRONCHIAL ANGIOGRAPHY AND EMBOLIZATION

Angiography has been proposed as the primary diagnostic procedure in place of bronchoscopy (Fig. 9.4). However, controlled comparisons of the two techniques demonstrated that bronchoscopy was superior, identifying 68% compared to 55% of bleeding sites. On this basis, bronchoscopy remains the primary diagnostic modality.[13] However, bronchial artery embolization is the established therapeutic technique for the control of haemoptysis.[14] It is initially successful in 70–100% of cases.[14,15] The best results are described in patients with dilated bronchial arteries (e.g. bronchiectasis). The frequency with which re-bleeding occurs is disputed. Some reports describe 80% recurrence within 10 days, others 22% recurrence over 1–48 months.[3,14] Recently published data described long-term control of haemoptysis (>3 months) in 45% of cases studied.[15] Embolization is associated with serious complications. Infarction of the anterior spinal artery with paraplegia has been reported in up to 5% of cases.[14] Other rare complications include ischaemic necrosis of the bronchus and arterial dissection. In general, embolization should be regarded as a temporary or palliative manoeuvre, when surgery is contraindicated or to stabilize a patient prior to definitive surgical therapy.

MEDICAL VERSUS SURGICAL TREATMENT

There is still dispute as to whether patients with massive haemoptysis should be treated conservatively (medically) or surgically. There are few comparative studies, most are retrospective and few take into account the aetiology of the bleeding. Most studies agree that surgical therapy is associated with the best long-term outcomes for isolated lesions.[9,16] In one such study, 5-year survival was 84% in surgically treated patients compared to 41% in medically treated patients.[16] Other studies report successful outcomes with surgery in 82–99% of patients.[4,9,16]

However, some respiratory physicians continue to advocate a conservative approach and suggest that surgical intervention is only justified if haemoptysis remains uncontrolled following arterial embolization or in patients with recurrent bleeding.[17] In two recent conservative studies, where surgery would have been feasible, the long-term success rates were 46% and 68%, respectively[4,7] Primary medical management may be mandatory because bleeding cannot be localized or is not amenable to the surgical resection of a pulmonary segment (Fig. 9.5). In other patients, surgery will be contraindicated because of end-stage lung disease (FEV_1 < 40% predicted), poor cardiac reserve, unresectable cancer or severe bleeding diathesis.

ASPIRATION SYNDROMES

To diagnose aspiration, a high index of suspicion is required in those at risk because it is often not witnessed.[18] Volume and type of fluid aspirated are critical and are usually related to the clinical scenario. In the peri-anaesthetic situation, the aspiration of large volumes of gastric contents rapidly progresses to aspiration pneumonia and acute respiratory distress syndrome (ARDS). In contrast, repeated microaspirations in the stroke patient with bulbar palsy cause nosocomial pneumonia. Examination of pharyngeal and tracheal aspirates may be helpful and arterial blood gases are essential to monitor the severity of aspiration syndromes.

High-risk groups for aspiration include those with:

- depressed levels of consciousness (head injury, drug overdose, epileptics and hypothermia),
- laryngeal incompetence (bulbar syndromes, cerebrovascular accident, myasthenia gravis, Guillain–Barré syndrome and multiple sclerosis),
- peri-operative, ICU and emergency room patients.

Risk factors for aspiration in ICU patients include:

- supine posture,
- nasogastric feeding,
- gastrointestinal haemorrhage,
- non-invasive ventilation: swallowed gas during continuous positive airways pressure (CPAP) or

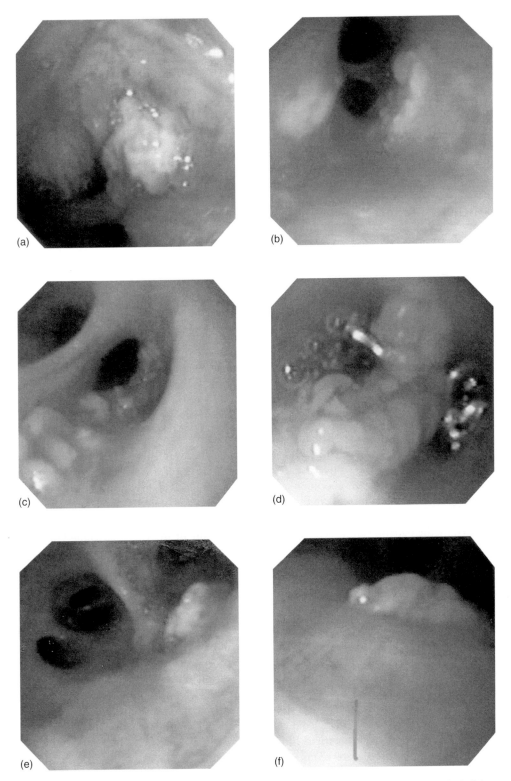

Figure 9.5 *Tracheobronchial aspergillosis affecting the right upper lobe (a, b), right lower lobe (c, d) and left lower lobe (e, f) in a 25-year-old, immunosuppressed patient with systemic lupus erythematosus and massive haemoptysis (see also Plate 3).*

non-invasive positive-pressure ventilation may cause vomiting and subsequent aspiration as airway clearance is impeded by the tight-fitting mask,

- mechanically ventilated patients with endotracheal or tracheostomy tubes,
- gastric lavage.

Tracheo-oesophageal fistulae may present with recurrent aspiration and most commonly are due to trauma or previously undiagnosed malignancy.

Solid particulate matter

A large variety of solid particulate matter may be aspirated, including confectionary, coins, teeth or rubber from balloons that burst while being inflated. However, the aspiration of partially masticated food during swallowing is the most common cause, giving rise to the 'café coronary'. Following the aspiration of a large particle that completely occludes the larynx or trachea, the subject is unable to speak or breathe and rapidly becomes cyanosed. If a sharp blow to the back of the chest fails to dislodge the particle, the Heimlich manoeuvre should be attempted. The attendant stands behind the patient with his or her arms around the upper abdomen, just adjacent to the costal margin, and the hands clenched below the xiphoid process. The hands are pulled sharply backwards, compressing the upper abdomen and lower costal margin. The sudden increase in thoracic pressure may dislodge the obstructing particle, which is exhaled by the patient. Continued obstruction rapidly leads to coma and death and, as a last resort, an emergency cricothyroidotomy should be attempted. This will only be successful if the obstruction is at the level of the larynx. If available, a large-bore needle should be inserted through the cricothyroid membrane, which is palpable just below the thyroid cartilage. Alternatively, a knife (or other sharp implement), with the blade in the horizontal axis, may be inserted at the same site and turned vertically to achieve an opening in the trachea. A pointed, hollow tube (straw, biro) may be equally effective in an emergency situation. Oxygen should be fed down the needle or tube, if available. Urgent rigid bronchoscopy and/or thoracic surgery are required to remove the obstruction.

Partial tracheal or bronchial obstruction by food or any other material causes symptoms common to all foreign-body aspiration, including stridor, cough, wheeze and tachypnoea. A history of recurrent pneumonia following an episode of aspiration is occasionally elicited and suggests that further exploration to recover an obstructing foreign body (e.g. a peanut) is necessary. Pneumonia, atelectasis and expiratory emphysema are common radiological findings in these circumstances. Small particles may be aspirated with gastric contents and initially only produce the characteristic inflammatory response of liquid aspiration. In the inadequately sedated ICU patient, endotracheal tubes may be 'bitten through' and the distal end of the tube aspirated.

Fluid aspiration

Gastric contents are the fluid most frequently aspirated.[18,19] Water (during drowning) and blood (during pharyngeal operations or haematemesis) may also be inhaled. Aspiration after accidental or deliberate self-poisonings with hydrocarbons, bleach and other toxic fluids usually occurs during vomiting or gastric lavage.

ASPIRATION OF GASTRIC CONTENTS

Aspiration of gastric contents or any other acidic fluid inhalation (pH < 2.5) is associated with severe lung damage.[18,19] The onset and severity of symptoms depend on the volume of gastric contents aspirated. Large-volume to moderate-volume aspiration (e.g. inadequate gastric emptying before intubation) can result in the rapid development of respiratory failure, with tachypnoea, wheeze, cyanosis, hypotension and hypoxaemia (Fig. 9.6). On occasions, frank pulmonary oedema or ARDS may develop. About two-thirds of aspirations are witnessed and the diagnosis is confirmed by the detection of gastric contents at tracheal suctioning and the demonstration of acidity by testing with litmus paper. In the remaining third, successful diagnosis depends on a high index of suspicion in high-risk patients. About 90% of patients who aspirate gastric contents will develop pulmonary infiltrates on CXR. However, radiographic changes are often delayed for 12–24 hours and initial films may be normal. The right main bronchus is the most direct path for aspirated material and the right lower lobe is the most commonly affected area when only one lobe is involved (in approximately 60% of cases). With large-volume

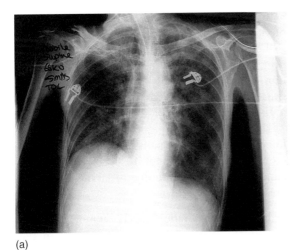

(a)

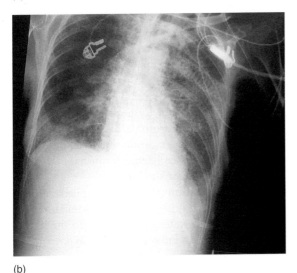

(b)

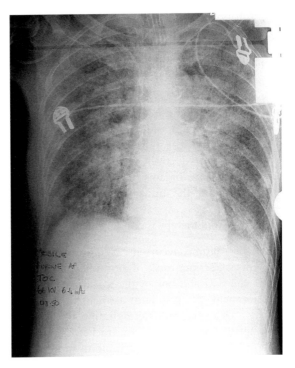

(c)

Figure 9.6 *Rapid development of aspiration pneumonia in a 79-year-old woman after a straightforward sigmoid volvulus repair. The patient vomited and aspirated gastric fluid immediately following extubation. The chest radiographs are at (a) 1 hour, (b) 3 hours and (c) 6 hours after the aspiration.*

aspiration, diffuse bilateral infiltrates may be observed. The development of ARDS secondary to aspiration pneumonia is associated with a high mortality (>80%).[19]

As treatment is ineffective, prevention is essential. When severe regurgitation occurs in the obtunded patient, immediate management involves the following.

1. Clearance of the upper airways of vomit, fluid and obstructing particles: suction should always be available when dealing with high-risk patients.
2. Positioning of the patient head down in the recovery position to reduce further lung 'soiling'.
3. The immediate administration of O_2.
4. Tracheal intubation may be necessary to secure the airway.

5. Neither tracheal suction nor bronchoscopy will prevent acid-induced lung injury, which is usually immediate, but will clear excess free fluid and remove particulate matter from the airways.[18,19]

Respiratory support will depend on the degree of lung damage.

- Aerosolized bronchodilators reduce aspiration-induced bronchospasm.
- CPAP may improve oxygenation and avoid the need for intubation in the alert, co-operative patient with even relatively severe diffuse acute lung injury. CPAP to 10 cmH$_2$O may be used, although above this pressure the lower oesophageal sphincter tone may be exceeded, with the risk of further vomiting and aspiration.

- Intubation and positive pressure ventilation will be required if the patient is obtunded or non-invasive support fails to maintain adequate oxygenation. Alveolar recruitment with high PEEP or prolonged inspiratory to expiratory ratios is often necessary.
- Antibiotic therapy is often instituted following gastric aspiration, although there is little evidence to support this practice. Traditionally, therapy should cover the Gram-positive and Gram-negative organisms colonizing the upper airways and the upper gastrointestinal tract anaerobes.
- Early steroid therapy is not beneficial.[20]

Smaller-volume, recurrent aspiration of gastric contents is a serious cause of morbidity and mortality in the ICU and one of the main factors in the development of ventilator-associated pneumonia.[21,22] This small-volume aspiration often occurs past inflated endotracheal or tracheostomy cuffs. The onset is slower and the symptoms more subtle, but the end result may be severe lung damage and a high mortality. Micro-aspiration in tube-fed patients may be detected by adding dye to the feed and observing for its appearance in tracheobronchial secretions or by using glucose oxidase reagent strips to test for glucose in tracheobronchial secretions, although, if negative, these tests do not necessarily exclude the diagnosis.

The management strategies used to reduce the incidence of small-volume aspiration in the ICU include:[21]

- nursing in the semi-recumbent position (30–45% head-up),[22]
- preventing gastric microbial overgrowth caused by stress ulcer prophylaxis, by early enteral feeding or sucrulfate, although further evidence-based data are required.
- Subglottic drainage did not reduce the incidence of Pseudomonas or Enterobacteriaceae respiratory tract colonization or infection in clinical studies.

NEAR-DROWNING AND WATER ASPIRATION

Aspiration of water and cases of near-drowning may present to any ICU. They are one of the commonest causes of accidental death in children and adults and are often associated with alcohol consumption. Although more frequent in areas with close proximity to natural water sources, deaths may occur in any home and in relatively small volumes of water (e.g. a shallow bath). Near-drowning is often secondary to a primary medical event, such as a myocardial infarction, occurring whilst the subject is in water. In this situation, the patient becomes suddenly motionless in the water, with little or no struggling.

The amount and type of water aspirated determine the severity and pathophysiology of the pulmonary lesion.[23,24] About 10% of near-drowning patients do not aspirate due to laryngospasm and breath holding.[24]

- Freshwater aspiration affects pulmonary surfactant and subsequent atelectasis results in pulmonary shunt, venous admixture and hypoxaemia.[24] Freshwater in alveoli is rapidly absorbed into the pulmonary circulation, and in large volumes may cause initial hypervolaemia. However, the patient may be hypovolaemic by the time he or she reaches hospital due to fluid redistribution and the development of pulmonary oedema. If sufficient freshwater is absorbed, the plasma becomes hypotonic, causing intravascular haemolysis. The resulting increase in plasma potassium and free haemoglobin has significant effects on the heart and kidneys.
- Seawater aspiration results in fluid-filled, perfused alveoli with shunting and venous admixture. The hypertonic sea water pulls fluid from the plasma into the lungs and may cause rapid hypovolaemia.

Mortality in freshwater and sea-water drowning is similar.[23,24] Those who survive the initial, short-lived pulmonary insult associated with water aspiration usually have no long-term respiratory impairment. In animal experiments, aspiration of as little as 2.5 mL kg^{-1} of water may increase the intrapulmonary shunt from the normal value of 10% to 75% ($PaO_2 < 8$ kPa) within 3 min. Typically, the respiratory symptoms (tachypnoea, wheeze and cyanosis) and the pulmonary oedema depend on the amount of water aspirated, the level of contamination by pollutants and the risk of secondary infection from sewage and other sources of infective organisms. Pulmonary oedema may be delayed by up to 12 hours after near-drowning incidents. For this reason, it is generally recommended that all conscious and asymptomatic cases of near-drowning should be admitted to a high dependency unit (HDU) for 12–24 hours' observation before discharge.

By reducing cerebral metabolism, profound hypothermia ($<30\,°C$) can prevent irreversible neurological damage, particularly in children, enabling them to survive protracted periods of asphyxia. However, cold-water immersion and hypothermia are major factors in the pathophysiology of near-drowning. Respiratory drive is inversely related to water temperature and, below $10\,°C$, uncontrollable hyperventilation increases minute ventilation tenfold and breath hold times are reduced to less than 10 s. This results in an increased risk of aspiration during escape from a submerged vehicle or when swimming in turbulent waters. Body temperatures $<28\,°C$ impair neuromuscular performance, making swimming difficult, and the conduction advantage of Purkinje tissue over normal ventricular tissue is lost. Rough handling of the hypothermic patient easily precipitates ventricular fibrillation.

The primary aims during the initial treatment of near-drowning[25,26] are to:

- reverse hypoxaemia,
- restore cardiovascular stability,
- prevent further heat loss,
- correct acidosis and electrolyte imbalance,
- prevent hypoxaemic brain injury.

At the scene of the accident, the victim must be retrieved from the water and cardiopulmonary resuscitation initiated as soon as possible. The American Heart Association does not recommend routine abdominal-thrust (Heimlich) manoeuvres to aid the drainage of fluid from the lungs because controlled studies demonstrated no benefit.[25] Gravitational drainage is equally effective and little water can be aspirated by direct suction within 5 min. In addition, arrhythmias or asystole may be induced, which are extremely difficult to reverse in the hypothermic patient. Gastric dilatation is often associated with near-drowning. Vomiting and aspiration may follow sudden increases in upper abdominal pressure.[25,26]

Victims who appear normal on arrival at hospital can deteriorate rapidly. Full resuscitative efforts should be attempted in all near-drowned patients and successful outcomes after several hours of manual resuscitation have been reported.[25,26] Hypothermic cases must be re-warmed before any decision is made to terminate resuscitation, because recovery after prolonged, cold submersion has been reported. Hypothermia may be associated with resistant arrhythmias. If initial attempts at defibrillation are unsuccessful, they should be discontinued until the core body temperature is $>29\,°C$. Re-warming techniques should aim to avoid shivering, which increases O_2 demand. Cardiovascularly stable patients should be rewarmed at $1\,°C\,h^{-1}$. This can be achieved using warm, humidified, inspired gas, warm intravenous fluids and warming blankets. Rapid re-warming should be considered when the core temperature is $<28\,°C$ because of the risk of ventricular arrhythmias. Extracorporeal rewarming with haemofiltration or cardiopulmonary bypass rapidly restores normothermia (up to $10.7\,°C\,h^{-1}$) and allows fluid removal in the presence of pulmonary oedema. When bypass is used, perfusion is re-instituted, regardless of the cardiac rhythm. Other techniques of rapid re-warming include peritoneal dialysis, bladder irrigation, gastric and pleural lavage.

Fluid resuscitation is essential and electrolyte imbalance, although infrequent, must be corrected. O_2 therapy should be given until hypoxaemia resolves. A normal CXR is present in up to 20% of cases at admission to hospital, although, in the majority, changes ranging from lobar infiltrates to bilateral pulmonary oedema are observed. Controlled studies have verified the effectiveness of CPAP, with either spontaneous or mechanical ventilation for hypoxaemia due to sea-water aspiration. In fresh-water aspiration, CPAP is more effective when combined with mechanical ventilation, which may reflect alterations in pulmonary surfactant after fresh-water aspiration.[23,24] Antibiotics should be withheld unless there is specific evidence of infection or the aspirated water was grossly contaminated. Although chest infections are most common, bacteraemia and brain abscesses have been reported following aspiration.

The degree of hypoxic brain injury often determines the outcome, but neither intracranial pressure monitoring nor corticosteroid therapy is beneficial.[23] Techniques including deliberate hypothermia and barbituate-induced coma do not improve survival and are not recommended. Prolonged submersion, delayed resuscitation, severe acidosis (pH <7.1), fixed, dilated pupils and a low Glasgow Coma Score (<5) are usually associated with death and brain injury, although none of these predictors is infallible.

HYDROCARBON ASPIRATION

The ingestion of petrol, furniture polish and other hydrocarbons accounts for about 15% of accidental poisonings in children. Pulmonary toxicity only occurs if there is inhalation during ingestion or following subsequent vomiting. The characteristic odour of hydrocarbon is usually readily detected and initially the patient experiences a burning sensation in the mouth and oropharynx. Central nervous system irritability with lethargy, dizziness, twitching and, less commonly, convulsions may occur. Non-infective fever is common. Laboured respiration and cyanosis follow symptoms of cough and choking. Progressive respiratory failure with hypoxaemia develops over the next 24 hours. Large aspirations may be associated with pulmonary oedema and haemoptysis. Patients with small aspirations usually recover over 2–5 days. Gastric lavage or induced emesis following the ingestion of hydrocarbons is not recommended because pulmonary aspiration, rather than gastrointestinal absorption of hydrocarbon, is the life-threatening event.

BLOOD ASPIRATION

Inhalation of blood may occur during haematemesis, intrapulmonary haemorrhage and surgery on the upper airways. Aspiration of blood mimics the acute phase of acid gastric content inhalation. Respiratory distress is associated with cyanosis if sufficient blood is inhaled to cause intrapulmonary shunting. However, unlike acid gastric content inhalation, these symptoms usually settle rapidly, with few long-term sequelae. Blood in the upper airways may also precipitate severe laryngospasm and this is a common and serious complication of upper airways surgery (see 'Large airways obstruction', below).

TRACHEO-OESOPHAGEAL FISTULA

Recurrent occult aspiration may be due to transoesophageal fistula (TOF) caused by tumour, trauma or mediastinal sepsis. The diagnosis can be difficult and may require bronchoscopy, oesophagoscopy, gastrograffin swallow and CT scan. The management will be determined by the underlying cause.

LARGE AIRWAYS OBSTRUCTION

In the critically ill patient, large airways obstruction is a common and life-threatening emergency.[27] It usually presents as sudden hypoxaemia and, if not rapidly corrected, cardiovascular instability and eventually cardiac arrest ensue. The causes of large airways obstruction include sputum plugs, blood clots, aspirated particulate matter, inhaled toxic gases, burns, trauma, anaphylactic attacks, laryngeal angioedema, severe laryngospasm and tracheal or other large airways stenoses. Rarely, childhood infections, including epiglottitis or diphtheria, may cause acute laryngeal obstruction (see below). Obstruction of the airways by the tongue in the unconscious patient should always be excluded and prevented with a pharyngeal airway. In the ICU, acute upper airways obstruction is often associated with the process of extubation or the complications associated with tracheostomy. Extubations should be undertaken with considerable care. Facilities for O_2 therapy, suction, nebulizers, re-intubation and non-invasive respiratory support should be immediately available.

Sputum plugs and blood clots

The commonest cause of large airways obstruction in the ICU is sputum plugs, which are often dislodged during physiotherapy. CXR reveals a collapsed lobe or segment. Physiotherapy with 'bagging' and gentle lavage and suctioning is usually sufficient to dislodge the obstruction, although bronchoscopy may be required to remove a viscid plug. Blood clots due to tracheal trauma during suctioning or following the insertion of a tracheostomy may result in obstructions. Viscid sputum or blood clots may also act as ball valves at the lower end of the tracheostomy or endotracheal tube, causing respiratory impairment and lung hyperinflation (Fig. 9.7).

Laryngospasm

Laryngospasm is an important but uncommon complication in the ICU. Irritation of the upper airways by blood, pharyngeal secretions, food or aspirated gastric

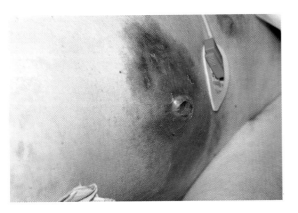

Plate 1 *A 41-year-old man with lung abscess presenting with haemoptysis. Subsequent development of empyema necessitans over left chest wall.*

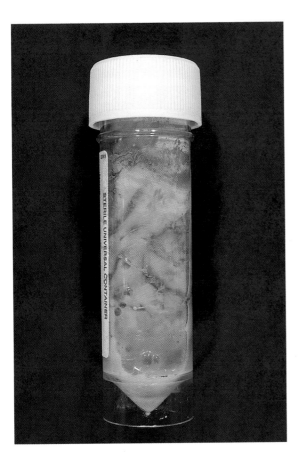

Plate 2 *A 41-year-old man with lung abscess presenting with haemoptysis. Subsequent discharge of pus from abscess.*

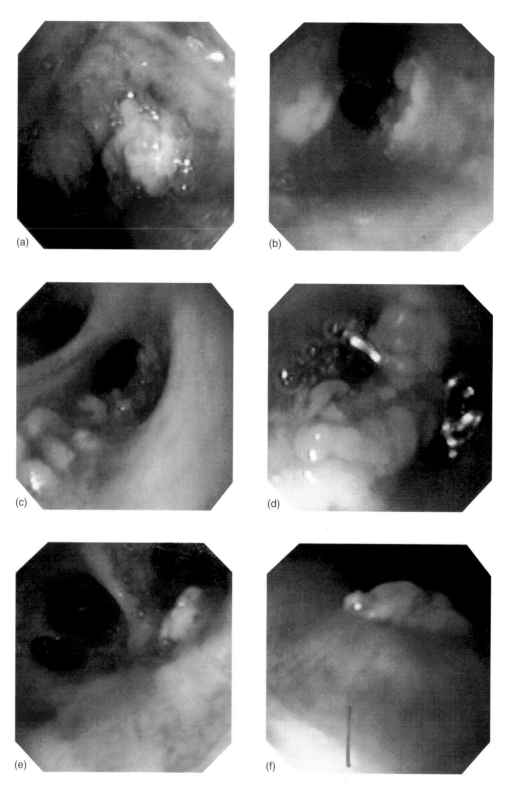

Plate 3 *Tracheobronchial aspergillosis affecting the right upper lobe (a, b), right lower lobe (c, d) and left lower lobe (e, f) in a 25-year-old, immunosuppressed patient with systemic lupus erythematosus and massive haemoptysis.*

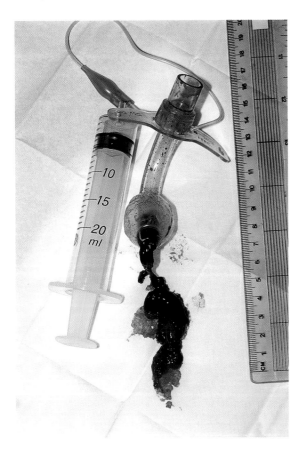

Plate 4 *Sudden, severe hypoxaemia and airways obstruction developed in a 26-year-old man 3 weeks following an episode of blunt chest trauma. A large blood clot was found occluding the tracheostomy at flexible bronchoscopy.*

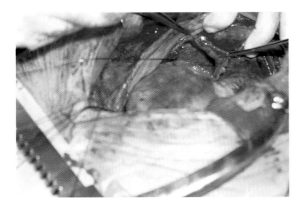

Plate 5 *A 27-year-old man sustained a severe blunt chest injury following a road traffic accident. His CXR and CT scan showed the heart to be displaced to the right. At thoracotomy, he was found to have a ruptured pericardial sac through which the heart had herniated.*

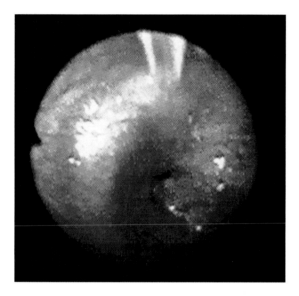

Plate 6 *Magnetic resonance imaging scan: bronchoscopic appearance looking down from the vocal cords. The stenosis developed 2 months after the insertion of a surgical tracheostomy in a 16-year-old boy ventilated for Guillain–Barré syndrome. Major tracheal surgery was required to repair the defect.*

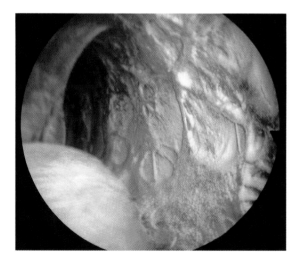

Plate 7 *Endoscopic view of thoracoscopic talc poudrage. Note the homogeneous distribution of talc powder across the entire left parietal pleura, adhering lung upper lobe on the left upper margin, free lower lobe at the left lower margin.*

Anaphylaxis and angioedema

The life-threatening anaphylactic response of a sensitized human appears within minutes of the administration of a specific antigen and usually presents as respiratory distress and cardiovascular collapse. Cutaneous manifestations include pruritis, urticaria and angioedema. A variety of materials may precipitate an attack, including foods, pollen, hormones and enzymes. In the ICU, drugs are the commonest cause, particularly antibiotics and contrast agents. Urticaria and angioedema may be associated with a variety of autoimmune or vasculitic diseases. Rarely, angioedema is a hereditary condition due to an autosomal dominant deficiency of C1 inhibitor, and it may also be acquired in certain lymphoproliferative disorders. The manifestations of anaphylaxis are attributed to the release of histamine, and levels of IgE are raised. Laryngeal oedema presents with hoarseness and stridor and bronchial obstruction with chest tightness and wheeze. The urticarial eruptions are intensely pruritic, may coalesce to form giant hives, but seldom persist for longer than 48 hours. A deeper, oedematous, cutaneous process – angioedema – may also be present. Angioedema of the larynx, epiglottis or upper trachea may cause severe obstruction and death.

The immediate treament of anaphylaxis includes intravenous adrenaline (0.5–1 mg), hydrocortisone (200 mg) and diphenhydramine hydrochloride (20 mg). Fluid resuscitation for hypotensive shock may be required. Bronchospasm is treated with O_2 therapy, nebulized salbutamol and, occasionally, intravenous aminophylline. Upper airways obstruction may require immediate intubation, but, if the situation is less critical, nebulized adrenaline may relieve largyngeal oedema and avoid the need for intubation. If intubation is not possible due to laryngeal deformity or oedema, an emergency cricothyroidotomy should be performed.

Trauma, toxic inhalational injury and burns

Inhaled toxins (sulphur dioxide, SO_2) and aspirated chemicals (bleach, acid, hydrocarbons) can cause injury, oedema and eventually obstruction to the upper airways.[28] Similarly, burns' victims who are

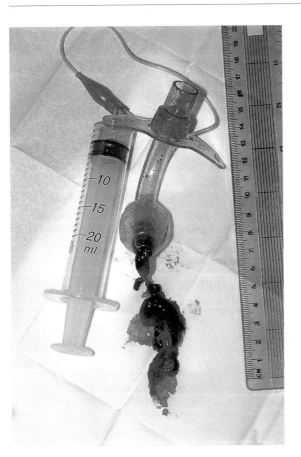

Figure 9.7 *Sudden, severe hypoxaemia and airways obstruction developed in a 26-year-old man 3 weeks following an episode of blunt chest trauma. A large blood clot was found occluding the tracheostomy at flexible bronchoscopy (see also Plate 4).*

contents can cause severe laryngeal spasm, presenting with stridor and respiratory distress. In the ICU, laryngospasm usually occurs immediately after extubation due to the oedema and stimulation of the upper airways associated with the removal of the endotracheal tube. In many cases, there may be bleeding in the pharynx due to trauma associated with the insertion of nasogastric tubes or following recent surgery. Severe respiratory distress requires immediate re-intubation. If the clinical situation is less critical, nebulized adrenaline (2–3 mL 1:1000 adrenaline), salbutamol and intravenous hydrocortisone (200 mg intravenously) may be administered to reduce laryngeal oedema, spasm and obstruction sufficiently to avoid re-intubation. Helium and O_2 mixes (Heliox) are often recommended as a temporary measure to improve gas flow through upper airways obstructions.

exposed to very high temperatures may develop serious injuries caused by the hot inspired gases.[29] Severe laryngeal or upper tracheal trauma may obstruct the upper airways. Immediate tracheostomy may be necessary in all these situations.

Many inhaled chemicals cause injury to the airway and alveolar epithelium (Table 9.1).[28] In general, chemicals are either direct respiratory toxins (NO_2, SO_2) or agents with systemic effects (CO, HCN). Toxic inhalational injuries depend on the properties of the inhaled gas, its concentration and the rate and depth of ventilation.

- Penetration of toxic particles is dependent on particle size, airways anatomy and breathing pattern. Particles > 10 μm are efficiently filtered by the nose, those between 2 and 10 μm are deposited in the tracheobronchial tree, and those <2 μm are deposited in the alveoli.
- Exercise and physical work increase the penetration of toxic gases into the lung and the 'total dose' of toxin.
- Highly soluble gases (such as SO_2) cause upper airways damage and oedema with localized

obstructive symptoms, whereas less-soluble gases (such as NO_2) penetrate deeply and cause parenchymal damage. Poorly soluble gases (e.g. CO) diffuse across the alveolar capillary membrane into the pulmonary circulation and may subsequently damage distant tissues.[30]

The clinical manifestations and timing of symptoms are dependent on the toxin, but include upper airways inflammation and oedema, laryngospasm, bronchospasm and pulmonary oedema. Whereas rapid death may occur with CO, delayed pulmonary oedema may occur at 24–48 hours with NO_2 or bronchiolitis obliterans at 2–7 days with smoke inhalation.

NITROGEN DIOXIDE

NO_2 causes peroxidation of lipid cellular membranes and subsequent tissue damage. Exposure occurs during welding, mining, fire fighting and in farmers. Gas stoves produce NO_2 and, when used in unventilated areas, may give rise to respiratory illness. Delayed pulmonary oedema and ARDS are

Table 9.1 *Inhalational toxins and sites of injury*

Type	Agent	Clinical effects
Direct respiratory toxins		
	Acetaldehyde	Upper airway irritation
	Acrolein	Upper airway irritation
	Ammonia	Upper airway irritation
	Bromine	ARDS
	Chlorine	Upper and lower airway damage
	Hydrogen chloride	Upper and lower airway damage
	Isocyanates	Increased airways responsiveness
	Nitrogen oxides	Airway responsiveness, ARDS, bronchiolitis obliterans
	Ozone	Airway responsiveness plus inflammation, ARDS
	Phosgene	Lower airway injury, ARDS
	Sulphur dioxide	Airway responsiveness, ARDS, bronchiolitis obliterans
	Cadmium	Emphysema, ARDS
	Manganese	Metal fume fever
	Mercury	ARDS
	Nickel	Asthma
Agents with systemic effect		
	Carbon monoxide	Tissue hypoxia
	Hydrogen cyanide	Tissue hypoxia, lactic acidosis
	Hydrogen sulphide	Tissue hypoxia
	Methane	Asphyxia

ARDS, acute respiratory distress syndrome.

the commonest clinical consequences of exposure. The concentration of gas is more important than the duration of exposure. In silo-filler's lung, NO_2 produced by grain fermentation can reach very high concentrations (200–2000 p.p.m.; safe range <8 p.p.m.) and, because NO_2 is heavier than air, it collects at the bottom of the silo. A single breath may be fatal and reported mortality varies between 20% and 65%.

CARBON MONOXIDE

CO poisoning is the commonest cause of acute fatal poisoning (3800 deaths per year in the USA). It is a colourless, odourless and tasteless gas, which is non-toxic to the lungs but displaces O_2 from haemoglobin and causes damage by reducing O_2 delivery to the tissues. Its affinity for haemoglobin is 220 times greater than that of O_2. By the Haldane equation, 0.1% CO in air would result in 50% carboxyhaemoglobin (COHb). Tissues with a high O_2 demand, including the brain and myocardium, are susceptible to CO poisoning. In the normal individual, breakdown of haemoglobin gives rise to a COHb level of less than 1%, although acute haemolysis can increase this level to 4–6%. Cigarette smoke contains 400 p.p.m. CO and cigarette smokers have COHb levels between 3% and 9%. CO poisoning results from poorly ventilated heating devices and the use of internal combustion engines in enclosed spaces. The clinical symptoms depend on the level of COHb:

- 10–20%: dizziness, headache,
- 20–30%: chest pain, reduced vision,
- 30–40%: nausea, vomiting, severe headache,
- 40–50%: confusion, ataxia, tachycardia,
- 50–60%: stupor, convulsions, coma,
- >60%: coma, death.

In general, patients who do not lose consciousness recover without permanent sequelae. Coma may be associated with basal ganglia or cerebellar damage, altered personality, memory loss, neuropsychiatric disorders and epilepsy. Treatment with high O_2 concentrations is essential. The half-life of COHb in room air is 240 min, compared to 30 min with 100% O_2 therapy. O_2 therapy should be continued until the COHb level falls below 7%. Hyperbaric O_2 therapy (100% O_2 at 3 atmospheres) reduces the half-life to <20 min. Although it has not been found to have any major benefit over 100% O_2 therapy, there is some evidence that it may reduce the long-term neurological sequelae. Limited availability and the time required for transport limit its practical use.

SMOKE INHALATION

Respiratory failure is the leading cause of death following burn injuries. The chemical composition of smoke depends on the material being burnt, but includes aldehydes, acrolein, ammonia, CO, HCN, NO_2, SO_2 and phosgene. Animal studies demonstrate that lung dysfunction is proportional to the mass of smoke inhaled and is independent of the tidal volume. Smoke directly injures the lung epithelial lining, causing pulmonary oedema, which is exacerbated by fluid therapy for the cutaneous burns. Early inactivation of surfactant leads to atelectasis and V/Q mismatch. Smoke inhalation is often associated with CO poisoning, burns to the upper airways and severe laryngospasm. The clinical features of upper airways obstruction following smoke inhalation can be delayed for several hours. Late-onset bronchiolitis obliterans may develop. Cyanide poisoning following smoke inhalation has been implicated as a cause of death and the use of sodium nitrite and thiosulphate therapy has been recommended.

NEUROMUSCULAR, INFECTIVE AND ENDOCRINE RESPIRATORY EMERGENCIES

There is an extensive list of neuromuscular, infective and endocrine diseases that may predispose to respiratory compromise and result in rapid respiratory impairment. Several factors may be present in the same patient.

- Central respiratory depression: coma, cerebrovascular accident, sedation during intubation or postoperatively.
- Self-poisoning: sedative drugs (benzodiazepines, neuroleptics) or neuromuscular poisons (strychnine) often result in progressive loss of respiratory drive and respiratory failure.
- Neurological disease: myasthenia gravis, ascending polyneuritis (Guillain–Barré syndrome) and restrictive chest-wall defects (kyphoscoliosis) are frequently referred to the ICU for monitoring of

respiratory function because of the potential risk of sudden respiratory failure. Progressive respiratory muscle weakness with inadequate cough may complicate myopathies or motorneuron disease. Atelectasis due to loss of mobility or laryngeal incompetence with aspiraton may occur.

- Infections: poliomyelitis, botulism, meningitis, miliary tuberculosis and tetenus may present as respiratory emergencies. ARDS complicating generalized sepsis is a frequent cause of respiratory failure on the general ward.
- Endocrine disorders: thyroid, adrenal and pituitary gland disorders may be complicated by respiratory failure due to central respiratory depression, muscle weakness or electrolyte imbalance.

Discussion of all the potential causes of respiratory impairment is not appropriate here, but those infective and neurological disorders that may result in rapid and potentially life-threatening respiratory failure and presentation to the ICU are reviewed in this section.

Infective respiratory emergencies

Although infective respiratory emergencies are rare in developed countries with advanced immunization and public health programmes, they remain a serious and relatively common cause for ICU admission in Third World countries.[31] The most serious include the following.

POLIOMYELITIS

Flaccid paralysis and respiratory failure may develop within hours of polio infection. Muscle weakness is usually asymmetric, widely distributed and initially involves the lower limbs and trunk. Upper-cord and brainstem lesions are associated with loss of diaphragmatic function and respiratory failure. Bulbar lesions cause speech and swallowing difficulties, with the risk of aspiration and secondary pneumonia. In a small proportion of cases, acute laryngeal obstruction or rapid respiratory failure may require urgent intubation. Therapy is supportive and, except in areas of complete paralysis, motor function recovers in the majority of patients. Persisting muscle weakness or paralysis may necessitate long-term ventilatory support.

BOTULISM

Botulism is a disorder of the myoneural junction caused by a Gram-positive anaerobic bacterium, *Clostridium botulinum*. Potent neurotoxins bind irreversibly to the presynaptic junction, preventing the release of acetylcholine. Symptoms develop within 1–24 hours of exposure to the neurotoxin, usually following ingestion of affected food or release from infected tissue. Decreased vital capacity, increased residual volume and hypoxaemia parallel severe respiratory muscle involvement and the need for mechanical ventilation. About 30% of patients develop respiratory failure severe enough to require mechanical ventilation. Aspiration is common. Therapy requires elimination of the neurotoxin from the gastrointestinal tract by gastric lavage and enemas, administration of trivalent antitoxin to neutralize circulating serum neurotoxin and of high-dose penicillin (3 MU 4 hourly intravenously) to eradicate the *C. botulinium* organisms and prevent further release of neurotoxin. Surgical debridement of infected wounds may be needed in some cases.

TETANUS

Tetanus is a toxin-mediated disease caused by *Clostridium tetani* . Usually, it presents as the generalized form, with diffuse muscle rigidity, generalized muscle spasms, respiratory failure and cardiovascular instability. Localized presentations, with rigidity around the site of injury, or the cephalic variant with trismus, dysphagia and paralysis of cranial nerves may occur. Both progress to the generalized form in 65% of cases. Appropriate management of the airways is the first priority in the treatment of tetanus. Patients with diffuse rigidity, generalized spasms or who are at risk of aspiration due to dysphagia should be intubated, even in the absence of respiratory compromise. A non-depolarizing neuromuscular blocking agent should be used to facilitate paralysis for intubation as depolarizing agents such as succinylcholine may cause hyperkalaemia and cardiac arrest. Muscular rigidity should be managed with high doses of intravenous benzodiazepine or morphine therapy. Paralysis with agents such as pancuronium, atracurium and vecuronium may be necessary to prevent spasms. Survival is improved by aggressive surgical debridement of necrotic wounds. Intramuscular human tetanus immune globulin

(3000–6000 IU) should be given as soon as possible and before any surgical debridement, which may be associated with the increased release of toxin. If the patient has not progressed to generalized spasms, intrathecal antitoxin (250 IU) may be more effective and is reported to reduce mortality. Antibiotics (penicillin, teracycline, chloramphenicol) are given to eradicate *C. tetani* and prevent further toxin formation. Cardiovascular instability is best controlled with deep sedation, but high-dose magnesium therapy may be required, with careful monitoring of the serum calcium levels and appropriate supplementation. Autonomic dysfunction is usually well controlled with bolus morphine therapy, although epidural bupivacaine may also be helpful. A successful outcome depends on meticulous intensive nursing care, which may be necessary for 6 weeks or more. If recovery occurs, immunity to tetanus is not guaranteed and primary immunization must start before the patient leaves hospital.

TUBERCULOSIS

In the majority of cases of both pulmonary and miliary tuberculosis, the presentation is slowly progressive. However, acute respiratory failure can occur when a large quantity of infected pus ruptures into the bronchial tree, or the vasculature, causing acute miliary tuberculosis. ARDS and disseminated intravascular coagulation can rapidly develop in these patients and signal a poor prognosis. Massive haemoptysis from active or healed disease may also result in aspiration and acute respiratory failure. The diagnosis is often missed in the ICU because of failure to consider advanced fibrocaseous or miliary tuberculosis in a patient presenting with acute respiratory failure. Assessment of potential risk factors and a high index of suspicion are essential. Cavitation on CXR is often suggestive, but both pulmonary and miliary tuberculosis may present with radiographic changes that may be confused with pneumonic consolidation or ARDS. A relatively normal white cell count should favour the diagnosis of tuberculosis. The detection of acid-fast bacilli (AFB) is diagnostic in pulmonary tuberculosis, but repeated sputum smears and bronchioalveolar lavage samples may be negative in miliary tuberculosis. In this situation, bone marrow, pleural, liver and lymph node biopsies or lumbar puncture may establish the diagnosis. Transbronchial biopsies in the mechanically ventilated patient have a relatively high risk of pneumothorax, and tuberculin skin testing is not often helpful in ICU patients. If AFB are detected, the species of *Mycobacterium* should be confirmed, the HIV status considered and, in the patient unable to give consent, the ethical guidelines regarding HIV testing should be addressed.

In acute respiratory failure due to tuberculosis, steroid therapy for 1–6 weeks is recommended, in conjunction with standard antimycobacterial drugs, unless there is a strong suspicion of co-existing bacterial infection. Steroids potentiate the resolution of tuberculous pneumonia, decrease exudative reactions and reduce systemic toxicity. In addition, steroids address the adrenocortical deficiency and hepatic enzyme induction associated with antituberculous medication, which result in low levels of endogenous steroid.

DIPHTHERIA

Diphtheria causes acute respiratory failure due to laryngeal obstruction or as a consequence of respiratory muscle failure due to polyneuritis. Several other pharyngeal and laryngeal infections, including epiglottitis, and peri-tonsillar abscesses (quinsy) may cause acute upper airways obstruction. Diphtheria is characterized by a local inflammatory lesion in the upper respiratory tract and remote effects resulting from the release of a toxin, which affects the heart and nerves. The characteristic pharyngeal membrane of diphtheria may spread over the posterior pharyngeal wall into the larynx, trachea and, less commonly, the bronchial tree. Bronchopulmonary diphtheria has a high mortality, not only because of the risk of obstruction, but also because of the large surface area from which the toxin can be absorbed.

Neuromuscular disorders

Many long-standing neurological diseases, including the myopathies, multiple sclerosis, motorneuron disease and post-polio syndrome, are associated with intermittent respiratory emergencies (muscle weakness, atelectasis, sputum retention). Acute ascending polyneuritis and myasthenia gravis are common neurological diseases that can cause a previously healthy person to develop paralysis and respiratory failure over the course of a few days.

GUILLAIN–BARRÉ SYNDROME (ACUTE ASCENDING POLYNEURITIS)

The most immediate threat to the patient is the development of respiratory failure from intercostal or diaphragmatic paralysis. This can occur very rapidly, with little previous distress or deterioration in blood gases. Arterial blood-gas monitoring is essential, but it must be emphasized that hypoxaemia and hypercapnia are late findings and indicate that respiratory arrest is imminent. Respiratory reserve is best monitored by serial determinations of forced vital capacity. Elective intubation should be performed when the vital capacity approaches $15 \, \text{mL kg}^{-1}$ (1 L) or sooner if pharyngeal paralysis impairs the handling of secretions. About 25% of patients ultimately require ventilation for periods ranging from 1 week to over 1 year. With good intensive care support, the mortality has been reduced to 5%, although about 15% of survivors have residual neurological deficits. Respiratory function will recover within 2 weeks in many patients, but a tracheostomy may be necessary if there is no sign of recovery after this time.

MYASTHENIA GRAVIS

Myasthenia gravis patients are often admitted to the ICU after thymectomy. Occasionally, confirmation of the diagnosis with the tensilon test may precipitate a 'cholinergic crisis', requiring immediate intubation. Rarely, myasthenia gravis may develop rapidly with severe, generalized muscle weakness and respiratory failure requiring urgent ventilation. Patients who complain of dyspnoea or difficulty swallowing should be admitted to hospital immediately for observation and monitoring of respiratory function. Use of the spirometer may be hampered by weak facial muscles, in which case monitoring negative inspiratory pressure is a useful alternative. A clear airway should be maintained by regular, gentle suctioning and postural drainage. Segmental atelectasis and hypostatic pneumonia may be prevented by intermittent positive pressure ventilation using a variety of techniques. Incentive spirometry may result in respiratory muscle fatigue and should be avoided. The patient should be transferred to the ICU if the vital capacity falls below 1.5 L, and serious consideration should be given to elective intubation if the vital capacity falls below 1 L. Early intubation may prevent a respiratory arrest due to mucous plugging or sudden fatigue. Mechanical ventilation is required in about 10% of patients with myasthenia gravis and may be precipitated by surgical stress, the administration of aminoglycosides, neuromuscular blocking agents or cholinergic agents. Infection may also precipitate respiratory failure, and these patients are at increased risk of infection due to immunosuppression (steroid/azothioprine therapy) or because respiratory muscle weakness impairs the ability to clear secretions. If ventilation is required, withdrawal of anticholinesterases (neostigmine, pyridostigmine) for 72 hours may improve their effectiveness when they are restarted.

REFERENCES

1. Thompson, AB, Teschler, H, Rennard, SI. Pathogenesis, evaluation, and therapy for massive haemoptysis. *Clin Chest Med* 1992; **13**: 69–82.
2. Cahill, BC, Ingbar, DH. Massive haemoptysis assessment and management. *Clin Chest Med* 1994; **15**: 147–68.
3. Garzon, AA, Cerruti, MM, Golding, ME. Exsanguinating hemoptysis. *J Thorac Cardiovasc Surg* 1982; **84**: 829–33.
4. Conlan, AA, Hurwitz, SS, Krige, L, Nicolaou, N, Pool, R. Massive hemoptysis. Review of 123 cases. *J Thorac Cardiovasc Surg* 1983; **85**: 120–4.
5. Hirshberg, B, Biran, I, Glazer, M, Kramer, MR. Hemoptysis; etiology, evaluation, and outcome in a tertiary referral hospital. *Chest* 1997; **112**: 440–4.
6. Patel, U, Pattison, CW, Raphael, M. Management of massive haemoptysis. *Br J Hosp Med* 1994; **74**: 76–8.
7. Crocco, JA, Rooney, JJ, Fankushen, DS, DiBenedetto, RJ, Lyons, HA. Massive haemoptysis. *Arch Intern Med* 1968; **121**: 495–8.
8. Gong, H, Salvatierra, C. Clinical efficacy of early and delayed fibreoptic bronchoscopy in patients with hemoptysis. *Am Rev Respir Dis* 1981; **124**: 221–5.
9. Bobrowitz, ID, Ramakrishna, S, Shim, YS. Comparison of medical vs surgical treatment of massive haemoptysis. *Arch Intern Med* 1983; **143**: 1343–6.
10. Conlan, AA, Hurwitz, SS. Management of massive haemoptysis with the rigid bronchoscope and iced saline lavage. *Thorax* 1980; **35**: 901–7.

11. Bense, L. Intrabronchial selective coagulative treatment of hemoptysis. *Chest* 1990; **97**: 990–6.

12. Saw, EC, Gottlieb, LS, Yokayama, T, Lee, BE. Flexible fibre optic bronchoscopy and endobronchial tamponade in management of severe haemoptysis. *Chest* 1976; **70**: 589–91.

13. Saumench, J, Escarrabil, J, Padro, L, *et al*. Value of fibreoptic bronchoscopy and angiography for diagnosis of the bleeding site in haemoptysis. *Ann Thorac Surg* 1989; **48**: 272–4.

14. Tan, RT, McGahan, JP, Link, DP, Lantz, BMT. Bronchial artery embolisation in management of haemoptysis. *J Intervent Radiol* 1991; **6**: 67–76.

15. Mal, H, Rullon, I, Mellot, F, *et al*. Immediate and long-term results of bronchial artery embolization for life-threatening hemoptysis. *Chest* 1999; **115**: 996–1001.

16. Jewkes, J, Kay, PH, Paneth, M, Citron, KM. Pulmonary aspergillosis: analysis of prognosis in relation to haemoptysis and survey of treatment. *Thorax* 1983; **38**: 572–8.

17. Jones, KD, Davies, RJ. Massive haemoptysis. *BMJ* 1990; **300**: 889–900.

18. Lomotan, JR, George, SS, Brandstetter, RD. Aspiration pneumonia. Strategies for early recognition and prevention. *Postgrad Med* 1997; **102**: 229–31.

19. Bynum, K, Pierce, AK. Pulmonary aspiration of gastric contents. *Am Rev Respir Dis* 1976; **114**: 1129–34.

20. Downs, JB, Chapman, RL, Modell, JH, et al. An evaluation of steroid therapy in aspiration pneumonitis. *Anaesthesiology* 1974; **40**: 129–34.

21. Drakulovic, MB, Torres, A, Bower, TT, Nicolas, JM, Nogue, S, Ferrer, M. Supine body position as a risk factor for nosocomial pneumonia in mechanically ventilated patients; a randomised trial. *Lancet* 1999; **354**: 1851–8.

22. Stoutenbeck, CP, van Saene, HK. Nonantibiotic measures in the prevention of ventilator-associated pneumonia. *Semin Respir Infect* 1997; **12**: 294–9.

23. Modell, HH. Drowning. *N Engl J Med* 1993; **328**: 253–6.

24. Golden, F, Tipton, MJ, Scott, RC. Immersion, near drowning and drowning. *Br J Anaesth* 1997; **79**: 214–25.

25. Standards and guidelines for cardiopulmonary resuscitation (CPR) and emergency cardiac care (EEC). *JAMA* 1986; **255**: 2905–84.

26. Ornato, JP. The resuscitation of near-drowning victims. *JAMA* 1986; **256**: 75–7.

27. Abdulmajid, OA, Ebeid, AM, Motaweh, MM, Kleibo, S. Aspirated foreign bodies in the tracheobronchial tree: report of 250 cases. *Thorax* 1976; **31**: 635–8.

28. Lentz, CW, Peterson, HD. Smoke inhalation is a multilevel insult to the pulmonary circulation. *Curr Opin Pulm Med* 1997; **3**: 221–6.

29. Frampton, MF, Utell, MJ. Inhalational injuries due to accidental and environmental exposures. *Curr Opin Crit Care* 1995; **1**: 246–52.

30. Jackson, DL, Menges, H. Accidental carbon monoxide poisoning. *JAMA* 1980; **243**: 172–4.

31. Christie, AB. *Infectious diseases: epidemiology and clinical practice* 4th edition. Edinburgh: *Churchill Livingstone*, 1987.

10

Respiratory emergencies II: chest trauma, air leaks and tracheostomy

RICHARD M LEACH AND DAVID A WALLER

CHEST TRAUMA

Chest trauma may be penetrating or blunt. Penetrating chest wounds are a surgical emergency and many patients will have had definitive treatment before they are admitted to the intensive care unit (ICU). However, while on the ICU they, must be monitored for secondary complications and problems that were not detected at admission. Chest trauma management requires a multidisciplinary approach involving the ICU team, cardiothoracic surgeons, radiologists and physicians. Frequently, life-threatening problems are neglected and the primary function of the ICU physician is to co-ordinate and oversee the management of these critically ill patients.[1–5]

General factors in chest trauma management

Chest injury is often a single component in the multiple-trauma victim.[1–5] Hypoxaemia, CO_2 retention and hypotension resulting from the chest damage can have profound detrimental effects on other organs. This is of particular importance when chest and head traumas occur together. Pain control is essential: inadequate analgesia results not only in an agitated patient, who will fight the ventilator and disconnect monitoring and intravenous lines, but also in poor ventilation, CO_2 retention and atelectasis.

Radiographic imaging, including chest radiography (CXR), chest computed tomography (CT) scan and screening techniques, is of particular importance in the management of thoracic trauma. An upright CXR should be obtained if possible because films taken in the supine position may not give an accurate estimation of the degree of pneumothorax or pleural fluid. The film should be assessed for the presence of soft-tissue and bony abnormalities, pulmonary infiltrates, pneumothorax, mediastinal shift or widening and thoracic fluid. The position of monitoring catheters, endotracheal and chest tubes should also be evaluated. Chest CT scans with contrast are invaluable in the assessment of intrathoracic damage and localization of abnormal air or fluid collections.

Penetrating chest trauma

Penetrating chest injuries are usually caused by sharp implements or gunshot wounds, which may be either low or high velocity.[1,4] Most low-velocity gunshot wounds and stab wounds to the pulmonary parenchyma will cause haemopneumothorax and can be managed with chest drainage alone. Chest drainage will re-expand the lung, evacuate blood and stop bleeding by tamponade of the low-pressure pulmonary vessels (Fig. 10.1). Bleeding from an intercostal vessel or a large pulmonary vessel may stop spontaneously, but often requires surgical control. Although an antero-apical drain to remove air and a postero-lateral drain to remove blood are frequently advocated, a single, correctly placed, large-bore postero-lateral chest drain is usually adequate. Multiple drains are only required for loculated collections.

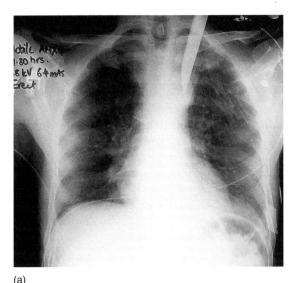

(a)

(b)

Figure 10.1 *An inebriated 64-year-old man walked into the casualty department complaining of 'stabbing' chest pain. Removal of his coat revealed a carving knife in his upper chest. His wife had stabbed him during a domestic dispute. When access to immediate surgical facilities was available, the knife was removed without complications and the patient was managed with a single left-sided chest drain. He made a good recovery. As his wife had stabbed him on a previous occasion, urgent marital counselling was advised!*

The indications for thoracotomy in penetrating chest trauma are:

- the initial amount of blood removed from the chest is greater than 1250 mL,
- chest drainage persists at more than 250 mL h^{-1} for 3 consecutive hours, suggesting damage to a large pulmonary or systemic vessel,
- an air leak sufficiently large to compromise ventilation,
- cardiac tamponade,
- transmediastinal stab wound: facilities for immediate surgery should be available before the implement is removed.

In high-velocity gunshot wounds, the enormous kinetic energy released causes cavitation, resulting in extensive lung and surrounding tissue damage. Early surgical intervention is usually required to evacuate blood clots, resect severely damaged lung and prevent air leaks, empyema and haemorrhage. Combat injuries often have to be managed initially with chest drainage alone, but many will develop complications that will require surgical intervention. High-velocity injuries are also more prone to air embolism than blunt or low-velocity injuries. This complication is more common than previously realized, potentially occurring in any patient with parenchymal injury. It may only become apparent when the patient is mechanically ventilated and the increased intrathoracic pressure forces air from a ruptured bronchus into pulmonary veins. Severe dysrhythmias may occur if air enters the coronary arteries, and neurological complications, particularly fitting, result if it enters the cerebral arteries. A large cerebral air embolus may mimic the appearance of a cerebrovascular accident. Multiple small air emboli result in confusion and a variety of focal symptoms and signs. Any patient who develops unexplained neurological or cardiac symptoms with penetrating chest trauma (including lacerations due to fractured ribs) should be assessed for air embolism. Chest auscultation may detect localized chest signs and air may be seen in the retinal arteries, which is diagnostic. Echocardiography may be particularly helpful in detecting air bubbles in the heart. If air embolism occurs, positive pressure ventilation should be stopped and the patient taken to theatre. Massive air embolism may require immediate thoracotomy in the ICU, with clamping of the affected hilum to prevent further air entering the bloodstream, after which mechanical ventilation may be restarted and definitive surgery arranged.

Blunt chest trauma

Blunt chest trauma is a common occurrence and relatively minor trauma may have serious consequences.[1–5] On chest examination, there may be few external signs, apart from bruising. Recognition of the resulting, and sometimes severe, intrathoracic damage is often delayed or missed.[4] Injury may affect any of the intrathoracic structures and many distant structures, such as the brain.

MECHANISMS OF INTRATHORACIC INJURY

The types of injury resulting from blunt chest trauma are direct (e.g. rib and sternal fractures, cardiac contusion and other soft-tissue injuries), shear and pressure related. All intrathoracic structures are tethered to adjacent tissues. Shear forces produced by differential organ motion may cause visceral or vascular tears. The most serious injuries of this type are deceleration-induced shear tears of the aorta and tracheobronchial tree. Other common injuries include pulmonary contusions and haematomas.

Sudden elevations of intrathoracic and intracavitary pressures may rupture air-filled or fluid-filled structures. Thus, oesophageal rupture may result in mediastinitis or empyema, and alveolar rupture may cause pneumothorax or pulmonary haemorrhage. The diaphragm may also tear, with herniation of abdominal contents into the thoracic cavity and restriction of ventilation.

Blunt trauma has also been classified according to the nature of the impact:[6]

- high-velocity impact (deceleration): fractured sternum/anterior flail segment, ruptured aorta, major airway injury,
- low-velocity impact (direct blow): unilateral fractured ribs, pulmonary and cardiac contusion,
- crush: fractured ribs/flail segments, ruptured bronchus/oesophagus.

CHEST-WALL INJURIES

Rib fractures occur more frequently in older patients. Chest-wall flexibility in younger patients often allows energy transfer to intrathoracic organs without rib fracture. Ribs six to nine are most fre-

quently broken, usually along the posterior axillary line, which is the site of maximum stress (Fig. 10.2). Ribs one and two are protected by the shoulder girdle, and fracture implies a very forceful blow and should raise the suspicion of potential damage to the airways and great vessels.[7] Ribs 10 to 12 are less prone to injury, but fracture indicates potential damage to the spleen, liver and kidneys. Rib fractures can cause direct lung damage with pneumothoraces, contusions, lacerations and haemothorax. The associated pain impedes breathing, causing hypoventilation and atelectasis.

A flail chest occurs in the self-ventilating patient when multiple rib fractures, usually in two sites, result in a free segment of chest wall or sternum with 'paradoxical motion' on inspiration. Dislocation of the costochondral junctions, which are not detected on chest films, may combine with posterior fractures to create a flail segment that may be missed. In this situation, careful palpation, in addition to radiography, is essential if the two sites of abnormal motion are to be detected. Even so, the flail segment may not be recognized for several hours due to 'splinting' by involuntary chest-wall muscle spasm. If the flail segment involves three ribs or more, the patient is at high risk of developing significant impairment of ventilation. Falls in vital capacity to 15 mL kg^{-1}

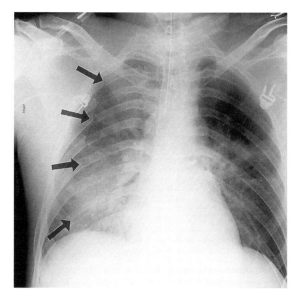

Figure 10.2 *Multiple right-sided (posterior axillary line) rib fractures and pulmonary contusion following severe, right-sided blunt chest trauma sustained during a road traffic accident by a 23-year-old motorcyclist.*

(normal 60 mL kg^{-1}) or blood-gas deterioration are independent indicators that mechanical ventilation may be required.

In patients with a 'mild to moderate' flail chest, the need for ventilation may be avoided with adequate pain control, drainage of air leaks, careful pulmonary toilet, nasotracheal suctioning and chest physiotherapy. Adequate analgesia will usually require a combination of oral, intravenous or patient-controlled opiate analgesia with intercostal nerve blocks. In general, intravenous analgesia will be required if more than two ribs are fractured. Nerve blocks with 0.25% bupivacaine and adrenaline 1:200 000 are extremely useful, but, if feasible, a thoracic epidural is more effective and provides easier long-term control.[8] These techniques have the advantages of causing less sedation than intravenous opiates, assisting physiotherapy and permitting mobility. The paradoxical motion of a 'severe' flail segment in combination with pulmonary contusions and other chest injuries will inevitably result in regional hypoventilation, retained secretions, shunting and severe hypoxaemia in some patients. Several studies have demonstrated that morbidity and mortality are improved with positive pressure ventilation, which overcomes the paradoxical motion of the chest wall and ensures adequate ventilation. Mechanical ventilation may be required for 7–14 days and patients with severe flail segments are usually more comfortable and easier to manage with an early tracheostomy. The important principle in the management of flail chest is that the underlying pulmonary contusion is more detrimental than any paradoxical movement and therefore therapy should be directed towards the underlying lung rather than the chest wall. In general, it is now accepted that external chest-wall stabilization (taping, sandbagging, fixation) is of little benefit in these patients.

TRACHEOBRONCHIAL INJURIES

Tracheobronchial injuries caused by blunt trauma are rare and often missed. A high index of suspicion is required in any patient with severe thoracic injury.[9,10] Fractures of the first and second ribs are associated with tracheobronchial disruption in 15% of cases.[7] The diagnosis should also be suspected in any patient with haemoptysis (10% of cases) or persistent air leaks (90% of cases), including bilateral pneumothoraces, pneumomediastinum and massive subcutaneous emphysema despite adequate chest drainage. Characteristic sites of injury are a longitudinal tear in the posterior membranous portion of the tracheal wall (15%) or a spiral tear in the main bronchi (80%), usually within 2.5 cm of the tracheal carina (Fig. 10.3). The injury occurs like a chicken wishbone breaking, with the force of the rotating heart forcing the bronchi apart. Tracheobronchial tears may not be recognized at the time of the injury and the process of repair is complicated by bronchial stenosis, secondary infection and the eventual development of irreversible bronchiectasis. Early rigid bronchoscopy will establish the diagnosis and allow the clearance of debris from the airway. If there is only a short longitudinal tear in the posterior membranous trachea or if the spiral tear is less than a third of the circumference and the lung is expanded, conservative management may be considered. A mini-tracheostomy may help by reducing intratracheal pressure and allowing air to escape from the mediastinum. Surgery, if necessary, should follow as soon as the patient has been stabilized. Complete separation of the lung from the trachea ('drop lung') due to transection of a main bronchus usually occurs within 2 cm of the carina. In contrast to bronchial tears, complete disruption is recognized early on the CXR. There are often no long-term complications following surgical repair.

LUNG INJURY AND FAT EMBOLISM SYNDROME

Pulmonary contusions are common after blunt chest trauma[11] and may occur in the absence of rib fractures. At the tissue level, localized bleeding and oedema occur, leading to ventilation–perfusion V/Q mismatching and hypoxaemia. Clinically, bruising at the site of chest trauma, haemoptysis and hypoxaemia are common. The CXR reveals ill-defined infiltrates or opacities in the path of the trauma, or contracoup, which usually develop within 6 hours (see Fig. 10.2). Opacification may increase for 24–48 hours and then gradually subsides over the next 7 days. However, progressive hypoxaemia in the absence of changes on the radiograph may be the first sign of pulmonary contusion. Pulmonary haematomas (1–6 cm) may develop, but are usually absorbed with minimal morbidity. If the trauma is severe, generalized pulmonary injury may lead to, or co-exist with, acute respiratory distress syndrome (ARDS). Ventilatory support may be required in the event of severe hypoxaemia, but the management of the pulmonary contusions is essentially supportive.

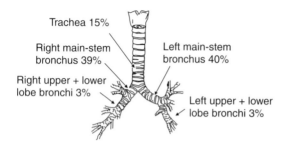

Trachea 15%

Right main-stem bronchus 39%

Left main-stem bronchus 40%

Right upper + lower lobe bronchi 3%

Left upper + lower lobe bronchi 3%

Figure 10.3 *The location of tracheobronchial tears following blunt chest trauma.*

Pulmonary torsion is a rare but life-threatening complication of blunt chest trauma. Early surgical correction is essential.

In cases of severe trauma, fat embolism syndrome (FES) may occur from 1 hour up to 3 days later. It is usually associated with multiple long-bone or pelvic fractures. Lipases hydrolyse neutral triglycerides to liberate fatty acids, which are toxic to the lung. In addition, fat emboli may pass through the pulmonary to the systemic circulation, causing infarctions in the retina, skin and brain. The characteristic clinical triad of FES is confusion, pulmonary dysfunction (with cough, dyspnoea and pleurisy) and a petechial rash over the upper torso. Initially, hypoxaemia may be associated with a normal CXR and reduced lung compliance and gas transfer. Eventually, ARDS may develop. Many patients also develop a coagulopathy, with disseminated intravascular coagulation and retinal infarcts. The diagnosis is established by detecting increased serum and urine lipase and fat globules in urine, sputum or serum.

CARDIOVASCULAR INJURY

Cardiac contusion

Cardiac contusion is a common, but frequently unrecognized, complication of non-penetrating blunt chest trauma.[12,13] Severe blows to the anterior chest wall involving the steering wheel or seat belt during road traffic accidents are the commonest cause. However, relatively mild chest trauma may cause severe myocardial injury (Fig. 10.4). At presentation, the patient may have little bruising or discomfort and recognition is again dependent on a high index of suspicion. Clinically, most cardiac contusions are mild, unrecognized and settle with supportive

therapy alone. Nevertheless, severe myocardial contusion is analogous to myocardial infarction, and cardiac arrhythmias are common but often delayed. Thus, cardiac monitoring is indicated for 24 hours after severe blunt chest injury. The anterior, thin-walled right ventricle is most commonly damaged, but the small amount of muscle involved at this site may not be sufficient to raise cardiac enzymes, despite significant dysfunction. Nevertheless, cardiac enzymes, troponin levels and serial electrocardiograms (ECGs) are usually monitored to assess progress. Technetium scans are non-specific but may be helpful (Fig. 10.4). Echocardiography is essential to assess the integrity of the valves, particularly when cardiac murmurs are detected. Coronary angiography is usually normal as the pathophysiological mechanism in cardiac contusion is thought to involve microvascular disruption secondary to tissue oedema. Treatment of arrhythmias and heart failure is as following myocardial infarction. Residual functional disability may occur (Fig. 10.4), but is rare: most cases are unrecognized and usually recovery is complete.

Aortic and great vessel injury

Abrupt deceleration injuries due to road traffic accidents account for most aortic injuries.[13,14] The aorta can withstand transmural pressures greater than 2000 mmHg, but it is less able to tolerate shear stresses. The majority of aortic injuries are fatal at the scene of the accident and therefore, in practice, this is an injury that is suspected much more often then it actually occurs. Characteristically, 80% of aortic ruptures occur just distal to the ligamentum arteriosum (the aortic isthmus) and 5% occur at the aortic root just above the aortic valve and may damage the valve and coronary arteries. Often there is no evidence of external trauma, and rib and sternal fractures are not always present. The diagnosis should be suspected when chest pain occurs in the intrascapular region, with signs of aortic valve regurgitation, pulse differentials or acute neurological changes after blunt chest trauma. The CXR may reveal a wide mediastinum, indistinct aortic arch, pleural fluid, a pleural cap or depressed left main bronchus. Angiography is the most sensitive technique to confirm the diagnosis. Evaluation of the aorta by helical CT scans with contrast is less sensitive because cross-sectional imaging may not demonstrate a transverse lesion. It has the advantages of speed and concurrent assessment of other intrathoracic structures in the

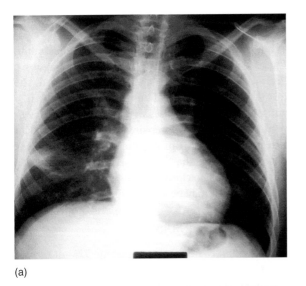

(a)

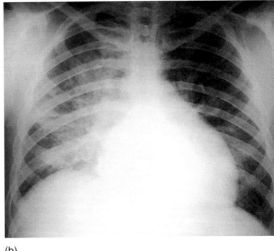

(b)

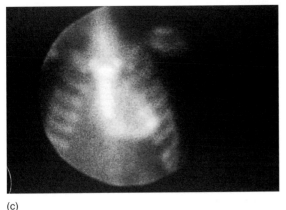

(c)

Figure 10.4 *Following arrest for suspected burglary, a 25-year-old man fell onto the back step of the police van, sustaining a blunt, central chest injury. The man presented to the casualty department 12 hours later with heart block (Mobitz 2) and ECG changes of an inferior myocardial infarction. His CXR at admission showed mild right-sided pulmonary contusion (a), but by 48 hours he had developed marked heart failure (b). A technetium scan (c) confirmed severe inferior and anterior myocardial damage, but coronary angiograms were normal. The man was discharged on diuretics with marked cardiomegaly.*

critically ill trauma patient, but surgery is unlikely to be undertaken without angiography.[15]

Traumatic injuries to the heart and pericardium

Traumatic damage to the heart can involve any of the chambers, valves, papillary muscles or the pericardial sac (Fig. 10.5).[13] In most cases (>80%), transmural rupture is rapidly fatal. Valve rupture is more common in older males. The aortic (60%) and mitral (30%) valves are most frequently affected. Diagnosis with transoesophageal echocardiogram and early repair is essential. Traumatic tamponade may be due to aortic root disruption, coronary artery laceration or rupture of the free ventricular wall. The clinical features are as for tamponade from any cause. Early surgical decompression reduces mortality, but pericardiocentesis may be attempted whilst preparing for surgery.

OESOPHAGEAL RUPTURE

Oesophageal injury in blunt chest trauma is uncommon.[1-5,16] However, in major thoracic trauma, the signs of a perforated oesophagus are often overlooked or attributed to other serious injuries. A perforated oesophagus implies violent deceleration and is usually associated with other life-threatening damage. The poor prognosis (approximately 60% mortality within 10 days of admission) is usually attributable to these accompanying injuries. The diagnosis should be suspected if major trauma is associated with rapidly developing pleural effusions, pneumothorax or mediastinal or subcutaneous emphysema. If the diagnosis has been missed, it may not be apparent until an empyema with associated pain, fever or hypotension develops. The CXR shows mediastinal widening with mediastinal or pleural

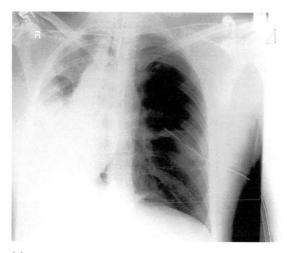

(a)

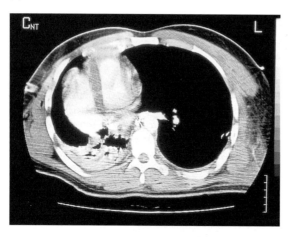

(b)

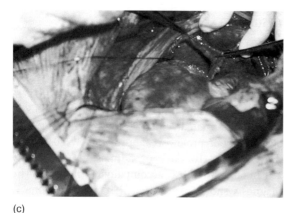

(c)

Figure 10.5 *A 27-year-old man sustained a severe blunt chest injury following a road traffic accident. His CXR (a) and CT scan (b) showed the heart to be displaced to the right. At thoracotomy (c), he was found to have a ruptured pericardial sac through which the heart had herniated (see also Plate 5).*

gas. The diagnosis should be established with a water-soluble contrast swallow, which reveals extravasation into the pleural cavity or mediastinum. Endoscopy and CT scans are unhelpful in diagnosis. Early diagnosis is essential because, untreated, the mortality of oesophageal rupture is about 2% h^{-1} and is fatal in 50% of cases within the first day due to mediastinitis. Surgical repair is usually undertaken within 24 hours of rupture, after which time surgery is reserved for mediastinal debridement and lavage. Rarely, oesophagectomy with primary or delayed reconstruction may be appropriate.

DIAPHRAGMATIC INJURY

Diaphragmatic injuries complicate 7% of severe thoracic trauma cases and are life threatening unless diagnosed and treated early (Fig. 10.6).[17] Mortality in patients with diaphragmatic injury due to blunt trauma is about 40% because it is commonly associated with rupture of the spleen or liver. About 80% occur on the left because the right hemidiaphragm is protected and supported by the liver. The diagnosis is often missed as positive pressure ventilation masks the respiratory distress and may relocate herniated bowel. The diagnosis may be confirmed by thoracoscopy, but treatment is best performed by a thoracotomy.

THE MANAGEMENT OF AIR LEAKS IN INTENSIVE CARE

Air leaks are a common and frequently serious problem in the ICU. The aetiology is extensive, but in the intensive care setting three situations are particularly important:

- ventilator-associated lung injury,
- cardiothoracic surgery (iatrogenic chest-wall penetration/parenchymal damage),
- blunt or penetrating chest trauma.

Many conditions predispose to air leaks, including necrotizing lung pathology, non-homogeneous parenchymal disease, prolonged ventilation and youth. As a general rule, all pneumothoraces in patients in the ICU require immediate tube drainage, whereas the management of pneumatocoeles and loculated pneumothoraces is less well defined. However, in our experience, drainage of most large air collections under radiological guidance may be life saving

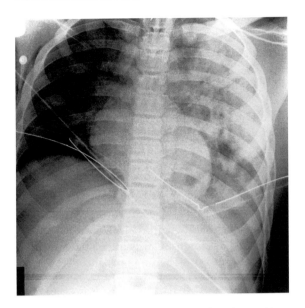

Figure 10.6 *Left-sided diaphragmatic rupture in a 33-year-old man following a road traffic accident. Characteristically, the diaphragm is not clearly visualized on the CXR. The left-sided chest drain had, in fact, been inserted into the abdominal cavity. This emphasizes the importance of performing a CT scan if this diagnosis is suspected.*

(Fig. 10.7) Drainage of other air leaks, including pneumomediastinum and subcutaneous emphysema, is not necessary, except in exceptional circumstances.

Pneumothorax

Pneumothorax[18,19] may be categorized into:

- primary spontaneous pneumothorax, usually occurring in a young adult without underlying lung disease,
- secondary pneumothorax, usually occurring in an elderly patient with underlying lung disease, e.g. chronic obstructive pulmonary disease (COPD),
- traumatic or iatrogenic pneumothorax caused by alveolar puncture due to a foreign body.

A tension pneumothorax may complicate all three types if air continues to accumulate in the pleural cavity faster than it can be removed or absorbed. The resulting increase in intrathoracic tension compresses the remaining functioning lung, inhibits venous return and reduces cardiac output. This condition is fatal if the tension is not rapidly relieved by drainage.

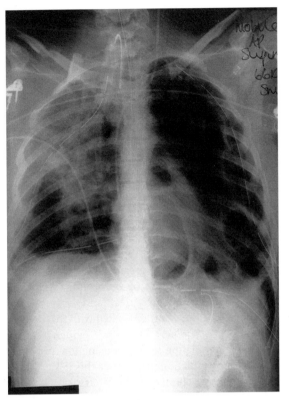

(a)

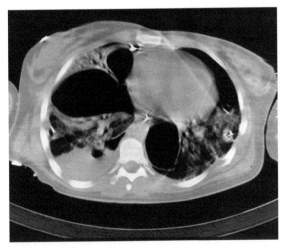

(b)

Figure 10.7 *Two weeks after admission, a 22-year-old woman with severe ARDS due to blunt chest injury had developed multiple loculated pneumothoraces and pneumatocoeles on CXR (a) and CT scan (b). The CT scan demonstrated that less than 30% of the lung tissue was ventilated. The woman's condition progressively deteriorated until the air collections were drained under radiological screening. At one stage, nine functioning chest drains were in place. She subsequently made a good recovery, with minimal long-term respiratory impairment.*

A small 'secondary' pneumothorax in a patient with emphysema may have more serious implications than a large 'primary' pneumothorax in an otherwise healthy young man because the respiratory reserve to compensate for the associated loss of ventilatory capacity is reduced in subjects with underlying lung disease.[19] The incidence of secondary pneumothorax increases with age and with the severity of the underlying lung disease. It is most commonly associated with COPD, but may affect a wide variety of other lung diseases that damage lung architecture or the pleura. The patient with a secondary pneumothorax is more likely to be admitted to the ICU, not only for management of the pneumothorax but also for management of the underlying lung disease. Ventilated patients with lung disease are also at greater risk of secondary pneumothorax as a result of 'barotrauma' (damage due to high airway pressures) and 'volutrauma' (alveolar over-distension) associated with mechanical ventilation.[20,21] There is now evidence that 'protective' ventilation strategies using low-pressure, low-volume ventilation may reduce this risk.[22] Blunt or penetrating chest trauma is associated with pneumothoraces due to direct penetration of the chest wall, increased intrathoracic pressure and shear stress causing tracheobronchial disruption or oesophageal rupture (see 'Chest trauma', above).

MANAGEMENT OF PNEUMOTHORAX IN INTENSIVE CARE

Most patients admitted with or developing a pneumothorax on the ICU will have either severe underlying lung disease or traumatic lung damage.[19] The majority will be ventilated and almost all will require intercostal tube drainage. Recognition and early drainage of significant air leaks can be life saving in such patients. Any pneumothorax that develops in a patient on positive pressure ventilation requires drainage before it enlarges and causes cardiorespiratory compromise. Prompt recognition of a tension pneumothorax, presenting with rapidly developing respiratory distress, hypoxaemia and cardiovascular instability, is essential. Clinical features include hyper-resonance on chest percussion, a shift in the trachea and apex beat and reduced breath sounds on auscultation over the affected lung. The detection of a tension pneumothorax is a clinical diagnosis and should be made *before* CXR

is performed. If a chest drain is not readily available, the largest available needle should be inserted through the chest wall in the third intercostal space in the mid-clavicular line into the pneumothorax, relieving tension and preventing the pneumothorax from increasing in size. Characteristically, a 'hiss of gas' escaping through the needle occurs as tension is relieved. A chest drain should be positioned as soon as practically possible. Bilateral pneumothoraces, often occurring after thoracic trauma, represent another situation in which immediate chest drainage is essential (Fig. 10.8).

The management of pneumothoraces in ventilated patients is a challenging problem. In experimental models, there is extensive evidence that high ventilatory pressures cause 'barotrauma', including pneumothoraces and other air leaks.[23,24] More recently, it has been postulated that high ventilatory volumes delivered to areas of lung unaffected by the disease process lead to damage by alveolar over-distension or 'volutrauma'.[24,25] This over-distension of relatively normal lung also results in air leaks, increased alveolar permeability and capillary damage. In animal studies, acute lung injury associated with air leaks has an increased mortality. In contrast, some studies of ARDS patients have reported that, although the incidence of air leaks varied from 0% to 92%, the correlation with airway pressure, ventilatory tidal volume

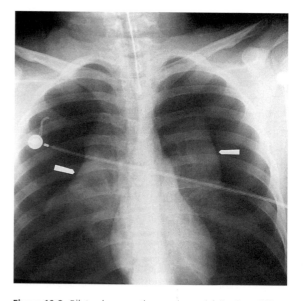

Figure 10.8 *Bilateral pneumothoraces (arrows) following a fall from a roof in a 33-year-old man.*

and mortality was poor.[21] However, these studies did not always differentiate between the early inflammatory and late fibroproliferative phases of ARDS and it is our experience that air leaks often develop in the late phase of the disease. Nevertheless, every effort must be made to reduce the risk of air leaks in mechanically ventilated patients, by avoiding high airways pressures and volumes, preventing secondary infection and by careful bronchial toilet. Recent studies have demonstrated that the early institution of low-pressure, low-tidal-volume ventilation improves both morbidity and mortality in ARDS.[22]

Once an air leak or pneumothorax has developed, high airways pressures associated with mechanical ventilation and alveolar recruitment strategies – positive end-expiratory pressure (PEEP) and reversed inspiratory:expiratory time (I:E) ratios – will encourage persistence of the leak. The appropriate strategy is to use the lowest peak, mean and end-expiratory airway pressures and I:E ratios compatible with adequate gas exchange and to ensure adequate drainage of any gas collection. Even a small pneumothorax may compromise gas exchange in the ventilated patient with severely damaged lung tissue, and conservative management or aspiration is inappropriate. Multiple intercostal drains inserted under screening may be required to ensure adequate lung re-expansion in patients with loculated pneumothoraces. However, this strategy requires early detection and precise localization of air spaces, which is not always possible with routine CXR. In this respect, serial CT scans and screening are an essential but insufficiently used diagnostic tool in the management of the critically ill patient with severe lung injury (Fig. 10.9).

In the mechanically ventilated patient with severe lung disease, air leaks may be large and difficult to manage.[26] If a large, persistent air leak develops, increased suction of up to 10 kPa may be applied to the drain with the aim of obliterating the pleural space. The correct pressure is that which opposes the lung and chest-wall pleural surfaces, allowing spontaneous pleurodesis. A high-flow, low-pressure system is essential. Wall suction is ideal and most portable pump systems are incapable of coping with a large flow rate and are potentially harmful because they may actually obstruct the air leak and produce a tension pneumothorax. Early thoracic surgical advice should be obtained if the pleural surfaces cannot be opposed in the presence of a large air leak.

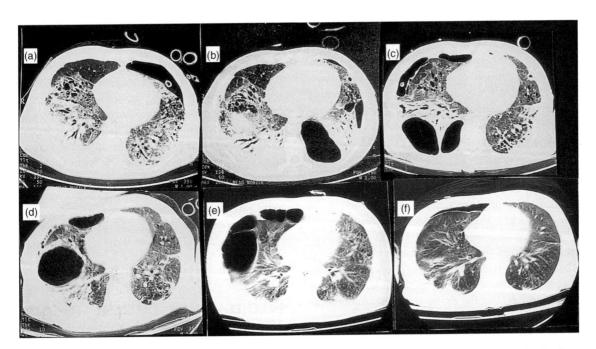

Figure 10.9 *Serial CT scans, at weekly intervals, in a 55-year-old man who developed severe postoperative ARDS with recurrent loculated pneumothoraces in different sites that compromised respiratory gas exchange. The loculated pneumothoraces could only be accurately located and drained with CT scanning.*

Initial bronchoscopy (preferably using the rigid scope) for bronchial toilet is valuable because the lung cannot re-inflate if the proximal bronchi are obstructed by blood or mucus. The decision then lies between surgical closure of the air leak or an attempt at chemical pleurodesis. There is no indication for introducing sclerosants if the pleural surfaces cannot be opposed and surgery is required. Now the treatment of choice is video-assisted thoracoscopy, which is as effective as thoracotomy but causes less respiratory dysfunction.[27,28] If the air leak persists but the lung is expanded, closed pleurodesis via the chest tube using a slurry of talc should be considered. The term bronchopleural fistula is frequently misused. It should be reserved for postoperative air leaks resulting from disruption of a bronchial suture line and is generally an indication for re-operation because the size of the air leak is so large.

Chest drains are often required to drain air or fluid from the traumatized chest to maintain both respiratory and cardiovascular function. They must be well positioned, secured and monitored to ensure proper functioning. All drains inserted without imaged guidance should be placed in the so-called 'triangle of safety' between the anterior border of latissimus dorsi and the posterior border of pectoralis major and above the level of the nipple. When inserting a drain in a ventilated patient, remember to disconnect the ventilator on insertion. High-flow wall suction of between 2 and 10 kPa negative pressure may be required to ensure complete lung expansion. Drain patency is enhanced by preventing kinking of the tube or pooling of secretions and subsequent clotting due to excessive length of tubing. Clamping of drains for transport or patient repositioning is not recommended because of the risk of tension pneumothorax.

Timing of chest drain removal depends on the clinical situation. In general, a chest drain can be removed when there is clinical and radiological evidence of lung re-expansion and there has been no air leakage (bubbling) through the drain for 12–24 hours. It is not necessary to clamp drains before removal, and this practice is discouraged. Before removal of the drain, the patient should be given adequate analgesic and anti-emetic cover. The drain should be pulled out when the patient is in inspiration or breath-holding, and the purse-string suture tied securely. The patient must be carefully observed for recurrence of the pneumothorax.

Other air leaks

Pneumomediastinum describes air dissecting along the mediastinal–pleural reflection, outlining the heart and great vessels with air. Air may also dissect along perivascular sheaths into the neck, causing subcutaneous emphysema, or around the heart, resulting in a pneumopericardium, which may cause tamponade. As with pneumothorax, the source of the air leak may be spontaneous, iatrogenic or traumatic. In the ICU, it can indicate on-going ventilator-induced 'barotrauma' or damage to the airways from intubation or percutaneous tracheostomy. More serious causes include injury to the trachea, bronchus and oesophagus, which require surgical repair.

Physical examination reveals subcutaneous emphysema at the root of the neck; a nasal quality to the voice and auscultation over the precordium may reveal a 'crunch' with each heart beat (Homan's sign). Paramediastinal air cysts are occasionally seen in young patients who experience severe chest trauma. Massive subcutaneous emphysema may occur over the entire body, leading to a grotesque, bloated appearance with closure of the eyelids and a characteristic crackling feeling on palpation.

In general, subcutaneous emphysema and pneumomediastinum are not associated with severe respiratory complications and both conditions usually resolve spontaneously. General management in the ICU includes low-pressure, low-tidal-volume, protective ventilation strategies and ensuring good drainage of existing air leaks. The failure of extensive subcutaneous emphysema to resolve, with progressive dyspnoea, usually indicates inadequate drainage of a large air leak and should prompt careful investigation, including bronchoscopy, for previously undetected leaks or problems that would decrease chest drain efficiency. Occasionally patients with severe surgical emphysema may require a superficial skin incision in the suprasternal notch (cervical mediastinotomy) to allow subcutaneous air to escape.

TRACHEOSTOMIES, TRACHEAL STENOSIS AND TRACHEOMALACIA

Prolonged endotracheal intubation causes progressive damage to the upper trachea as a result of cuff pressure and movement.[29] Prevention requires the use of appropriate cuffed tubes, low cuff pressures and the prevention of movement. The longer the endotracheal tube is to be left in place, the more important is each of the components. Large-volume, low-pressure or foam cuffs are available that will maintain a good seal at low pressure and prevent aspiration. Cuff pressures should be measured and maintained at the lowest levels that ensure no leaks or aspiration. Patient movement can be minimized by securely fixing the endotracheal tube and ensuring adequate sedation and analgesia. Appropriate endotracheal tube position, with the tip 3–5 cm above the carina, is confirmed at CXR. It is important to note that the tip will move between 2 and 4 cm from full extension to full flexion of the neck and chin. Failure to prevent damage may lead to the development of tracheomalacia or tracheal stenosis. In addition to local tracheal considerations, it is becoming increasingly apparent that there are a number of other factors that may be important in determining the timing of a tracheostomy. Early tracheostomy may be associated with reduced requirements for sedation, improved intestinal motility and enteral nutrition (less sedation), early weaning and earlier discharge from the ICU.[30]

The timing, method used and care of tracheostomies vary amongst units. To a large extent, the time at which a tracheostomy is fashioned depends upon the individual case and varies from 10 to 35 days. At 7–10 days, we assess whether extubation is likely within the next week. If extubation is considered possible, we continue translaryngeal intubation, but, if not, a tracheostomy is formed. The recently introduced technique of percutaneous tracheostomy, using a Seldinger technique with progressive dilatation, has reduced the cost, need for surgical personnel and theatre facilities for fashioning tracheostomies, thus expediting the process by an average of nearly 3 days.[31] In general, this new technique is safe and easily performed by appropriately trained clinicians who can manage the life-threatening complications.[32,33] Deaths have been reported during the procedure, due either to the loss of adequate upper airway control or to massive bleeding. The prompt availability of anaesthetic and surgical back-up is essential. The addition of fibreoptic bronchoscopy facilitates the midline placement of the guide wire and dilators and may reduce the chance of fashioning a false track in the pre-tracheal space or the oesophagus and of tears to the posterior wall of the trachea.[32,33] The primary complication is bleeding, which affects 6% of first-time percutaneous tracheostomies and up to 25–30% of subsequent tracheostomies placed through a previous tracheostomy scar. Bleeding may be torrential if any of the major vessels close to the trachea are damaged, and deaths due to rupture of the brachiocephalic vein have been reported. The larger thyroid veins and arteries are often involved and, if the tamponade associated with insertion of the tracheostomy fails to stem the bleeding, surgical exploration may be required. Infection is rare with percutaneous tracheostomy.

Surgical tracheostomy has become much less common with the advent of the technique of percutaneous tracheostomy. Surgical tracheostomy may be advisable for patients with abnormal neck anatomy or recent upper airways or neck surgery and in those patients at significant risk of bleeding. Infection rather than bleeding is the primary complication, affecting about 10% of surgical tracheostomies. The development of significant (>75%) late subglottic (tracheal) stenosis appears to be very low (<1–2%) with both procedures, although minor stenosis at the site of the stoma occurs more frequently and is in some part related to the degree of laryngeotracheal injury prior to tracheostomy (Fig. 10.10).

Once inserted, tracheostomy care involves maintaining a clear, clean and humidified airway. Clots of blood formed at the time of procedure may cause severe obstructions shortly after the insertion of the tracheostomy. Similarly, tracheal drying and the formation of thick viscid secretions due to the loss of nasal and pharyngeal humidification during ventilation may lead to episodes of obstruction and desaturation. If the patient cannot be weaned off ventilatory support within 10 days, the initial tracheostomy tube should be replaced with a long-term tracheostomy tube with a removable inner tube that can be cleaned regularly. These tubes should be changed every 4 weeks because secretions accumulate on the outer surface of the tube and may form ball valves that subsequently obstruct the lumen. Humidification of the inhaled gas will prevent the formation of sputum plugs and, during the weaning process, a 'Swedish nose' will reduce water loss by as much as 70%. As respiratory independence returns, the tracheostomy cuff may be deflated for periods and the tracheostomy can eventually be replaced with a non-cuffed tube. The tracheostomy lumen can be reduced with each change of tracheostomy tube. The tube is eventually capped to ensure independent breathing prior to removal.

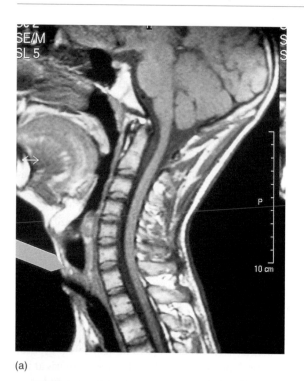

(a)

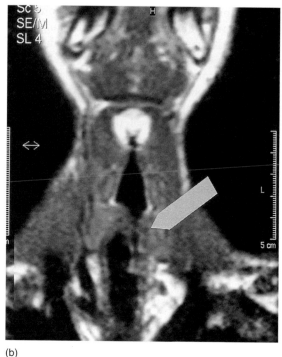

(b)

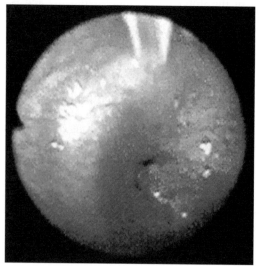

(c)

Figure 10.10 *Magnetic resonance imaging scan: sagittal section (a); coronal section (b); and bronchoscopic appearance looking down from the vocal cords (c); see also Plate 6 of a subglottic tracheal stenosis, indicated by the arrow in (b). The stenosis developed 2 months after the insertion of a surgical tracheostomy in a 16-year-old boy ventilated for Guillain–Barré syndrome. Major tracheal surgery was required to repair the defect.*

REFERENCES

1. Sabbe, MB. Recent advances in the diagnosis and treatment of thoracic injury. *Curr Opin Crit Care* 1995; **6**: 503–8.

2. Kshettry, V, Bolman, R. Chest trauma: assessment, diagnosis, and management. *Clin Chest Med* 1994; **15**: 137–46.

3. Anderson, DR. The diagnosis and management of non-penetrating cardiothoracic trauma. *Br J Clin Pract* 1993; **47**: 97–103.

4. Wall, MJ, Soltero, E. Damage control for thoracic injuries. *Surg Clin North Am* 1997; **77**: 863–78.

5. Ferguson, M, Luchette, FA. Management of blunt chest injury. *Respir Care Clin North Am* 1996; **2**: 449–66.

6. Westaby, S, Brayley, N. ABC of major trauma. Thoracic trauma I. *BMJ* 1990; **300**: 1639–43.

7. Gupta, A, Jamshidi, M, Rubin, JR. Traumatic first rib fracture: is angiography necessary? A review of 730 cases. Cardiovasc Surg 1997; **5**: 48–53.

8. Luchette, F, Radafshar, S, Kaiser, R, *et al*. Prospective evaluation of epidural versus intrapleural catheters for analgesia in chest wall trauma. *J Trauma* 1994; **36**: 865–70.

9. Guest, JL, Anderson, JN. Major airway injury in closed chest trauma. *Chest* 1977; **72**: 63–6.

10. Huh, J, Milliken, JC, Chen, JC. Management of tracheobronchial injuries following blunt and penetrating trauma. *Am Surg* 1997; **63**: 896–9.

11. Hoff, S, Shotts, S, Eddy, V, Morris, J. Outcome of isolated pulmonary contusion in blunt trauma patients. *Am Surg* 1994; **60**: 138–42.

12. Kumar, S. Myocardial contusion following non-fatal blunt chest trauma. *J Trauma* 1983; **23**: 4–9.

13. Pretre, R, Chilcott, M. Blunt trauma to the heart and great vessels. *N Engl J Med* 1997; **336**: 626–32.

14. Ahrar, K, Smith, DC. Trauma to the aorta and aortic arch branches. *Curr Opin Cardiol* 1998; **13**: 355–68.

15. Unsworth-White, MJ, Buckenham, T, Treasure, T. Traumatic rupture of the thoracic aorta: computed tomography may be a dangerous waste of time. *Ann R Coll Surg Engl* 1994; **76**: 381–3.

16. Stothert, JC, Buttorff, J, Kaminski, DL. Thoracic oesophageal and tracheal injury following blunt trauma. *J Trauma* 1980; **20**: 992–5.

17. Steinau, G, Bosman, D, Dreuw, B, Schumpelick, V. Diaphragmatic injuries; classification, diagnosis and therapy. *Chirurg* 1997; **68**: 509–12.

18. Millar, AC, Harvey, JE, on behalf of Standards of Care Committee, British Thoracic Society. Guidelines for the management of spontaneous pneumothorax. *BMJ* 1993; **307**: 114–16.

19. Marini, JJ, Wheeler, AP. *Chest trauma, pneumothorax and barotrauma in critical care medicine*. Baltimore: Williams & Wilkins, 1989; 257–70.

20. Gammon, RB, Shin, MS, Groves, RH, *et al*. Clinical risk factors for pulmonary barotrauma: a multivariate analysis. *Am J Respir Crit Care Med* 1995; **152**: 1235–40.

21. Weg, JG, Anzueto, A, Balk, RA, *et al*. The relation of pneumothorax and other air leaks to mortality in acute respiratory distress syndrome. *N Engl J Med* 1998; **338**: 341–6.

22. The Acute Respiratory Distress Syndrome Network. Ventilation with lower tidal volumes as compared with traditional tidal volumes for acute lung injury and the acute respiratory distress syndrome. *N Engl J Med* 2000; **342**: 1301–8.

23. Kolobow, T, Morretti, MP, Fumagalli, R, *et al*. Severe impairment in lung function induced by high peak airways pressure during mechanical ventilation: an experimental study. *Am Rev Respir Dis* 1987; **135**: 312–15.

24. Dreyfuss, D, Soler, P, Basset, G, Saumon, G. High inflation pressure pulmonary edema: respective effects of high airway pressure, high tidal volume, and positive end-expiratory pressure. *Am Rev Respir Dis* 1988; **137**: 1159–64.

25. Dreyfuss, D, Saumon, G. Role of tidal volume, FRC, and end-inspiratory volume in the development of pulmonary edema following mechanical ventilation. *Am Rev Respir Dis* 1993; **148**: 1194–203.

26. Powner, DJ, Grenvik, A. Ventilatory management of life-threatening bronchopleural fistulae – a summary. *Crit Care Med* 1981; **9**: 54–8.

27. Waller, DA, Forty, J, Morritt, GN. Video-assisted thoracoscopic surgery versus thoracotomy for spontaneous pneumothorax. *Ann Thorac Surg* 1994; **58**: 372–7.

28. Waller, DA. Video-assisted thoracoscopic surgery for spontaneous pneumothorax – a 7 year learning experience. *Ann R Coll Surg Engl* 1999; **81**: 387–92.

29. Gaynor, ER, Greenberg, SB. Untoward sequelae of prolonged intubation. *Laryngoscope* 1985; **95**: 1461–7.

30. Grower, ER, Bihari, DJ. The role of tracheostomy in the adult intensive care unit. *Postgrad Med J* 1992; **68**: 313–17.

31. Friedman, Y, Fildes, J, Mizock, B, *et al*. Comparison of percutaneous and surgical tracheostomies. *Chest* 1996; **110**: 480–5.

32. Griggs, WM, Myburgh, JA, Worthly, LIG. A prospective comparison of a percutaneous tracheostomy technique with standard surgical tracheostomy. *Intensive Care Med* 1991; **17**: 261–3.

33. Ciaglia, P, Graniero, KD. Percutaneous dilational tracheostomy: results and long-term follow-up. *Chest* 1992; **101**: 464–7.

11

Pathophysiology of acute lung injury

S JOHN WORT AND TIM W EVANS

DEFINITIONS

Acute respiratory distress syndrome and acute lung injury

Acute respiratory distress syndrome (ARDS) was first described over 30 years ago in 12 patients who developed acute respiratory failure in association with a variety of serious surgical and medical pathologies, not all of which involved the lung directly. Seven of the 12 patients died.[1] In 1988, Murray proposed an expanded definition of ARDS that attempted to quantify the extent of lung injury as well as including information about possible causes and the presence of non-pulmonary organ dysfunction. Unfortunately, this lung injury score (LIS) proved unable to predict outcome and therefore had limited clinical usefulness (Table 11.1). It was not until 1994 that a Consensus Definition of the syndrome finally emerged, by which time it was recognized that ARDS probably represents only the extreme end of a spectrum of lung injury[2] Consequently, a lesser degree of acute lung injury (ALI) was also formally defined by the Consensus group (Table 11.2). However, the significance of ALI

as a separate entity, or as a predictor of progression to 'full-blown' ARDS, remains far from clear. Although a declared goal of the Consensus Conference was to bring clarity and uniformity to the definition of ARDS, important problems remain.

- When applied to large populations of hypoxaemic patients, the only difference between ALI and ARDS appears to be the severity of oxygenation impairment at the time of assessment, although it may be that more patients develop ARDS in certain predisposing groups and more develop ALI in other 'at-risk' groups.
- The present definitions of ALI and ARDS still have serious shortcomings because ARDS attributable to a direct pulmonary insult, such as pneumonia, differs both in evolution and physiological characteristics from lung injury attributable to indirect insults, such as intra-abdominal sepsis.
- Neither definition takes into account the nature of the precipitating cause, or the presence of non-pulmonary organ dysfunction, both of which are known to influence outcome.
- The variation in interpretation of chest radiography (CXR) of patients with lung injury is considerable, even amongst experts.

Table 11.1 *Components of the Murray Lung Injury Score*

	Value
Chest radiograph score	
No alveolar consolidation	0
Alveolar consolidation in one quadrant	1
Alveolar consolidation in two quadrants	2
Alveolar consolidation in three quadrants	3
Alveolar consolidation in all four quadrants	4
Hypoxaemia score	
$PaO_2/FiO_2 \geq 300$	0
PaO_2/FiO_2 225–299	1
PaO_2/FiO_2 175–224	2
PaO_2/FiO_2 100–174	3
$PaO_2/FiO_2 < 100$	4
Respiratory system compliance	
≥ 80	0
60–79	1
40–59	2
20–39	3
≤ 19	4
Positive end-expiratory pressure (PEEP) score when ventilated (cmH_2O)	
≤ 5	0
6–8	1
12–14	3
≥ 15	4

The final value is obtained by dividing the
   aggregate sum by the number of
   components used

Score

No injury	0
Mild to moderate injury	0.1–2.5
Severe injury (ARDS)	>2.5

Adapted from Murray *et al.* (1988).[25]

EPIDEMIOLOGY OF ACUTE LUNG INJURY/ACUTE RESPIRATORY DISTRESS SYNDROME

Variation by definition

At least ten epidemiological studies have shed light on the incidence of ALI and ARDS. Figures derived from these studies suggest an incidence from 1.5 to 13.5 cases per 100 000 inhabitants per year for ARDS. This wide range may be attributed to a lack of unified and agreed definitions, the variety of ther-apies applied at the time the defining criteria are sought, and the failure to define the population within which patients with ARDS are detected. However, two recent investigations applying the ARDS/ALI definitions of the 1994 American–European Consensus Conference suggest that 16% and 18% respectively of all mechanically ventilated patients had ARDS.[3,4] Surprisingly, only 4–5% of these subjects had ALI, a markedly lower figure than that previously published.

Influence of precipitating conditions

The most important precipitating conditions for lung injury are sepsis, gastric aspiration, major trauma and multiple blood transfusions. The likelihood of a patient with any individual condition developing lung injury is also variable. The incidence of ARDS associated with cardiopulmonary bypass surgery is 1–2%, but it is 30–40% in patients with gastric aspiration. Although the extent to which the individual response to an inflammatory insult influences

Table 11.2 *Criteria for the diagnosis of acute lung injury (ALI) and acute respiratory distress syndrome (ARDS)*

	Timing	Oxygenation	Chest radiograph	Pulmonary artery wedge pressure
ALI criteria	Acute onset	PaO_2/FiO_2 ≤ 300 mmHg	Bilateral infiltrates seen on frontal chest X-ray	≤ 18 mmHg when measured or no clinical evidence of left atrial hypertension
ARDS criteria	Acute onset	PaO_2/FiO_2 200 mmHg	Bilateral infiltrates seen on frontal chest X-ray	≤ 18 mmHg when measured or no clinical evidence of left atrial hypertension

Adapted from Bernard *et al.* (1994).[26]

progression to ARDS is unknown, high levels of interleukin-8 (IL-8) in broncho-alveolar lavage (BAL) fluid taken from trauma victims predict the development of ARDS with reasonable accuracy.[5] A wide variety of endogenous defence mechanisms, including redox balance, may also influence individual susceptibility.[6,7] The extent to which the endogenous responsiveness to inflammatory insults correlates with the precipitating insult remains unclear, but the manifestation of lung injury probably differs amongst patients suffering indirect, as opposed to direct, pulmonary insults.[8]

Cause of death

The precipitating condition also influences clinical outcome. Trauma victims have a better prognosis than those who develop ARDS secondary to gastric aspiration. Although the severity of respiratory failure has been shown to predict mortality, patients with ARDS rarely succumb to respiratory failure, but rather to multiple-organ dysfunction. Multivariate analysis in a recent study indicated mortality to be associated with septic shock, high severity of illness scores and immunosuppression.[3]

Trends in mortality

Single European and American centres have reported mortality amongst patients with ARDS varying from 25–70%. Recently, two long-term studies controlled for case-mix severity and performed in major referral centres on either side of the Atlantic showed significant falls in mortality rates.[9] However, a recent meta-analysis evaluating 101 peer review articles published between 1967 and 1994[10] did not detect a trend towards decreased mortality rates and, world wide, any improvement is undoubtedly patchy: the reported mortality in Spain is 43%, whereas it remains around 60% in France.[3] Such outcome variation is difficult to explain, but it is possible that reduced mortality may be achieved by specialized centres, which have defined admission criteria. In addition, many of the published studies cited above found similar mortality rates for ALI and ARDS, suggesting that the severity of lung injury itself may not be relevant.

Impact on the conduct and outcome of clinical trials

The failure of the majority of the large-scale clinical trials of therapeutic interventions in ARDS/ALI to demonstrate any mortality benefit may be explained by

- variation in the definitions used and case-mix with regard to the precipitating cause of the ALI/ARDS,
- the intervention is ineffective under the circumstances of the investigation or it has been applied inappropriately, e.g. used too late, or given to patients in whom the intervention cannot work because the underlying condition is irreversible,
- the influence of lung injury and respiratory failure on patient outcome in patients with ARDS may be small relative to other factors,
- critically ill patients are, by definition, an inhomogeneous group, and are therefore often treated with a number of co-interventions that may influence the end-point under evaluation, e.g. the use of muscle relaxants and sedative agents in a trial using ventilator days as an outcome measure.

The relationship between ALI/ARDS, sepsis and multiple organ dysfunction syndrome

Sepsis and its associated syndromes (Table 11.3) affect more than 1% of hospital patients and in up to 40% of cases cause circulatory failure. An identifiable microbiological source of infection is found in less than 50% of patients, the remainder displaying the systemic inflammatory response syndrome (SIRS). Many authorities consider that sepsis, SIRS and septic shock represent a continuum in the severity of the host response to non-infective and infective insults and the extent of this response influences prognosis. Thus, the mortality for patients with SIRS is approximately 7%, but rises to 50–90% for those with septic shock and multiple organ dysfunction syndrome (MODS).[11,12]

ARDS is now widely regarded as the pulmonary manifestation of MODS. Pulmonary hypertension with increased pulmonary vascular resistance is common, even in the setting of the lowered systemic vascular resistance that characterizes SIRS and sepsis. From the late 1980s, ARDS was known to be

Table 11.3 *Definitions of the systemic inflammatory response syndrome, sepsis, septic shock and multiple organ dysfunction/failure*

Systemic inflammatory response syndrome
Two or more of the following clinical signs of systemic response to endothelial inflammation:
- a temperature of >38 °C or <36 °C
- an elevated heart rate >90 beats min^{-1}
- Tachypnoea, manifested by a respiratory rate of >20 breaths min^{-1} or hypoventilation ($PaCO_2$ <4.25 kPa)
- an altered white blood cell count (>12×10^9 L^{-1}, or <4×10^9 L^{-1}, in the presence of more than 10% immature neutrophils)

In the setting (or strong suspicion) of a known cause of endothelial inflammation, such as:
- infection (Gram − or Gram +ve bacteria, viruses, fungi, parasites, yeasts or other organisms)
- pancreatitis
- ischaemia
- multiple trauma and/or tissue injury
- haemorrhagic shock
- immune-mediated organ injury

Sepsis
The systemic response to infection, manifest by two or more of the following as a result of infection:
- a temperature of >38 °C or <36 °C
- an elevated heart rate >90 beats min^{-1}
- tachypnoea, manifested by a respiratory rate of >20 breaths min^{-1} or hypoventilation ($PaCO_2$ <4.25 kPa)
- an altered white blood cell count (>12×10^9 L^{-1}, or <4×10^9 L^{-1}, in the presence of more than 10% immature neutrophils)

Septic shock
Sepsis-induced hypotension (systolic blood pressure <90 mmHg or a reduction of >40 mmHg from baseline) despite adequate fluid resuscitation

Multiple organ dysfunction syndrome
Presence of altered organ function in an acutely ill patient such that homeostasis cannot be maintained without intervention

Adapted from reference 27.

associated with endothelial dysfunction and disruption and this has recently been characterized *in vivo* using non-invasive radioisotopic techniques.[13] The recognition that the refractory hypoxaemia of ARDS was attributable to a loss of hypoxic pulmonary vasoconstriction in these patients highlighted the importance of vascular control mechanisms in determining the clinical characteristics of the syndrome and possibly also the development of multiple organ failure. Indeed, changes in vascular control have been documented in both experimental models and patients with sepsis uncomplicated by ARDS, and are characterized by systemic hypotension unresponsive to pressor agents and inotropes, possibly mediated through changes in the production of endothelially derived vasomotor agents. The hypothesis that such substances (Table 11.4) play a significant role in modulating both systemic and pulmonary vascular tone under physiological conditions was proven by the early 1990s. This emphasized the importance of the barrier and endocrine functions of the endothelium in determining the clinical manifestations of SIRS/sepsis and particularly in the development of MODS.

The way forward: epidemiology

There are a number of initiatives that may improve our understanding of the relevance of epidemiology in determining outcome in ALI/ARDS and the way in which the definition might be modified to benefit the conduct of clinical trials.

- The issues that influence outcome need to be more precisely identified, so that the influence of population homogeneity in determining trial inclusion criteria can be minimized.
- The extent to which defining criteria for ARDS might be modified by the provision of an optimal regimen of mechanical ventilation and general

Table 11.4 *Substances produced by the endothelium*

Thrombomodulatory
Thrombomodulin
Tissue plasminogen activator
Heparan sulphates
Von Willebrand factor
Ecto ADPases
Tissue factor

Vasoactive
Prostacyclin, thromboxane and other prostanoids
Nitric oxide
Endothelins

Adhesion molecules
E-selectin
ICAM-1 and ICAM-2
VCAM

Inflammatory molecules
Platelet-activating factor
Cytokines: IL-6, IL-8, MCP-1
Class II MHC molecules

ICAM, intercellular adhesion molecule; VCAM, vascular cell adhesion molecule; IL, interleukin; MCP, monocyte chemoattractant protein, MHC, major histocompatibility molecules.

supportive measures (e.g. fluid balance, prone positioning, use of nitric oxide (NO) etc.) needs to be identified. Recruiting patients to clinical trials who may meet ALI/ARDS criteria merely because they are receiving suboptimal care at the time of assessment is clearly inappropriate. Standardization of care and the use of agreed management protocols might obviate this problem.

- The influence of inter-observer variability in applying physiological and radiographic definitions of ALI/ARDS needs to be recognized and addressed.
- The therapeutic and prognostic significance of dividing patients into ALI and ARDS categories needs to be established before ALI can reasonably be considered to be a relevant and separate entity: ALI will therefore not be discussed in the remainder of this chapter.
- Criteria that define appropriate end-points for clinical trials must be agreed.

HISTOLOGICAL CHANGES WITHIN THE LUNG

The response of the lung to injury is stereotypical, and histological examination rarely identifies either the initiating event or the pathogenetic mechanisms. Characteristically, there is disruption of the alveolar-capillary unit, described as 'diffuse alveolar damage', comprising three overlapping stages: exudative, proliferative and fibrotic.

The exudative stage (Fig. 11.1) occurs within the first 48 hours and is characterized by the development of non-specific intra-alveolar oedema associated with epithelial and endothelial cell damage. After 24 hours, hyaline membranes are detected lining the alveoli and alveolar ducts, together with fibrin thrombi. Hyaline membranes are distinctive features of early ARDS and are composed of condensed plasma proteins mixed with cell debris. Although there is evidence of early damage to the endothelium, there is often extensive necrosis of type I pneumocytes.

The second, or proliferative, stage (>7 days) is more variable and is characterized either by resolution of the changes already occurring or by organization of the intra-alveolar and interstitial exudates. The latter course involves formation of intra-alveolar granulation tissue from fibroblasts and myofibroblasts, which eventually develops into dense fibrosis. Vascular remodelling begins at this stage and may contribute to pulmonary hypertension.

The last, or fibrotic, stage is characterized by increased fibrosis and collagen deposition, although collagen and its precursor proteins can be identified much earlier. The lung consists of microcystic areas and irregular scarring together with larger cystic areas characteristic of chronic ARDS. There is extensive vascular remodelling with muscularization of pre-acinar and intra-acinar vessels, leading (rarely) to irreversible pulmonary hypertension.

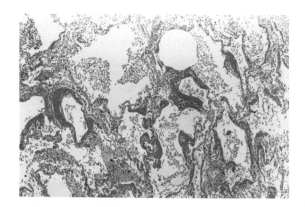

Figure 11.1 *Histopathology of the 'exudative' early phase of ARDS, demonstrating distorted alveolar spaces filled with inflammatory cells and lined with hyaline membranes.*

PATHOGENESIS

The precipitating causes of ARDS can be divided into those causing a direct insult to the lung and those in which the lung injury complicates a more remote disease process. This highlights two important points. First, although the response of the lung to injury may be uniform in a histopathological sense, there is unlikely to be a single pathogenetic pathway. Second, circulating inflammatory mediators are likely to be important in modulating these processes, at least as far as distant insults are concerned. Inflammatory mediators, such as cytokines, are known to induce an acute inflammatory response in the microvasculature of the lung and other organs. Cells activated by such a process in turn produce more inflammatory mediators, leading to endothelial and epithelial cell damage and ultrastructural changes that cause increased permeability of the alveolar capillary membrane. Vasoactive mediators, including NO, cyclo-oxygenase (COX) products and endothelin-1 (ET-1), regulate vascular tone at a local level under physiological conditions, but alterations in their generation and site of release have been described in animal models of sepsis/ARDS, leading to disordered vascular control. In addition, activation of platelets and the complement and coagulation

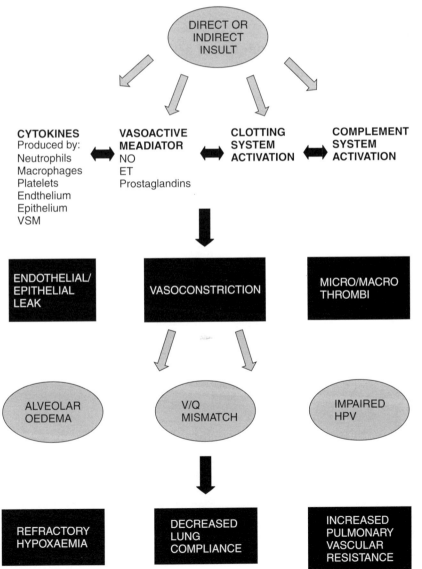

Figure 11.2 *Overview of the pathogenesis of ALI/ARDS. VSM, vascular smooth muscle; NO, nitric oxide; ET, endothelin; V/Q, perfusion/ventilation; HPV, hypoxic pulmonary vasoconstriction.*

cascades leads to the formation of microthrombi. The clinical consequences of these events are impaired hypoxic pulmonary vasoconstriction and ventilation – perfusion relationships leading to refractory hypoxaemia, alveolar oedema formation and increased pulmonary vascular resistance (Fig. 11.2).

Neutrophil-dependent lung injury

Histological specimens from the lungs of patients dying with ARDS demonstrate sequestration and subsequent migration of neutrophils into lung tissue. In addition, BAL fluid taken from patients early in the course of the syndrome demonstrates neutrophilia,[14] the extent of which correlates with levels of granulocyte colony stimulating factors (G-CSF) and dictates disease progression and severity. Increased levels of the neutrophil secretory products elastase and collagenase have also been described. *In vitro*, neutrophil-mediated cell injury can only occur when the cell is in close proximity to the capillary endothelium. In the pulmonary capillary, this is likely to occur by two mechanisms (Fig. 11.3):

- neutrophils become rigid, inhibiting flow through smaller capillaries,

- increased adhesion between the neutrophil and the endothelium develops, secondary to up-regulation of adhesion molecules on both cells (see the section on endothelial activation).

Once activated and in the presence of high applied oxygen concentrations (FiO_2), neutrophils and macrophages release reactive O_2 species, leading to the production of the toxic hydroxyl radical, which, in the presence of reactive iron species, causes oxidative damage to lipids and proteins.

Despite such evidence suggesting a central role for the neutrophil in the evolution of ARDS, neutropenic patients can develop ARDS, and increasing circulating neutrophil numbers with G-CSF does not lead to more severe lung injury.

Endothelial activation

The endothelial cell exerts active control over vascular tone, thrombosis and permeability, through the synthesis and release of a wide variety of substances (Table 11.4, Fig. 11.4). Under inflammatory conditions, the endothelial cell is activated, leading to a loss of vascular integrity, increased expression of leucocyte adhesion molecules, HLA molecules and cytokines, and becomes pro-thrombotic. Two stages

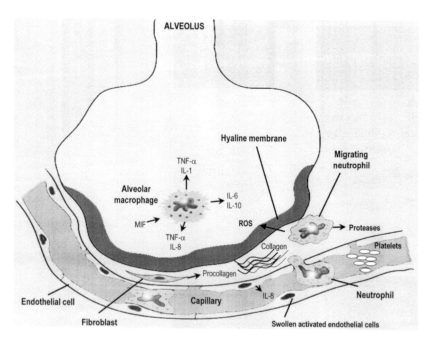

Figure 11.3 *Early events in the pathogenesis of ARDS, with particular reference to neutrophil-mediated lung injury. IL-1, IL-6, IL-8, IL-10, interleukins 1, 6, 8, 10; TNF-α, tumour necrosis factor-α; ROS, reactive oxygen species; MIF, macrophage inhibitory factor.*

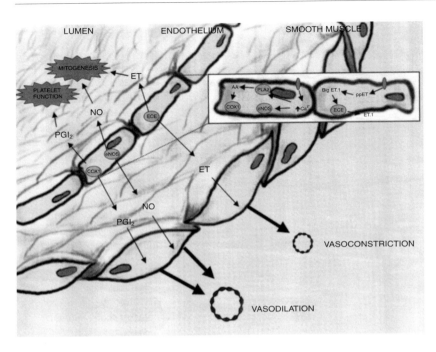

Figure 11.4 *The maintenance of vascular homeostasis by the tonic release of mediators such as nitric oxide (NO), prostacyclin (PGI$_2$) and endothelin-1 (ET-1). AA, arachidonic acid; PLA2, phospholipase A2; COX1, cyclo-oxygenase 1; ppET, endothelin; ECE, eicoanoids; eNOS,*

of activation occur. Type I activation does not require either *de-novo* protein synthesis or genotypic up-regulation. Endothelial cells retract from each other, express P-selectin leading to increased neutrophil adhesion, and release von Willebrand factor, which regulates platelet adherence to the subendothelium. By contrast, Type II activation requires up-regulation of mRNA expression and *de-novo* protein synthesis, particularly of cytokines and adhesion molecules.

There appear to be common intracellular control mechanisms involved in both processes, such as those mediated through the intracellular messenger nuclear factor-κB (NF-κB). The endothelium produces vascular cell adhesion (VCAM-1) and intercellular adhesion (ICAM-1 and ICAM-2) molecules and E-selectin, facilitating the binding of leucocytes. Simultaneously, activated neutrophils express a complementary sequence of surface adhesion molecules termed integrins, the most significant of which is a CD11/CD18 complex that determines the migration of neutrophils into the interstitium. This adhesion cascade is reviewed in detail elsewhere,[15] but is associated with increased expression of endotoxin/cytokine-inducible genes that are significant in determining vasomotor control, particularly those encoding for the production of NO, ET-1 and COX products (Fig. 11.5). These

mediators and their role in modulating the vascular control under inflammatory conditions have recently been reviewed.[16] Recent work has demonstrated that the underlying smooth muscle can be an important source of vasoactive mediators under inflammatory conditions,[17] and human systemic and pulmonary artery smooth muscle can both produce ET-1 and COX products when stimulated with cytokines *in vitro*.[17–19] These cells may be particularly important if the endothelial layer is dysfunctional or missing. Additionally, autocrine mechanisms may cause vasoconstriction, cellular proliferation and vascular remodelling.

Epithelial injury

The acute phase of ARDS is characterized by the presence of protein-rich fluid in the alveolar space. Consequently, there must be increased permeability of the alveolar-capillary membrane due to breaches of both endothelial and epithelial cells. The degree of epithelial cell damage is increasingly recognized as clinically significant and is an important predictor of outcome.[14] The normal epithelium is composed of both type I and type II pneumocytes. Type I cells are more prevalent under normal conditions

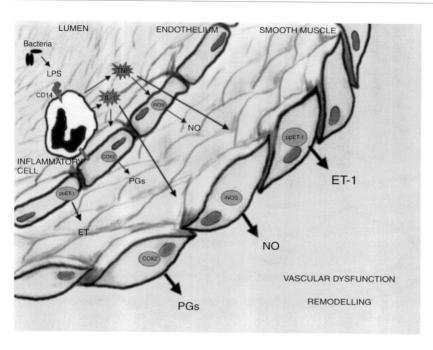

Figure 11.5 *Disruption of vascular control mechanisms in sepsis. Under these conditions the smooth muscle itself is an important producer of these mediators. The relative proportions of the vasodilators nitric oxide (NO) and prostacyclin (PGI₂) and the vasoconstrictor and mitogen, endothelin-1 (ET -1), determine the vascular response in the affected area. LPS, lipopolysaccharide; CD14, cluster of differentiation 14; ppET-1, prepro-endothelin 1; TNF, tumour necrosis factor; COX2, cyclo-oxygenase 2; IL-1, interleukin 1; iNOS, inducible nitric oxide synthase.*

(90:10), but type II cells are more resistant to injury, as well as having important functions such as surfactant production, ion transport and differentiation to type I cells after injury. Damage to type II cells may:

- disrupt fluid transport, leading to impaired fluid removal,
- impair surfactant production,
- influence the repair process, increasing the likelihood of fibrosis developing.

Resolution

Enhancing natural resolution processes may be as important as attenuating early inflammation. Alveolar oedema is cleared by an active process involving sodium transport from the distal airways into the interstitium, followed by movement of water across the epithelium. It now appears that this process involves specialized water channels termed aquaporins, located on type I cells. However, little is known about the regulation of these channels. The ability to clear fluid appears to be associated with a better prognosis. Soluble protein is removed by passive diffusion, whereas insoluble protein is removed by endocytosis across epithelial cells and phagocytosis by macrophages. Epithelial integrity is restored

by type II cells, which re-epithelialize the denuded alveolar epithelium by differentiating into type I cells. This process presumably requires adhesion, spreading, migration and proliferation of the type II cells. Although this is an area of active research, such processes require cell–cell and cell–matrix interactions, which are probably mediated by epithelial integrins. In addition, such processes need modulators such as cytokines and growth factors. Tumour growth factor-β (TGF-β) is of particular interest as it has the ability to regulate the expression of epithelial integrins, as well as being a potent inhibitor of epithelial cell proliferation.

Resolution of accumulated cellular infiltrate and fibrosis must also occur. Apoptosis, or 'programmed cell death', may be involved in clearing neutrophils. Certainly, markers of apoptosis are high in the pulmonary oedema fluid of patients and such fluid induces epithelial cell apoptosis *in vitro*. This is likely to represent an important area for future research.

Fibrosis

In those patients in whom resolution does not occur, progression to the late stage of ARDS, characterized by intra-alveolar and interstitial fibrosis, is inevitable. Interestingly, fibrosis appears to occur rapidly and is present as early as the first week. The development of fibrosis is associated with hypoxaemia, reduced lung compliance, ventilator dependence and a poor outcome. N-terminal procollagen III (N-PCP-III), a precursor of collagen III, is actively synthesized in the normal lung. N-PCP-III levels are raised in BAL fluid and in the serum of ARDS patients as early as 24–48 hours after ventilation.[20,21] In addition, BAL fluid taken from ARDS patients within 48 hours is also intensely mitogenic for fibroblasts. Such data suggest that the mechanisms capable of producing fibrosis are in place early in the course of the disease. Although epithelial, endothelial and smooth muscle cells can produce collagen, the principal source is the fibroblast. Cytokines released from these cell types may also stimulate collagen synthesis and fibroblast proliferation. In addition, macrophages are an important source of TGF-β, insulin-like growth factor (IGF-1) and ET-1, which are all important pro-fibrotic cytokines.

Cytokines

Cytokines are released by cells under stress and may be involved in the initiation and progression of ARDS. Broadly, there are pro-inflammatory cytokines, such as tumour necrosis factor-α (TNF-α), interleukin-1β (IL-1β), interferon-γ (IFN-γ) and IL-8, and anti-inflammatory cytokines, such as IL-10, IL-11 and macrophage inhibitory factor (MIF), as well as related molecules such as IL-1 receptor antagonist (IL-1 Ra) and soluble TNF receptor and antibodies against IL-8.[14] In inflammatory conditions, there seems to be a local or systemic imbalance of these cytokines. The balance may change with the progression of the disease. Clearly, in studying the role of cytokines in ARDS, biological activity is of paramount importance, rather than simply the levels.

Other cells implicated in acute respiratory distress syndrome

EOSINOPHILS

Eosinophil activation has been related to lung damage in ARDS. Levels of eosinophil cationic protein (ECP) are higher in the BAL fluid taken from patients with ARDS than in that from controls and the levels relate to severity of the disease.

MAST CELLS

Mast cells have been detected in 50% of cases of progressive ARDS studied by immunohistochemical methods. Although appearing after the onset of fibrosis, tryptase, stored in mast cell granules, is a mitogen for fibroblasts in vitro and may contribute to the propagation of the process.

PLATELETS

Progressive thrombocytopenia occurs in 50% of patients with non-traumatic ALI, its severity paralleling the development of worsening hypoxaemia. At least some of these platelets appear to be trapped in the lung microvasculature, as autopsy specimens demonstrate thrombi containing enmeshed platelets, neutrophils and fibrin. Platelets, once activated, release the contents of their granules, which have the potential to participate in the pathogenesis of lung injury. Serotonin and thromboxane can cause vasoconstriction, whereas TGF-α, TGF-β and platelet-derived growth factor (PDGF) are mitogens and may therefore take part in vascular remodelling and fibrosis. However, despite many animal and clinical studies, it is still not known whether the changes in platelet numbers and function are directly related to the pathogenesis of ARDS or merely an epiphenomenon.

MACROPHAGES

Macrophages produce pro-inflammatory cytokines such as IL-1β and TNF-α as well as growth factors such as PDGF, TGF-β, IGF and ET-1. They may therefore play a key role in both the initiation and propagation of ARDS. However, whereas high neutrophil counts in BAL fluid from patients with ARDS are associated with more severe disease and a worse outcome, an increase in BAL fluid macrophage count is associated with the resolution of lung injury and improved survival. Thus, the macrophage appears to be capable of both pro-inflammatory and anti-inflammatory actions.

Ventilator-induced lung injury

Substantial interest has recently been directed at the role of mechanical ventilation in the development and propagation of lung injury. Studies have demonstrated that ventilation at low tidal volumes, compared with traditional tidal volumes, can improve outcome for patients with ARDS. Lower plasma levels of IL-6 were also found in those patients ventilated at lower tidal volumes.[22] Several animal experiments have indicated that ventilation at high tidal volumes leads to damage to the epithelium and endothelium, with consequent inflammation, oedema formation, atelectasis, hypoxaemia and the release of cytokines. Alveolar over-distension, together with repeated collapse and re-opening of atelectatic alveoli, also results in an increase in systemic cytokine levels and this may contribute to the development and propagation of MODS. A recent report demonstrated that the use of a 'lung-protective' ventilatory strategy reduced both the pulmonary and systemic cytokine responses.[23]

PULMONARY AND SYSTEMIC MARKERS OF LUNG INJURY

Three reasons exist for measuring systemic markers in ARDS:

- they may identify patients likely to develop the syndrome in an 'at-risk' population,
- they may provide information concerning the pathogenesis of ARDS,
- they might represent a method for monitoring progress and predicting outcome.

Samples for analysis may be collected from blood (plasma/serum) or from the distal airways (pulmonary oedema or BAL fluid). The pros and cons of sampling oedema fluid or BAL fluid will not be discussed further, except to say that BAL is more widely performed but suffers from the complication of an unknown dilution factor of the alveolar fluid.

CD14 and lipopolysaccharide

CD14 is a pattern-recognition molecule present on the cell surface of macrophages and neutrophils. It is a receptor for lipopolysaccharide (LPS) complexes and LPS binding protein (LBP). In turn, CD14 employs 'toll-like' receptors for signal transduction. A soluble form of CD14 (sCD14) is released from cell membranes and complexes with LPS and mediates LPS-dependent response in CD14-negative cells, such as endothelial and epithelial cells. Soluble CD14 and LBP levels are significantly increased in BAL fluid from

patients with ARDS. In addition, the levels correlate with BAL total protein and neutrophil number, both major indices of lung inflammation. However, neither sCD14 nor LBP levels alone predict mortality. LPS itself has been measured in the plasma of patients at risk of and with ALI/ARDS. Unfortunately, there were conflicting results with regard to the predictive value of raised levels, although there were problems with patient selection and measurement methodology.

Early-response cytokines

TNF-α and IL-1β are early response cytokines produced by macrophages and neutrophils. They can induce epithelial and endothelial cells, fibroblasts and smooth muscle cells to produce further cytokines, thereby initiating the inflammatory cascade (see section on pathogenesis). TNF-α is produced initially in a membrane-associated 26-kD form, which is cleaved by TNF-α converting enzyme (TACE) into the soluble 17.5-kD cytokine.

TUMOUR NECROSIS FACTOR-α

Soluble TNF-α levels are increased in the plasma and BAL fluid of patients with ARDS. Studies have tried to establish a link between levels of plasma-soluble TNF-α and the risk of the development of ALI or ARDS. Disappointingly, the results have been mixed. It appears that circulating levels of TNF-α are more indicative of the extent of lung injury than of the actual diagnosis. In addition, the administration of anti-TNF-α receptor antibody does not reduce mortality in patients with sepsis. More recently, increased functionally active membrane-associated TNF-α on alveolar macrophages has been identified in patients with ARDS, suggesting that surface expression of functionally active TNF-α may be an important mechanism for TNF-α-mediated lung injury. This may partly explain the disappointing results from studies investigating the use of soluble TNF-α.

INTERLEUKIN-1β

IL-1β levels are increased and are biologically active in the BAL fluid from patients at risk from and in the early stages of ARDS. These levels are sustained throughout the course of the syndrome and persistently high concentrations are predictive of a poor outcome. Increased levels in BAL fluid from these patients are in part due to increased production by alveolar macrophagess. Plasma levels of IL-1β do not predict those patients at risk of developing ARDS.[14] IL-1β receptor antagonist (IL-1 Ra) is the naturally occurring antagonist of IL-1β and is elevated in patients with ARDS, but IL-1β is tenfold in excess of this, so that the equilibrium is shifted favouring a pro-inflammatory state. Low concentrations of IL-1 Ra and IL-10 (another anti-inflammatory cytokine) in the BAL fluid of patients in the early phase of ARDS are associated with a poor prognosis. IL-1β is able to initiate a cascade of inflammatory events, including the release of prostaglandins, increased synthesis of collagenases and the migration of neutrophils through the endothelium and the production of other inflammatory cytokines such as IL-8 and macrophage inflammatory protein-1 (MIP-1).

Chemokines

Chemokines are molecules that direct leucocyte migration. Two major classes exist: the α or CC chemokines, such as MIP-1, and the β or CXC chemokines, such as IL-8 and ENA-78, which are potent neutrophil chemotactic agents. Of these, IL-8 is by far the most studied in ARDS. IL-8 is detectable in the BAL fluid of patients at risk of developing ARDS and may be predictive of those who subsequently develop the established syndrome.[5] Alveolar macrophages are an abundant source of this chemokine when exposed to LPS, although other cells are able to produce it when exposed to cytokines such as TNF-α and IL-1β. IL-8 measured in BAL fluid correlates with its neutrophil concentrations, but not with the severity of the lung injury. Although early studies found that IL-8 levels were highest in the BAL fluid of non-survivors, subsequent studies suggest that levels do not predict an adverse clinical course. IL-8 cannot be easily measured in blood because of binding to red blood cells. Moreover, inhibitory factors such as endogenous immunoglubulin G (IgG) auto-antibodies and α2-macroglobulin bind and neutralize the molecule.

Interleukin-6

IL-6 was originally described as a B-cell growth factor although, in the context of inflammatory conditions, it is believed to be an 'orchestrator', stimulating acute-phase responses in the liver. It is produced by activated alveolar macrophages in response to other cytokines such as IL-1β and TNF-α. IL-6 could also be directly involved in the pathogenesis of ARDS by stimulating neutrophils to release elastase. IL-6 levels are raised in the BAL fluid of patients at risk for ARDS, and remain elevated throughout the course of the disease. However, concentrations do not predict the onset or outcome of ARDS. In addition, a soluble receptor, IL-6R, is raised in the BAL fluid of patients at risk and during the course of ARDS. Interestingly, this receptor is an agonist, unlike IL-1Ra. Recently, IL-6 levels in the plasma of patients with ARDS have been shown to be lower in those ventilated with protective, lower tidal volumes, suggesting a possible role for this cytokine in ventilator-induced lung injury.[22]

Interleukin-10

IL-10, as already mentioned, is an anti-inflammatory cytokine that is believed, like IL-4 and IL-13, to counteract or balance the pro-inflammatory cytokines. IL-10 is present in the BAL fluid of patients with ARDS, although in low quantities. Indeed, patients who die with ARDS appear to have very low levels of IL-10 in their BAL fluid.

Macrophage inhibitory factor

Macrophage inhibitory factor (MIF) has a complex role, antagonizing the effect of cortisol on cytokine production by alveolar macrophages. As such, MIF may act to sustain the inflammatory response. It is present in the BAL fluid of patients studied on the first day of ARDS, and immunoreactive MIF is detectable in isolated macrophages. MIF is also present in the BAL fluid of patients at risk of ARDS, and the concentration rises as the disease progresses.

Growth factors and collagen

Transforming growth factor-α (TGF-α) increases fibroblast collagen production and may be important in the development of fibrosis in ARDS. Indeed, TGF-α is present in the BAL fluid of patients with sustained ARDS, and high levels in BAL fluid on day 7 are associated with a poorer prognosis. TGF-α is also a mitogen for epithelial cells *in vitro*. Procollagen peptide III (PCP III) is a marker of collagen synthesis and is detectable in BAL fluid at the onset of ARDS, with high levels being associated with a poor prognosis. In addition, PDGFs are present that stimulate fibroblast proliferation *in vitro* and also the production of an angiogenic factor that is present in the BAL fluid in 70% of patients with ARDS. Clearly, more work is needed in this area as these and other growth factors are probably key mediators in the remodelling processes that occur in the lung during the course of the disease.

Coagulation cascade

Coagulation cascade activation is a feature of ARDS. However, conventional laboratory measurements of coagulation parameters do not distinguish between patients with and without ALI. Despite this, there is a wealth of evidence for coagulation abnormalities in the pathogenesis of ARDS. Fibrin deposition is found in the lungs as well as micro-emboli in the vasculature of patients with ARDS. The BAL fluid of patients with ARDS is pro-coagulant, containing tissue factor–factor VII/VIIa complexes, and it is therefore capable of activating the extrinsic coagulation cascade via the generation of factor X. This pro-coagulant property increases for 3 days following diagnosis and then decreases over a 2-week period. Although fibrin is present in the lungs of patients with ARDS, it has not been possible to detect thrombin in the BAL fluid of patients with ARDS. However, thrombin levels are increased in the lungs of patients with pulmonary fibrosis associated with systemic sclerosis. Apart from its pro-coagulant properties, including platelet aggregation, thrombin is also capable of increasing vascular permeability, inducing pro-inflammatory cytokines and promoting fibrosis, by inducing fibroblast proliferation and the production of growth factors. There is also evidence for reduced fibrinolysis, encouraging extravascular fibrin deposition. Plasminogen levels are higher in patients with ARDS compared to controls and those at risk of ARDS, although most plasminogen appears to be bound to local inhibitors. In addition, there appear to be reduced amounts of naturally occurring anticoagulants such as antithrombin III, protein C and protein S. There is also

evidence of increased antifibrinolytic activity in the BAL fluid of ARDS patients, with increased levels of urokinase inhibitors such as plasminogen activator inhibitor (PAI-1). However, another study found that plasma levels of PAI-1 (and factor VIII) were not predictive of the development of ARDS in patients at risk.

Reactive oxygen species

Once activated, and in the presence of the high O_2 concentrations frequently necessary to support patients with ARDS, neutrophils and macrophages release ROS, leading to the production of the hydroxyl radical, which, in the presence of reactive iron species, causes oxidative damage to lipids and proteins. Xanthine oxidase is a key enzyme in the production of ROS, and its enhanced production as well as the increased production of its substrates xanthine and hypoxanthine are seen in non-survivors of ARDS, suggesting that they experience more oxidative stress than survivors.[7] Increased levels of the free radical species hydrogen peroxide (H_2O_2), formed by the action of O_2 radicals and water, have also been demonstrated in urine in the first 48 hours in patients with ARDS compared to controls. As these pro-oxidant molecules are generally unstable, and therefore difficult to measure, it is sometimes easier to measure anti-oxidant molecules in patients with ARDS. Plasma levels of catalase, an enzyme that scavenges H_2O_2, are higher in septic patients with lung injury than in those without. In addition, increased serum levels of catalase and manganese superoxide dismutase (SOD) have been shown to predict the development of lung injury in an at-risk population. Furthermore, plasma iron-binding anti-oxidant activity is lower in patients with ARDS than in controls and this correlates with the percentage iron saturation of transferrin.[6] Indeed, in patients with ARDS and abnormal liver function, low-molecular-mass iron has been detected in plasma, and transferrin was shown to be fully saturated with iron, resulting in greatly decreased anti-oxidant protection. Caeruloplasmin is another primary plasma anti-oxidant and acute phase protein, capable of binding to iron and therefore regulating iron-dependent oxidative reactions. Both proteins are raised in BAL fluid and in the serum of patients at risk of and with established lung injury. However, despite high levels of caeruloplasmin in the BAL fluid of patients with ARDS, the ferroxidase activity appears diminished, perhaps due to proteolytic activity.

Selectins

Neutrophils migrate from the vascular compartment by a multistage process (discussed above in the section on pathogenesis). Selectins form a family of molecules that are important in the early attachment of neutrophils. E-selectin and P-selectin are expressed on the surface of the endothelium, whereas L-selectin is expressed only on leucocytes. Soluble L-selectin (sL-selectin) inhibits neutrophil binding to endothelial cells *in vitro* in a concentration-dependent manner. Plasma levels of sL-selectin are lower in patients at risk of or who develop ARDS. In addition, low values are associated with an increased mortality. Reduced levels of sL-selectin may therefore represent a marker of panendothelial activation in ARDS.

THE WAY FORWARD: INVESTIGATING 'AT-RISK' POPULATIONS

Predicting which patients are at risk of developing ALI or ARDS is potentially important for future studies of both the pathogenesis of ARDS and potential therapeutic interventions. This may be particularly relevant to the identification of genetic polymorphisms that increase the likelihood of a patient developing lung injury following a specific insult. However, there are several problems with defining the 'risk' or 'latent' period:

- only 5% of patients with a risk factor for ARDS develop the full syndrome,[24]
- this period may be very variable and can range from hours to days if the insult is distant from the lung,
- studies examining this risk period may select their data from different times, often very late in this period.

Studies into the subclinical lung damage will nevertheless provide opportunities for defining the early disease mechanisms. In support of this last point, reports have been published describing altered pulmonary levels of IL-8[5] and blood levels of sL-selectin and neutrophil elastase within 90 min of multiple trauma, pancreatitis and perforation of a viscus, identifying a group of patients at very high risk of ARDS.

CONCLUSIONS

Despite 30 years of interest in ARDS, its precise pathogenesis remains elusive. Many different cells and mediators are involved. Consequently, manipulation of a single mediator is unlikely to produce major therapeutic benefit. Determining which patients are at risk of developing ARDS may prove to be of particular importance. This will involve not only measuring markers in BAL fluid and plasma as early as possible in the course of the disease, but also determining which patients are genetically predisposed to develop the syndrome.

REFERENCES

1. Ashbaugh, DG, Bigelow, DB, Petty, TL, *et al.* Acute respiratory distress in adults. *Lancet* 1967; **2**: 319–23.
2. Bernard, GR, Artigas, A, Brigham, KL, *et al.* The American–European Consensus Conference on ARDS. Definitions, mechanisms, relevant outcomes, and clinical trial coordination. *Am J Respir Crit Care Med* 1994; **149**: 818–24.
3. Roupie, E, Lepage, E, Wysocki, M, *et al.* Prevalence, etiologies and outcome of the acute respiratory distress syndrome among hypoxemic ventilated patients. SRLF Collaborative Group on Mechanical Ventilation. *Société de Reanimation de Langue Française*. Intensive Care Med 1999; **25**: 20.
4. Luhr, OR, Antonsen, K, Karlsson, M, *et al.* Incidence and mortality after acute respiratory failure and acute respiratory distress syndrome in Sweden, Denmark, and Iceland. The ARF Study Group. *Am J Respir Crit Care Med* 1999; **159**: 1849–61.
5. Donnelly, SC, Strieter, RM, Kunkel, SL, *et al.* Interleukin-8 and development of adult respiratory distress syndrome in at-risk patient groups. *Lancet* 1993; **341**: 643–7.
6. Gutteridge, JM, Quinlan, GJ, Mumby, S, *et al.* Primary plasma antioxidants in adult respiratory distress syndrome patients: changes in iron-oxidizing, iron-binding, and free radical-scavenging proteins. *J Lab Clin Med* 1994; **124**: 263–73.

7. Quinlan, GJ, Lamb, NJ, Tilley, R, *et al.* Plasma hypoxanthine levels in ARDS: implications for oxidative stress, morbidity, and mortality. *Am J Respir Crit Care Med* 1997; **155**: 479–84.

8. Gattinoni, L, Pelosi, P, Suter, PM, *et al.* Acute respiratory distress syndrome caused by pulmonary and extrapulmonary disease. Different syndromes? *Am J Respir Crit Care Med* 1998; **158**: 3–11.

9. Abel, SJ, Finney, SJ, Brett, SJ, *et al.* Reduced mortality in association with the acute respiratory distress syndrome (ARDS). *Thorax* 1998; **53**: 292–4.

10. Krafft, P, Fridrich, P, Pernerstorfer, T, *et al.* The acute respiratory distress syndrome: definitions, severity and clinical outcome. An analysis of 101 clinical investigations. *Intensive Care Med* 1996; **22**: 519–29.

11. Rangel-Frausto, MS, Pittet, D, Costigan, M, *et al.* The natural history of the systemic inflammatory response syndrome (SIRS). A prospective study. *J Am Med Assoc* 1995; **273**: 117–23.

12. Marshall, JC, Cook, DJ, Christou, NV, *et al.* Multiple organ dysfunction score: a reliable descriptor of a complex clinical outcome. *Crit Care Med* 1995; **23**: 1638–52.

13. Sinclair, DG, Braude, S, Haslam, PL, *et al.* Pulmonary endothelial permeability in patients with severe lung injury. Clinical correlates and natural history. *Chest* 1994; **106**: 535–9.

14. Pittet, JF, Mackersie, RC, Martin, TR, *et al.* Biological markers of acute lung injury: prognostic and pathogenetic significance. *Am J Respir Crit Care Med* 1997; **155**: 1187–205.

15. Albelda, SM, Smith, CW, Ward, PA. Adhesion molecules and inflammatory injury. *Faseb J* 1994; **8**: 504–12.

16. Wort, SJ, Evans, TW. The role of the endothelium in modulating vascular control in sepsis and related conditions. *Br Med Bull* 1999; **55**: 30–48.

17. Woods, M, Mitchell, JA, Wood, EG, *et al.* Endothelin-1 is induced by cytokines in human vascular smooth muscle cells: evidence for intracellular endothelin-converting enzyme. *Mol Pharmacol* 1999; **55**: 902–9.

18. Jourdan, KB, Evans, TW, Lamb, NJ, *et al.* Autocrine function of inducible nitric oxide synthase and cyclooxygenase-2 in proliferation of human and rat pulmonary artery smooth-muscle cells: species variation. *Am J Respir Cell Mol Biol* 1999; **21**: 105–10.

19. Wort, SJ, Mitchell, JA, Woods, M, *et al.* The prostacyclin-mimetic cicaprost inhibits endogenous endothelin-1 release from human pulmonary artery smooth muscle cells. *J Cardiovasc Pharmacol* 2000; **36**: S410–13.

20. Marshall, RP, Bellingan, G, Webb, S, *et al.* Fibroproliferation occurs early in the acute respiratory distress syndrome and impacts on outcome. *Am J Respir Crit Care Med* 2000; **162**: 1783–8.

21. Chesnutt, AN, Matthay, MA, Tibayan, FA, *et al.* Early detection of type III procollagen peptide in acute lung injury. Pathogenetic and prognostic significance. *Am J Respir Crit Care Med* 1997; **156**: 840–5.

22. The Acute Respiratory Distress Syndrome Network. Ventilation with lower tidal volumes as compared with traditional tidal volumes for acute lung injury and the acute respiratory distress syndrome. *N Engl J Med* 2000; **342**: 1301–8.

23. Ranieri, VM, Suter, PM, Tortorella, C, *et al* Effect of mechanical ventilation on inflammatory mediators in patients with acute respiratory distress syndrome: a randomized controlled trial. *J Am Med Assoc* 1999; **282**: 54–61.

24. Baumann, WR, Jung, RC, Koss, M, *et al.* Incidence and mortality of adult respiratory distress syndrome: a prospective analysis from a large metropolitan hospital. *Crit Care Med* 1986; **14**: 1–4.

25. Murray, JF, Matthay, MA, Luce, JM, Flick, MR. An expanded definition of the adult respiratory distress syndrome. *Am Rev Respir Dis* 1988; **138**: 720.

26. Bernard, GR, Artigas, A, Brigham, KL, *et al.* The American European Consensus Conference on ARDS. Definitions, mechanisms, relevant outcomes, and clinical trial coordination. *Am J Respir Crit Care Med* 1994; **149**: 818–24.

27. American College of Chest Physicians/Society of Critical Care Medicine Consensus Conference. Definitions for sepsis and organ failure and guidelines for the use of innovative therapies in sepsis. *Crit Care Med* 1992; **20**: 864–74.

12

Management of acute lung injury

KEITH G HICKLING AND ANDREW BERSTEN

INTRODUCTION

Until recently the mortality (50–60% in most studies) amongst patients with the acute respiratory distress syndrome (ARDS) has remained unchanged since the condition was first described, despite increased understanding of its pathophysiology and the use of specific treatments directed at these pathological processes. The recognition that mechanical ventilation can itself cause acute lung injury (ALI), and may have actually contributed to the high mortality rate, has led to the development of 'lung-protective' ventilation strategies that have resulted in improved outcome. A number of uncontrolled studies report mortality rates of 12–30% using lung-protective ventilation (Table 12.1), a mortality lower than historical controls. Two randomized trials have shown marked reductions in mortality in patients managed with lung-protective ventilation, from 71% to 38%, $p < 0.001$,[11] and from 39.8% to 31%, $p = 0.007$.[12] However, three other randomized trials have not been able to demonstrate a reduction in mortality, although the explanation may be that the control groups were not exposed to sufficient levels of lung distension to be injurious. As the potential for causing ventilator-induced lung injury (VILI), and its

associated morbidity, has been recognized, the goal of mechanical ventilation in ARDS has shifted from achieving optimum oxygenation to the avoidance of VILI. The extent to which these goals differ is, however, unclear.

VENTILATOR-INDUCED LUNG INJURY

Animal studies have shown that mechanical ventilation produces an acute parenchymal lung injury that is histologically very similar to that seen in ARDS. This is associated with an inflammatory response in the lung, characterized by granulocyte infiltration, the release of pro-inflammatory and anti-inflammatory cytokines and chemokines into the alveolar spaces,[13] and increased microvascular permeability in the lung and systemic tissues. Studies have also shown that VILI results in the release of cytokines into the systemic circulation in both animals and patients with ARDS.[13] In animals, following the instillation of bacteria into the trachea, injurious ventilation resulted in a high frequency of positive blood cultures (termed 'bacterial translocation' from the lung), whereas blood cultures were negative in most animals ventilated with non-injurious ventilation.

Table 12.1 *Uncontrolled studies of outcome in ARDS managed with lung-protective ventilation and permissive hypercapnia*

n	Patients	Management	Mortality (%)	Reference
50	ARDS, LIS > 2.5	PH, PIP < 30–40 cmH$_2$O always <40 cmH$_2$O	16	Hickling *et al.* (1990)[1]
9	ARDS	PH	22	Toth *et al.* (1992)[2]
49	Severe ARDS referred for ECCO$_2$R	PH < ECCO$_2$R (24), NO (7), FPC	24	Lewandowski *et al.* (1992)[3]
53	ARDS, LIS > 2.5	PH, PIP < 30–40 cmH$_2$O	26	Hickling *et al.* (1994)[4]
20	ARDS, ECMO crit LIS 3.6 ± 0.2	PH, NO, TGI, prone positioning	30	Levy *et al.* (1995)[5]
53	ARDS, LIS > 2.5	Mild PH, PH > 7.3, PPL 39 ± 15, PIP 44 ± 16	40	Thomsen *et al.* (1994)[6]
40	Children with ARDS	PH, PCV, PIP < 35–40 PaCO$_2$ 71 ± 23 mmHg	30	Nakagawa and Bohn (1995)[7]
23	Children with ARDS LIS > 2.5	PH, PIP < 35 cmH$_2$O, PaCO$_2$ 39–94 mmHg	17.4	Botero *et al.* (1995)[8]
54	Children, burns	PIP < 40 cmH$_2$O, PaCO$_2$ 39–111 mmHg	0	Sheridan *et al.* (1995)[9]
25	Trauma/sepsis	Consensus criteria LIS ≥ 2.5	12	Stocker *et al.* (1997)[10]

PH, permissive hypercapnia; LIS, lung injury score; NO, nitric oxide inhalation; TGI, tracheal gas insufflation; FPC, frequent body position changes; PCV, pressure-control ventilation; PIP, peak inspiratory pressure; 1979 ECMO study criteria, criteria used for selecting patients for entry to the 1979 randomized trial of extracorporeal membrane oxygenation in severe ARDS.

> Ventilation-induced lung injury may lead to a systemic inflammatory response, organ dysfunction and even sepsis.

These findings have led to speculation that VILI may result in the systemic inflammatory response syndrome (SIRS). This could cause, or contribute to, the development of the multiple organ dysfunction syndrome (MODS) and thus to increased mortality from MODS and associated sepsis. A *post-hoc* analysis of data from one trial[14] showed that patients with ARDS randomized to lung-protective ventilation developed significantly less remote organ dysfunction (especially renal dysfunction) than controls. The number of organs failing during the study period correlated with the change in plasma interleukin-6 (IL-6), tumour necrosis factor-α (TNF-α) and IL-1β concentrations, lending further support to this hypothesis. These findings are important because most deaths of patients with ARDS are due to MODS, often associated with sepsis, rather than to respiratory failure. If VILI can contribute to the development of MODS, then modified ventilation strategies designed to avoid VILI could result in a substantial reduction in mortality rate. These findings provide a plausible mechanism to explain the substantial reduction in mortality rate seen with lung-protective ventilation strategies.

> The aspects of mechanical ventilation resulting in VILI in animal models are end-inspiratory overdistension or end-expiratory collapse and tidal reinflation.

It is important to understand that it is regional lung volume, not high airway pressure, that is important in causing injury. The term volutrauma has therefore been suggested, rather than barotrauma, to describe such injury. When chest and abdominal strapping is applied to prevent thoracic hyperinflation, the ventilation of animals with very high airway pressures does not result in VILI. In contrast, when the animals were ventilated with negative-pressure ventilation, high peak lung volume resulted in VILI, even with low (atmospheric) airway pressure. This is not surprising and simply illustrates that it is the *transpulmonary* pressure, not the airway pressure alone, that determines lung distension and associated injury. This is important in considering the effects of spontaneous respiratory muscle activity and abnormal chest wall compliance during mechanical ventilation (see below).

The detailed mechanisms resulting in VILI have not yet been determined, but it is thought that excessive stretch of alveolar walls, and perhaps of small airways, may provide signals for the release of cytokines. It has also been shown that lung capillary stress failure, resulting from high lung microvascular pressure, occurs to a greater extent when lung volume is high. Capillary wall stress is a composite determined by both transmicrovascular pressure and alveolar wall stretch. This process may also be important in causing VILI and may account for the 'bacterial translocation' from the lung. Accordingly, therefore, high microvascular pressure may contribute to VILI during injurious ventilation. High alveolar wall stress occurs with excessive peak lung volume (regional or global) at end-inspiration. High tissue stresses during inflation may occur at the interfaces between atelectatic and aerated lung, even in the absence of high airway pressures, if end-expiratory collapse and tidal re-inflation occur with each breath.

In animal models, VILI associated with such end-expiratory collapse can be prevented by using sufficient PEEP to prevent collapse.

In most studies, for any degree of peak lung distension, higher positive end-expiratory pressure (PEEP) – and higher end-expiratory volume and therefore lower tidal volume – has been associated with less VILI. This has suggested that the goals in mechanical ventilation should be to use sufficient PEEP to prevent end-expiratory collapse and to limit tidal volume to avoid end-inspiratory over-distension. However, the best method of selecting an appropriate tidal volume and PEEP level has not yet been agreed. The physiological basis for making this selection is discussed below.

THE LUNG IN ACUTE RESPIRATORY DISTRESS SYNDROME

The compliance of aerated lung in ARDS appears to be normal.

Using computerized tomography (CT) scans, Gattinoni and colleagues have demonstrated that the reduced lung compliance usually seen in early ARDS is not a result of a uniform increase in elastic recoil of lung, but a reduced amount of aerated lung. The remaining lung is non-aerated and does not contribute to ventilation. The amount of aerated lung may be only half to one-third of normal, but its specific compliance (defined as compliance per unit weight of aerated lung tissue) is probably relatively normal. The use of a tidal volume of 10–15 mL kg^{-1}, as recommended in the past, will therefore result in over-distension of aerated lung, indicated by increased peak inspiratory pressure (PIP) and end-inspiratory plateau pressure (P_{PL}), and may result in VILI. If the specific compliance is indeed normal, then the highest level of P_{PL} that can safely be applied in ARDS without over-distending the aerated lung should be the same as in a normal lung. It has been recommended that P_{PL} should be limited to 35 cmH$_2$O in ARDS.[15] It is perhaps surprising that the specific compliance of aerated lung is normal, because it is known that surfactant is dysfunctional in ARDS. If the specific compliance was overestimated, and is actually reduced, it is possible that a higher P_{PL} could be acceptable. However, preliminary data (unpublished) suggest that a $P_{PL} > 32$–35 cmH$_2$O is associated with worse outcome, suggesting that a higher P_{PL} may be injurious and that specific compliance is relatively normal. Other evidence suggests significant surfactant dysfunction, both in ARDS and animal models of ALI. Perhaps inhomogeneity of surfactant distribution and function in ARDS may account for this conflicting evidence. Further studies are clearly needed.

Some of the non-aerated lung can be re-inflated when exposed to a sufficient transpulmonary pressure. This occurs predominantly in the dependent regions (i.e. posteriorly in supine patients) and redistributes rapidly when patients are placed in the prone position. The collapse of the dependent lung regions appears to be a result of compression by the weight of the overlying lung; the amount of PEEP required to prevent end-expiratory collapse at any lung level is similar to the superimposed pressure from the weight of the lung above this level.[16] The lung thus behaves like a wet sponge: the distribution of water is relatively uniform throughout, but the lower regions are compressed by those above.

The amount of PEEP required to prevent end-expiratory collapse should be equal to the hydrostatic pressure resulting from the overlying lung. This is usually not more than 15–20 cmH$_2$O, although some additional PEEP may be required to overcome surface tension forces favouring collapse. The prevention of end-expiratory collapse is the main mechanism by which PEEP improves oxygenation in ARDS. An important implication of these findings is that, if sufficient PEEP is applied to prevent collaps, the non-dependent regions will be moderately distended even at end-expiration. A low tidal volume is thus required to prevent over-distension injury. In the later stages of ARDS, the pathophysiology changes and inflammation and fibrosis are more prominent and PEEP less effective in achieving lung aeration and improving oxygenation. PEEP is also less effective in ARDS due to direct pulmonary insults (such as pneumonia) rather than to extrapulmonary causes of ARDS. Unilateral lung involvement, with pneumonia or other processes, also frequently results in a poor or even paradoxical response to PEEP. PEEP may cause little recruitment of the affected lung and over-distension of the relatively normal lung may increase pulmonary vascular resistance and divert pulmonary blood flow to the consolidated lung, thus increasing intrapulmonary shunt. Lateral positioning, with the consolidated lung downwards, may also increase blood flow to the consolidated lung and increase shunt.

VENTILATION STRATEGIES

VILI develops rapidly, within minutes to hours, so it is important that lung-protective ventilation is applied from the start. Although supporting spontaneous breathing is preferred, controlled mechanical ventilation, and even muscle paralysis, may be required. Pressure support should be titrated to reduce excessive work. However, there is no agreement about what represents excessive respiratory work, but tachypnoea (>35–45 min^{-1}) associated with excessive intercostal in-drawing and accessory muscle use should probably be avoided. Tachycardia, hypertension and sweating may also indicate excessive respiratory work, but may simply result from hypercapnia without necessarily a high workload. Dyspnoea, in conscious patients, may require the use of sedation or increased ventilatory support. If increased support in these circumstances results in an excessive tidal volume, further respiratory depression or paralysis should be considered (see below).

Lung recruitment and the open-lung approach

As discussed above, the role of PEEP is to prevent end-expiratory collapse. However, as expected from LaPlace's Law, alveoli or small airways that have collapsed require a higher pressure to re-inflate them (the opening pressure) than to keep them open. Re-inflation may also occur only gradually over several minutes. Even in normal lungs, a sustained inflation of 30–40 cmH$_2$O is required to achieve re-inflation after collapse has occurred during thoracotomy. In ALI, the opening pressure in some lung regions may be as high as 45–60 cmH$_2$O. Therefore, once dependent collapse has occurred, the application of PEEP alone may not result in complete re-inflation.

It may be necessary to apply various 'recruitment manoeuvres' to achieve additional re-inflation and thus to improve oxygenation.

Different recruitment manoeuvres can be employed, such as:

- sustained inflation at 35–60 cmH$_2$O in the paralysed patient,
- continuous positive airway pressure (CPAP) at 30–50 cmH$_2$O, with pressure-support ventilation (PSV) of only 5–10 cmH$_2$O, during spontaneous breathing,
- a period of ventilation with a higher tidal volume and an end-inspiratory pause with a resulting P_{PL} of 35–60 cmH$_2$O.

These manoeuvres are usually applied for 30s to 2 min whilst monitoring the patient for hypotension and subsequently for a pneumothorax. Alternatively, the use of 'sighs' (the intermittent delivery of larger tidal volumes by the ventilator on a continuous basis) may be effective. Such manoeuvres are reasonably safe, but clinical experience is limited, particularly with airway pressures of 50–60 cmH$_2$O. In some patients, the result is a marked improvement in oxygenation. The use of recruitment and sufficient PEEP to prevent end-expiratory collapse has been called the 'open-lung approach' and the PEEP used to maintain full recruitment the 'open-lung PEEP'. Following a recruitment manoeuvre, a higher PEEP level may be required to maintain the recruitment and improved oxygenation than previously used.

Whether such 'open-lung' strategies result in less VILI, or in improved outcome, compared with approaches limiting P_{PL} but using PEEP in a more traditional manner (to provide adequate oxygenation with an inspired O_2 concentration of 60% or less) is unknown.

At present, recruitment manoeuvres should possibly be restricted to patients with moderate or severe hypoxaemia.

Similarly, 'de-recruitment' may occur when the airway pressure is allowed to fall during ventilator disconnection or suctioning. Such drops in tracheal pressure should be prevented as far as possible. Chest-wall compression during physiotherapy or loss of pressure when suctioning may also cause de-recruitment and may account for the hypoxaemia frequently observed following physiotherapy.

Expiratory muscle activity in patients with tachypnoea may oppose the effect of PEEP and decrease end-expiratory volume. Paralysis may then improve oxygenation.

Selection of tidal volume

Having used sufficient PEEP to prevent end-expiratory collapse, the tidal volume should be limited to achieve a safe P_{PL},[15] which is probably between 32 and 35 cmH_2O. This usually requires a tidal volume of <8 mL kg^{-1}, and often <6 mL kg^{-1}. However, in a trial of low tidal volume ventilation,[12] there was no significant interaction between tidal volume and static compliance, suggesting that a tidal volume of 6 mL kg^{-1} was associated with better outcome than in patients in whom the P_{PL} remained <35 cmH_2O but with a higher tidal volume. This requires confirmation.

Interpretation of end-inspiratory plateau pressure with abnormal chest-wall compliance

The P_{PL} required to produce a particular degree of end-inspiratory lung distension (with relaxed respiratory muscles) depends on both lung and chest-wall compliance. If chest-wall compliance is reduced (for example by pre-existing chest-wall abnormalities, chest-wall oedema or abdominal distension with high diaphragms), a higher P_{PL} will be required and end-inspiratory pleural pressure will be increased by the same amount.

Chest-wall compliance is reduced in many patients with ARDS, probably as a result of chest-wall oedema, abdominal distension or pleural effusions.

Thus, a higher P_{PL} may be acceptable in such patients. It is the transpulmonary pressure that determines lung distension and, in patients with abnormal chest-wall compliance, estimation of transpulmonary pressure using an oesophageal balloon may be helpful. The goal is to limit regional peak lung distension to a safe level.

Estimation of lung distension during spontaneous breathing

In the presence of spontaneous breathing, the interpretation of airway pressure traces is difficult and lung over-distension can occur with airway pressures in an apparently acceptable range. During volume-controlled ventilation (VCV), inspiratory muscle activity results in lower airway and pleural pressures than would otherwise occur, but transpulmonary pressure and lung volume are unaffected. Thus, an excessive tidal volume resulting in lung over-distension may be associated with a relatively low PIP or P_{PL}. During pressure-control ventilation (PCV) and PSV, spontaneous breathing will result in a lower pleural pressure and an increase in transpulmonary pressure and peak lung volume while airway pressure remains unchanged; again, lung over-distension may occur. If the ventilator settings are initially made during paralysis, subsequent breathing during VCV will not result in increased tidal volume (but, rather, the PIP and P_{PL} will decrease), whereas, with PCV, increased tidal volume and over-distension will occur. Even with low levels of PSV or PCV, a tidal volume >6 mL kg^{-1} commonly occurs. In the trial of Amato et al.,[11] tidal volume was limited to 6 mL kg^{-1} during spontaneous breaths; this may be important, although it can be difficult to accomplish in patients with high respiratory drive and may require a reduction in the inspiratory airway pressure to much less than 30 cmH$_2$O and the use of sedatives.

In our experience, the use of paralysis for 24–48 hours often allows adaptation to hypercapnia, and paralysis can then be discontinued and spontaneous breathing resumed with much lower respiratory drive, tidal volume and respiratory work. Amato *et al.* have used partial paralysis, with controlled infusions of muscle relaxants, with careful monitoring of expired tidal volume.[11] The interpretation of airway pressures during spontaneous breathing can be facilitated using an oesophageal balloon or by temporarily abolishing respiratory muscle activity using neuromuscular blockade or opiates. The expired tidal volume should be monitored and limited to that producing an acceptable P_{PL} during paralysis, and preferably to ≤6 mL kg^{-1}. Basic principles suggest that this is just as important as the limitation of P_{PL} during paralysis and therefore should be attempted at all times during ventilation, although this is not commonly the practice.

Selection of positive end-expiratory pressure and the pressure–volume curve

The best method of selecting open-lung PEEP is not clear. Collapse can be visualized on CT scans, but it is not feasible to perform frequent CT scans for this purpose. The respiratory inflation pressure–volume curve in ARDS usually has a sigmoid shape (as shown in Fig. 12.1), with lower and upper inflexion points (Pflex). It was previously believed that the lower Pflex indicates the pressure and volume range over which

re-inflation (recruitment) of collapsed lung units occurs and that no further recruitment occurs on the 'linear' portion above the lower Pflex because further recruitment would result in a continued increase in slope (upwards concavity). It has also been assumed that the upper Pflex indicates the beginning of lung over-distension. It has therefore been recommended that tidal ventilation should occur over a pressure range between the lower and upper Pflex.

However, a mathematical model of the ARDS lung[17] suggests that recruitment of previously collapsed lung units can continue over the whole length of the PV curve, that an upper inflection point can occur as recruitment stops or diminishes (without necessarily implying alveolar over-distension) and that the lower Pflex may not be closely related to open-lung PEEP.

The mathematical model incorporates gravitational superimposed pressure increasing from zero in the non-dependent regions to 15 cmH$_2$O in the dependent regions, in keeping with Gattinoni's concept. These findings have been supported by clinical studies and suggest that previous interpretations of the pressure–volume curve are incorrect.[18]

Figure 12.1 shows an example of a pressure-volume curve produced by a modified version of the mathematical model. As the pressure increases during inflation, collapsed alveoli in the non-dependent lung regions become inflated (recruited) when their opening pressure is exceeded, resulting in a greater number of aerated alveoli and therefore increasing compliance (i.e. pressure–volume slope) to produce

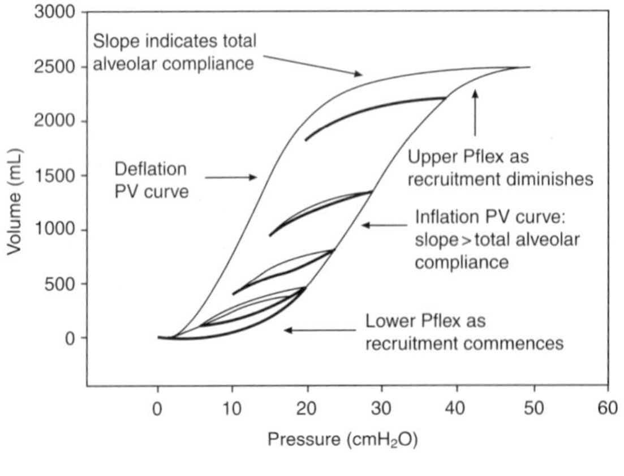

Figure 12.1 *Inflation and deflation static pressure–volume (PV) curve generated using a mathematical model of ARDS lungs. The lower and upper inflection points (Pflex) on the inflation curve are indicated. Recruitment continues during inflation over the whole length of the plot and the upper Pflex occurs as recruitment diminishes. Inflation (bold lines) and deflation tidal PV plots are also shown with tidal volume of 400 mL at incremental PEEP levels of 0, 5, 10, 15 and 20 cmH$_2$O. Opening pressures were normally distributed and varied from 5 to 35 cmH$_2$O. (See reference 17 for details of the model.)*

the lower Pflex. As each alveolus is recruited, it 'snaps' open and suddenly increases its volume from zero to that appropriate to its new transalveolar pressure. With each increment of pressure, the increase in volume in newly recruited alveoli is much greater than that of alveoli that were already aerated prior to the pressure increment. On the steep portion of the pressure–volume curve above the lower Pflex, most of the volume increment with each pressure increment (i.e. slope) is a result of these large volume increases as newly recruited alveoli snap open (i.e. to recruitment). The slope of this portion of the curve is much greater than the total compliance (sum of the individual compliances, or 'total alveolar compliance') of all of the inflated alveoli. When the rate of recruitment diminishes and finally stops, the slope decreases to that of the total alveolar compliance, causing an upper Pflex. The total compliance of all alveoli that were inflated at end-inspiration is shown by the slope of the deflation pressure–volume curve over the upper pressure range. When the pressure during deflation falls below open-lung PEEP, the dependent lung regions start to collapse, resulting in sudden decrements in volume as each alveolus collapses; this again results in a steepening of the curve. However, it is not possible to identify open-lung PEEP on the deflation curve, either with the model or in patients. If the assumptions of this model are correct, the lower Pflex indicates the commencement of recruitment and is unlikely to be closely related to open-lung PEEP, and the upper Pflex may also be greatly influenced by recruitment. Inflation and deflation tidal pressure–volume plots are shown in Figure 12.1 within the envelope of the inflation and deflation pressure–curves.

A method that has been widely used to determine 'optimum PEEP' is to increase PEEP progressively until the 'effective compliance' (tidal volume/[$P_{PL} - $ PEEP]) reaches a maximum. It was suggested that, when PEEP is increased above the lower Pflex of the pressure–volume curve, ventilation would occur on the steep portion, increasing effective compliance. Some data suggest that this is true in those who show no recruitment (i.e. upwards displacement on the volume axis) with PEEP; PEEP then simply moves the end-expiratory point further up on the same pressure–volume curve. However, such patients also show little improvement in oxygenation with PEEP. In patients showing recruitment with PEEP and improved oxygenation, there may be little change or

even a decrease in effective compliance as PEEP is increased (Fig. 12.2). As PEEP increases, there is little change in the tidal pressure–volume slope (effective compliance) because the end-expiratory volume increases (due to prevention of end-expiratory collapse by PEEP) by a similar amount to the end-inspiratory volume. As PEEP approaches open-lung PEEP, eliminating end-expiratory collapse, the effective compliance may decrease slightly. With a low tidal volume, the effective compliance may further increase with PEEP well above open-lung PEEP, because the P_{PL} continues to increase as PEEP increases, causing more end-inspiratory recruitment. This increases the number of aerated alveoli and therefore compliance.

An incremental PEEP trial with a low tidal volume is really testing the recruiting ability of the end-inspiratory pressure rather than the ability of PEEP to prevent end-expiratory collapse. Therefore, even oxygenation during an incremental PEEP trial, theoretically, would not be expected to be a good indicator of open-lung PEEP, and limited clinical and experimental data support this.

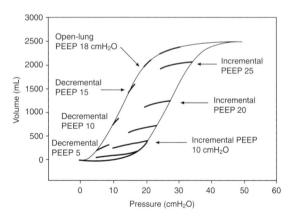

Figure 12.2 *Inflation and deflation pressure–volume (PV) curve generated by mathematical model of ARDS lungs. Inflation tidal PV plots are shown with tidal volume of 150 mL and incremental and decremental positive end-expiratory pressure (PEEP) from 0 to 25 cmH$_2$O in 5-cmH$_2$O steps. Opening pressures were normally distributed and varied from 5 to 35 cmH$_2$O. With decremental PEEP, the tidal PV plot remains superimposed on the deflation PV curve until PEEP falls below open-lung PEEP. The PV slope is much higher with decremental PEEP, and the maximum tidal PV slope occurs at a PEEP level several cmH$_2$O below open-lung PEEP.*

In contrast, if a recruitment manoeuvre is performed and then a *decremental* PEEP trial is performed, both oxygenation and effective compliance are likely to better indicate open-lung PEEP. In the mathematical model, effective compliance during a decremental PEEP trial always underestimates open-lung PEEP, but is related to it more predictably than during an incremental PEEP trial. As PEEP is reduced, the effective compliance initially increases because each alveolus moves onto a more compliant portion of its pressure–volume curve. The tidal PV plot moves downwards superimposed on the deflation PV curve (see Fig. 12.2). When PEEP is reduced below open-lung PEEP, some end-expiratory collapse occurs. Some alveoli remain collapsed at end-inspiration, because their opening pressures are not exceeded, so the end-inspiratory point is no longer superimposed on the deflation pressure–volume curve, but is below it. The reduced number of aerated alveoli tends to reduce effective compliance, but this is opposed by the increasing compliance of each alveolus as PEEP is reduced and compliance continues to increase. Some tidal recruitment (alveoli that are inflated at end-inspiration but collapse at end-expiration) also tends to increase compliance, but this occurs less than during incremental PEEP. As PEEP is reduced further, more alveoli collapse and eventually this has a greater effect on effective compliance than the continuing increase in compliance of each alveolus; effective compliance therefore falls. The maximum value of effective compliance in the model with a low tidal volume (in most circumstances) occurs at a PEEP level 3–6 cmH_2O below open-lung PEEP. Thus, during *incremental PEEP*, the PEEP giving the highest effective compliance is highly dependent on tidal volume, opening pressures and 'lung mechanics' and can be well above or below open-lung PEEP. These factors have much less effect during a *decremental PEEP* trial, which is therefore more reliable in indicating open-lung PEEP. The same principles suggest that the best oxygenation would also indicate open-lung PEEP more reliably during a decremental rather than during an incremental PEEP trial. Clinical data concerning the use of decremental PEEP trials in ARDS are very limited and the use of effective compliance during decremental PEEP to determine open-lung PEEP cannot currently be recommended. However, the limitations of incremental PEEP trials (especially with a low tidal volume) are being recognized. Limited data concerning oxygenation during a decremental PEEP trial suggest that this may be a useful method to determine open-lung PEEP. Further studies will be required, however.

Figure 12.3 shows the effect of different tidal volumes with the same PEEP level (15 cmH_2O) generated by the model. As tidal volume is increased, the end-expiratory volume increases, because most of the additional lung units recruited at the higher end-inspiratory pressure remain inflated at end-expiration. The figure shows a simulated recruitment manoeuvre followed by a return to a low tidal volume, demonstrating a large increase in lung volume and effective compliance during subsequent tidal ventilation and a shift towards the deflation limb of the pressure–volume curve. A higher level of PEEP may be subsequently required to maintain this increased lung volume and the associated improvement in oxygenation.

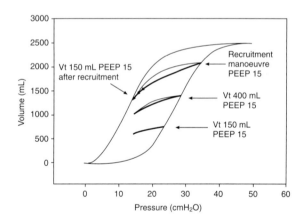

Figure 12.3 *Inflation and deflation pressure–volume (PV) curve and inflation (bold lines) and deflation tidal PV plots with two tidal volumes (150 and 400 mL) and a simulated recruitment manoeuvre with a volume of 1000 mL. The positive end-expiratory pressure (PEEP) level is 15 cmH_2O in each case, but the end-expiratory volume is greater with the higher end-inspiratory pressures, because more lung units have been recruited at end-inspiration, and most remain inflated at end-expiration because PEEP is higher than their closing pressure. The tidal PV slope is also much greater with a high tidal volume (Vt) because of more end-inspiratory recruitment. The plot shown as black triangles indicates the inflation tidal PV plot with Vt of 150 mL and PEEP 15 cmH_2O following the recruitment manoeuvre. Effective compliance is much higher and the plot has moved towards the deflation PV curve, as occurs during a decremental PEEP trial. Opening pressures were normally distributed and varied from 5 to 35 cmH_2O*

Pressure-control versus volume-control ventilation

The main differences between these two modes relate to the effect of spontaneous breathing, as discussed above. Either mode can be used to generate any desired peak lung volume and flow rate. There is little evidence that the de-accelerating flow profile that occurs during PCV offers any real benefit; indeed, the higher early-inspiratory flow rate may cause greater VILI. The high peak pressure during coughing with VCV is not associated with high transpulmonary pressure, so it does not result in volutrauma. Using the same tidal volume, the slightly higher peak pressure that occurs during VCV (with constant flow) rather than PCV is a result of continuing flow at end-inspiration and the associated pressure drop across the airways; the alveolar pressure (and the potential for VILI) does not differ. Studies comparing PCV and VCV in ARDS at equivalent levels of total (applied plus intrinsic) PEEP have shown no benefit in terms of oxygenation.

High-frequency ventilation

Theoretically, high-frequency ventilation (HFV) offers the advantage of maintaining lung recruitment with a lower tidal volume yet maintaining adequate CO_2 elimination. The results in neonatal respiratory distress syndrome (RDS) appear encouraging, but outcomes also appear to be improving with modified conventional ventilation. No trials have adequately compared HFV and optimum modified conventional ventilation, either in neonates or adults.

Inverse ratio ventilation

Extended ratio ventilation occurs when the inspiratory to expiratory (I:E) ratio is increased above the commonly used 1:2 and inverse ratio ventilation (IRV) when the I:E ratio is >1:1. IRV increases the mean airway pressure and this may be associated with improved oxygenation. It has been suggested that IRV may facilitate lung recruitment, but no studies have compared it with current strategies using the open-lung approach. When the expiratory time is decreased sufficiently, expiration remains incomplete and dynamic hyperinflation and intrinsic PEEP (PEEPi)

occur. This has a similar effect to applied PEEP and may improve oxygenation. If excessive, it may result in hypotension and barotraumas. During VCV, PEEPi results in increased end-inspiratory lung volume and P_{PL} (unless tidal volume is reduced), whereas during PCV the end-inspiratory pressure is unchanged and tidal volume decreases. It has therefore been suggested that PCV is safer than VCV during IRV, but either approach is acceptable providing that the tidal volume and P_{PL} are carefully monitored. Preliminary data suggest that there may be greater regional over-distension during IRV at equivalent tidal volume and total PEEP levels, suggesting more heterogeneous distribution of ventilation related to the shorter expiratory time (unpublished data, Bersten A *et al.*). The role of IRV therefore remains uncertain; it has no proven benefit and this possible disadvantage.

Newer modes of ventilation

A number of new ventilation modes have been developed, a full discussion of which is beyond the scope of this chapter. However, none has been shown to have a real advantage over optimum conventional ventilation in ARDS. It is now possible to achieve the optimum peak and end-expiratory lung volume and flow rates using several different modes and with different contributions to respiratory work from the ventilator and the respiratory muscles. There are no data showing an advantage of any particular mode.

Permissive hypercapnia

The protective ventilation strategies described above frequently result in hypercapnia. This is usually well tolerated, especially if it occurs gradually, allowing compensation of the resulting acidosis. The physiological effects of acute hypercapnia are complex and only a few aspects will be discussed here. Most of the effects are thought to be caused by the associated intracellular acidosis and this is corrected quite rapidly (within a few hours, as opposed to 1–2 days for the renal compensation of the extracellular acidosis) by cell membrane ion transporters that protect intracellular pH. Thus, the direct depression of myocardial contractility caused by acute hypercapnia in denervated heart preparations is largely corrected within a few hours. During sustained hypercapnia, therefore, the extracellular (blood) pH may not provide a good indication of the physiological effect of hypercapnia. In intact animals and humans, myocardial contractility and cardiac output increase because of increased sympathetic activity. Pulmonary artery pressure frequently increases in ARDS during hypercapnia and, when severe, this may be associated with a fall in cardiac output. The pulmonary hypertension can be reduced by buffering the acidosis or by inhaled nitric oxide. Hypercapnia may rarely precipitate arrhythmias.

> Even in critically ill patients requiring inotropic drug infusions, cardiac output increases during hypercapnia, although blood pressure may fall from systemic vasodilatation.

The effects of hypercapnia on gas exchange are complex but, in ARDS, there is usually little change or a slight increase in PaO_2 and an increase in mixed venous O_2 (PvO_2) as a result of an increase in cardiac output and a right-shift of the haemoglobin–O_2 dissociation curve. The overall effect, therefore, is likely to be beneficial to tissue O_2 uptake. However, higher levels of PEEP may be required to maintain recruitment when tidal volume is reduced. Hypercapnia has a direct vasodilator effect on pulmonary arterioles. This is offset by the potentiation of hypoxic vasoconstriction caused by acidosis. In an animal model, buffering of the acidosis resulted in a marked increase in intrapulmonary shunt and a decrease in arterial O_2 saturation by removing the acidosis-induced potentiation of hypoxic vasoconstriction and leaving the vasodilator effect of CO_2 unopposed.[19] The effect of buffering during hypercapnia on gas exchange in ARDS has not been adequately studied.

Therapeutic hypercapnia

> Part of the improved outcome resulting from lung-protective ventilation strategies may be due to the hypercapnia *per se* rather than solely to the ventilation strategy.

Acute hypercapnia has a number of poorly understood effects, including the suppression of cytokine release and the oxidative burst *in vitro*. Intracellular acidosis has been shown to prevent cell death during anoxia in cultured cells and, in an isolated perfused heart model, hypercapnic acidosis resulted in better cardiac function following cardioplegic ischaemia. A series of studies in isolated perfused lungs and, more recently, in intact rabbits,[20] showed that hypercapnic acidosis is protective against ischaemia–reperfusion injury. The protection is probably mediated by the inhibition of xanthine oxidase and it was therefore speculated that part of the improved outcome resulting from lung-protective ventilation strategies may be from the hypercapnia itself, rather than solely from the ventilation strategy – hence the term 'therapeutic hypercapnia'. These observations are intriguing and merit further study. At present, hypercapnia should be regarded as an undesirable side effect of lung-protective ventilation, and severe hypercapnia should be avoided, when possible, whilst meeting the targets for P_{PL} and PEEP. The use of alkali to correct the acidosis has not, as yet, been adequately studied.

Hypercapnia should be avoided in patients with, or at risk of, intracranial hypertension and should be allowed cautiously in ischaemic heart disease. In such patients, measures should be taken to reduce the $PaCO_2$, which may include an increase in the ventilator rate, tracheal gas insufflation, and high-fat enteral feeding. If possible, the tidal volume and PEEP levels should be maintained at 'protective' levels.

Extracorporeal support

Extracorporeal support has been used to improve oxygenation in patients with refractory hypoxaemia. However, a trial of extracorporeal membrane oxygenation (ECMO) in ARDS showed no benefit. Lung tissue ischaemia may have resulted from the veno-arterial bypass, which reduces pulmonary blood flow, and the continuation of mechanical ventilation with a high tidal volume may have resulted in VILI. In 1980, Gattinoni and colleagues used extracorporeal CO_2 removal (ECCO$_2$R). They used veno-venous extracorporeal perfusion (perfusing the lung with a normal flow of well-oxygenated blood) and emphasized lung rest, using a low tidal volume. Initial experience suggested an improved outcome, but a further trial in the USA[21] showed a similar mortality rate in the ECCO$_2$R and control groups. This study has been criticised because the investigators had limited experience of the technique. The role of ECCO$_2$R therefore remains controversial and unproven. Outcomes with conventional ventilation appear to be improving and fewer patients are being considered for $ECCO_2R$.

Liquid ventilation

Ventilation with perfluorocarbons is usually administered as partial liquid ventilation, in which tidal gas volumes are delivered to the perfluorocarbon-treated lung. It is a promising novel therapy. A volume of perfluorocarbon equivalent to the functional residual capacity is administered via the endotracheal tube. Its high O_2 and CO_2 solubility, reduction in surface tension (a surfactant like effect) and ability to recruit dependent lung offer improved oxygenation coupled with reduced volutrauma. Because the perfluorocarbons are denser than water, they may be viewed as a form of 'liquid PEEP'. They increase the transalveolar pressure preferentially in the dependent regions, reducing the gravitational gradient of transpulmonary pressure caused by the weight of the lung, and may also redirect blood flow away from dependent areas, thereby improving oxygenation. When external PEEP is applied, the dependent lung could become over-distended.

Clinical studies[22] have confirmed laboratory data showing improved gas exchange and lung mechanics after the administration of perfluorocarbons.

Although this has not been accompanied by improved survival or ventilator-free days, the studies have been inadequately powered. However, a significant incidence of pneumothorax was reported and, while this may just reflect the severity of the underlying disease, appropriate ventilatory strategies will be crucial to the design of further clinical trials.

POSTURE

Although it has been traditional to manage critically ill patients supine, other approaches to body positioning should be considered. The two important issues in patients with ARDS are the prone and semi-recumbent positions.

Prone positioning

Turning a patient with ARDS prone from the supine position increases oxygenation in approximately 80% of patients and this may be sustained for some hours when returned to the supine position.

Although there are no published phase II or phase III studies using the prone position, the improvement in oxygenation may be dramatic and this manoeuvre should be considered when there is severe hypoxaemia despite adequate PEEP and recruitment manoeuvres.

Complications include accidental removal of tubes and lines, facial oedema, skin abrasion and apical atelectasis. The prone position is relatively contraindicated following recent sternotomy or during haemodynamic instability, and the turning procedure requires time, personnel and preparation (See Chapter 6).

The mechanisms behind the effect are debated. On turning prone, there is a significant change in transpulmonary pressure that allows dorsal inflation without an equivalent degree of ventral collapse. Ventilation becomes more uniform and aeration of lung in the posterior diaphragmatic recess is improved. Because pulmonary blood flow is relatively unchanged, there is an immediate improvement in pulmonary shunt. A number of factors have been proposed to contribute to this differential effect, including the shape of the chest wall and diaphragm and compression by the heart. Prone positioning may also reduce VILI through the recruitment of collapsed air spaces.

Semi-recumbent position

Although not specific to ARDS patients, the semi-recumbent position reduces nosocomial pneumonia (but not mortality) in critically ill patients, presumably through reduced aspiration. Factors such as haemodynamic instability, multiple trauma or the requirement for postural drainage limit the number of patients that can be managed entirely semi-recumbent, but it is otherwise the preferred position when supine.

SURFACTANT REPLACEMENT THERAPY

Pulmonary surfactant is essential for normal lung function. It is a complex mix of phospholipids, neutral lipids and proteins that lines the gas/liquid interface, reduces surface tension and allows it to vary directly with alveolar radius. Consequently, the work of breathing is reduced and alveoli of different sizes are able to co-exist. In addition, surfactant plays an important role in fluid balance and host defence within the lung.

Surfactant is synthesized primarily by alveolar type II cells and is stored in lamellar bodies. In response to a number of stimuli, in particular physical distortion of the type II cells, lamellar bodies are exocytosed into the hypophase, where they unravel to form tubular myelin, which in turn supplies the surface active monolayer. The monolayer constantly becomes inactive and, coupled with the re-uptake of inactive surfactant, release of fresh surfactant is essential for maintaining a viable lung.

Although pulmonary surfactant is not deficient in ARDS, it is dysfunctional and this correlates with the degree of lung damage. The surface tension hysteresis is decreased and the minimum surface tension is increased up to twofold in patients at risk of developing ARDS and fourfold in ARDS patients. Samples obtained from patients with ARDS by bronchoalveolar lavage have abnormal surfactant composition (Table 12.2), which, together with surfactant inactivation by plasma proteins, reactive O_2 species and phospholipases, results in surfactant dysfunction.

These changes probably make important contributions to both alveolar instability and collapse, with consequent shunt and hypoxaemia, and to decreases in specific lung compliance. In addition, because dysfunctional surfactant exaggerates the heterogeneity of air-space ventilation, it will contribute to regional over- inflation and to the opening and closing of alveoli during tidal ventilation, leading to further lung damage.

Despite the important role that surfactant abnormality plays in the pathogenesis and pathophysiology of ARDS, promising results in animal models of lung injury, and the proven efficacy of exogenous surfactant replacement therapy (ESRT) in infants with established RDS, it has not yet been shown to be of benefit in ARDS. A number of small studies have reported improved oxygenation and compliance with ESRT, but neither outcome nor physiological benefit was found in a large, multi-centre, prospective, randomized trial of ESRT in patients with sepsis-induced ARDS.[23] There are a number of reasons why this may have occurred. The surfactant preparation used may not have reached the air spaces or may have modified the composition and surface tension of the alveolar epithelial lining fluid. The dose of surfactant administered was probably an order of magnitude less than optimal. It was administered as an aerosol, which results in preferential distribution to well-ventilated areas; bronchoscopically administered surfactant can reach poorly ventilated regions, where it will be most useful. The surfactant preparation used is sensitive to protein inhibition and does not contain surfactant proteins that improve its surface-tension-reducing

Table 12.2 *Changes in surfactant composition in ARDS*

Component		Comment
Phosphatidylcholine	↓	The major phospholipid class
Disaturated phospholipids	↓	The main surface active phospholipids
Phosphatidlyglycerol	↓	
Phosphatidylinositol	↑	
Sphingomyelin	↑	Probably a cell membrane component
Lysophosphatidylcholine	↑	The first catabolic product of PC
		Directly interferes with the surface active properties of surfactant
Surfactant protein-A	↓	Important for reducing surface tension and host defence
Surfactant protein-B	↓	Essential for reducing surface tension
Tubular myelin-rich aggregates	↓	Functionally active component
Tubular myelin-poor aggregates	↑	Functionally inactive component

properties. Ventilatory strategies were not controlled and recent data suggest that a low tidal volume maintains a greater proportion of tubular myelin-rich aggregates following ESRT. Finally, these patients were enrolled with established ARDS, whereas ESRT will be most beneficial if delivered early.

> Although ESRT has not proven to be of clinical benefit in ARDS, there are sound reasons for believing that, with improved preparations, administration techniques and study design, ESRT may find a role in management. Techniques such as intermittent lung stretch or biological variability in tidal volume may also prove useful through enhanced release of endogenous surfactant.

MANIPULATION OF THE PULMONARY VASCULATURE

Hypoxic pulmonary vasoconstriction causes some redistribution of pulmonary blood flow away from the dependent atelectatic areas to better-ventilated lung. Inhaled nitric oxide (iNO), prostacyclin (PGI_2) and intravenous almitrine may be used to manipulate the pulmonary circulation to further reduce shunt. Both iNO and PGI_2 are potent vasodilators. When delivered by inhalation, they are distributed to aerated lung regions and vasodilate the local pulmonary circulation, further increasing pulmonary blood flow to well-ventilated lung and improving oxygenation. Almitrine is a selective pulmonary vasoconstrictor that reinforces hypoxic pulmonary vasoconstriction. It may improve oxygenation alone, but has usually been trialled with iNO. The effects are additive, allowing a lower dose of almitrine to be used, thereby reducing the risk of pulmonary hypertension and polyneuropathy that has been reported with long-term almitrine use.

Inhaled NO and PGI_2 also reduce right ventricular after-load, which is often increased in ARDS. This may result in improved cardiac output and O_2 transport, especially during permissive hypercapnia. In patients with severe primary or secondary pulmonary hypertension, these agents may also be effective. Intravenously administered PGI_2 improves cardiac output in ARDS, but widespread pulmonary vasodilatation results in increased intrapulmonary shunt and worse oxygenation.

Inhaled nitric oxide

Most clinical experience has been with iNO. NO is an endothelium-derived smooth-muscle relaxant, but has other crucial physiological roles, including neurotransmission, host defence, platelet aggregation, leucocyte adhesion and bronchodilatation. Doses as low as 60 parts per billion iNO may improve oxygenation, although concentrations of 1–40 parts per million (p.p.m.) are often used in ARDS. A higher dose may be required to reduce pulmonary artery pressure. Delivery is usually as medical-grade NO/N_2, and this should be adequately mixed to avoid variable NO concentrations. It is recommended that inspiratory NO and NO_2 concentrations are measured. The electrochemical method is accurate to 1 p.p.m. (adequate for clinical use) and is less expensive than the more accurate chemoluminescence method. Environmental levels of NO and NO_2 during iNO therapy are usually low and predominantly influenced by atmospheric concentrations. However, it is still common practice to scavenge expired gas. Binding to haemoglobin in the pulmonary circulation rapidly inactivates NO, and systemic effects are only reported following high concentrations. Systemic methaemoglobin levels may be monitored and are generally less than 5% during clinical use. NO may cause lung toxicity through combination with O_2 free radicals and through the metabolism of NO to NO_2, but these do not appear to cause major clinical problems.

Only 40–70% of patients with ARDS sustain improved oxygenation with iNO (responders), probably because active hypoxic pulmonary vasoconstriction has already minimized intrapulmonary shunt in the remainder. Two large trials of iNO[24,25] have shown no improvement in the mortality or reversal of ALI, although the requirement for ECMO was reduced in infants with persistent pulmonary hypertension. However, iNO was safe and improved oxygenation initially. This was not sustained beyond 12–24 hours, however, and some patients receiving placebo had an increase in $PaO_2 \geq 20\%$ at 4 hours. Consequently, the role of iNO in patients with ARDS remains uncertain.

> In severe hypoxaemia, perhaps in combination with almitrine, iNO may provide temporary rescue.

ANTI-INFLAMMATORY DRUGS

A complex inflammatory response is central to the development of diffuse alveolar damage (see Chapter 11). Consequently, a number of anti-inflammatory pharmacological interventions have been examined, but, in general, promising laboratory data have not held up in clinical trials.

Glucocorticoids

Glucocorticoids inhibit several aspects of alveolar inflammation through inhibition of the transcription of many of the involved cytokines (including IL-1, IL-2, IL-6, TNF-α, and interferon-gamma [IFN-γ]), inhibition of complement-mediated neutrophil aggregation, the synthesis of the arachidonic acid metabolites, platelet-activating factor and NO. Although short-term glucocorticoid therapy was ineffective in early ARDS and in septic at-risk patients, there is renewed interest in its use later in ARDS when it may modify persistent alveolar inflammation and fibroproliferative obliteration of the blood-gas membrane.

> Encouraging small case series have been followed by a small, prospective, randomized trial in which ICU and hospital mortality rate and remote organ dysfunction were reduced.[26]

Because pneumonia frequently occurrs in the absence of fever, surveillance using bronchoalveolar lavage is recommended. Further trials are required before the routine use of glucocorticoids can be confidently recommended in this situation.

Ketoconazole

This antifungal has anti-inflammatory properties, including inhibition of both thromboxane synthase and 5-lipoxygenase – enzymes that are necessary in the production of thromboxane A_2 and leukotriene B_4. Because both are involved in alveolar inflammation, ketoconazole has been trialled in ARDS. Small studies of ketoconazole in at-risk patients have shown a reduction in the development of ARDS and

possibly mortality. However, in a large trial in early ALI and ARDS, ketoconazole did not affect the mortality rate or lung function.[27] Consequently, it cannot be recommended at present.

Prostaglandin E$_1$ and prostacyclin

These prostaglandins are potent vasodilators and inhibit platelet and neutrophil function. They cause reduced expression of the CD11b/CD18 neutrophil adhesion complex, and decreased neutrophil activation due to increased c-AMP, with attenuated release of O_2 radicals and leukotriene B_4. Although their intravenous administration may result in hypotension, and worsen hypoxaemia by causing pulmonary vasodilatation, they have been trialled in ARDS. Prostaglandin E$_1$ is metabolized in the lung and so causes less systemic vasodilatation than prostacyclin. It has therefore been used in most studies, often as a liposomal mixture to enhance intracellular penetration. Despite encouraging animal data, in a phase III trial involving 350 ARDS patients, liposomal prostaglandin E$_1$ did not reduce mortality, although the time to a $PaO_2/FiO_2 > 300$ was decreased.[28] Hypotension and hypoxia were common reasons for altering drug infusion in the liposomal prostaglandin E$_1$ arm (59% versus 15% in control patients).

Cytokine antagonism

Elevated levels of both pro-inflammatory and anti-inflammatory cytokines are present in the lung and in plasma in ARDS, but their role is uncertain. In patients with indirect risk factors for ARDS, such as non-pulmonary sepsis, elevated circulating cytokines fail to predict the development of ARDS and, in patients with a direct risk factor, such as pneumonia or aspiration of gastric contents, the initial increase in circulating cytokines may simply be attributable to leakage from the alveolus because of damage to the alveolar-capillary membrane.

Most studies of cytokine antagonism have targeted sepsis, rather than ARDS. Overall, no outcome advantage has been shown, although, in some studies, an improved or worse outcome occurred in *post-hoc* subgroup analysis. Various factors should be considered when interpreting these data, including the heterogeneous populations, the timing of therapy, possible effects of the drug and its efficacy. For example, although TNF-α plays a role in increased capillary permeability in ALI, it increases alveolar epithelial fluid clearance in models of pneumonia via a non-catecholamine-dependent mechanism and also promotes the clearance of bacteria in pneumonia. Consequently, the effect of an anti-TNF-α antibody may be influenced by the precise risk factor for ARDS and a number of other factors. Without further clinical data, antagonism of cytokines cannot be recommended in ARDS.

Other anti-inflammatory drugs

A number of other agents have been examined as anti-inflammatory agents in ARDS, but none has lived up to the promising results in animal models. Pentoxyfilline inhibits (i) TNF-α release following endotoxin, (ii) polymorph deformability, (iii) the release of O_2-derived free radicals, and (iv) responsiveness to platelet-activating factor. However, lisophylline, a related drug, does not appear to influence outcome in ARDS. Non-steroidal anti-inflammatories reduce thromboxane A_2 and prostacyclin through inhibition of cyclo-oxygenase, but fail to reduce the incidence of shock or ARDS in septic

> Although the results of anti-inflammatory therapy in animal models have been encouraging, clinical trials have so far been disappointing.

patients.[29] Whereas anti-oxidants such as N-acetyl-cysteine and its analogues have not proven useful, the central role of O_2-derived free radicals in generating lung injury suggests that further clinical research is warranted. A platelet-activating factor antagonist also failed to alter mortality in ARDS.

FLUID THERAPY

There is general agreement that intravenous fluids should be limited to the minimum necessary to maintain adequate cardiac output and tissue perfusion. Elevated pulmonary microvascular pressure, as well as increasing pulmonary oedema, may interact with alveolar stretch to augment VILI, providing a further reason to maintain lung microvascular pres-

sure as low as possible. However, there is still no easy method of determining the adequacy of intravascular volume (see Chapter 8). Regional tissue hypoxia may be present with normal indices of global perfusion and tissue oxygenation. Therefore, fluid therapy remains controversial. It is important to recognize the effects of cardiovascular changes on gas exchange. A low cardiac output results in a low mixed venous O_2 saturation and, in the presence of high levels of intrapulmonary shunt, this may result in a fall in arterial O_2 saturation. Fortunately, a reduction in cardiac output often causes a reduction in intrapulmonary shunt, opposing this effect. Nevertheless, it is important to ensure that any hypovolaemia is corrected. CVP may be elevated in the presence of pulmonary hypertension and right ventricular dysfunction and does not correlate well with PA wedge pressure in ARDS. It is also important to consider the effect of variations in intrathoracic pressure, including intrinsic and applied PEEP, on the measured vascular pressures. The preference for colloid or crystalloid therapy remains controversial, although several meta-analyses have failed to show any benefit of colloids.

SUMMARY

Rapid and adequate treatment of the underlying conditions causing ALI, including definitive surgical treatment of sepsis or excision of necrotic tissue when required, and early recognition and treatment of secondary infection remain of fundamental importance. In association with current ventilation strategies, mortality rates appear to be falling. A greater understanding of lung mechanics is helping to develop improved ventilation and recruitment strategies, but there are still many unresolved issues. Anti-inflammatory agents, cytokine modulation and surfactant replacement have, so far, been disappointing, but may eventually yield additional treatments and lead to even greater improvements in outcome.

REFERENCES

1. Hickling, KG, Henderson, SJ, Jackson, R. Low mortality associated with low volume pressure limited ventilation with permissive hypercapnia in severe

adult respiratory distress syndrome. *Intensive Care Med* 1990; **16**: 372–7.

2. Toth, JL, Capellier, G, Walker, P, Winton, T, Marshall, J, Demajo, W. Lung emphysematous changes in ARDS. *Am Rev Respir Dis* 1992; **145**: A184.

3. Lewandowski, K, Falke, KJ, Rossaint, R, Slama, K, Pappert, D, Kuhlen, R. Low mortality associated with advanced treatment including V-V ECMO for severe ARDS. *Intensive Care Med* 1992; **19**: S42.

4. Hickling, KG, Walsh, J, Henderson, S, Jackson, R. Low mortality rate in adult respiratory distress syndrome using low-volume, pressure-limited ventilation with permissive hypercapnia: a prospective study. *Crit Care Med* 1994; **22**: 1568–78.

5. Levy, B, Bollaert, PE, Bauer, P, *et al.* Therapeutic optimisation including inhaled nitric oxide in adult respiratory distress syndrome in a polyvalent intensive care unit. *J Trauma* 1995; **38**: 370–4.

6. Thomsen, GE, Morris, AH, Pope, D, *et al.* Mechanical ventilation of patients with adult respiratory distress syndrome using reduced tidal volumes. *Crit Care Med* 1994; **22**: A205.

7. Nakagawa, S, Bohn, D. Pressure controlled ventilation with limited peak inspiratory pressure below 35 to 40 cm H_2O may improve survival of pediatric acute respiratory failure. *Am J Respir Crit Care Med* 1995; **151**: A77.

8. Botero, C, Reda, Z, Mendoza, P, Davis, A, Harrison, R. Pressure limited ventilation with permissive hypercapnia (PH) in children with ARDS. *Crit Care Med* 1995; **23**: A188.

9. Sheridan, RL, Kacmarek, RM, McEttrick, MM, *et al.* Permissive hypercapnia as a ventilatory strategy in burned children: effect on barotrauma, pneumonia and mortality. *J Trauma* 1995; **39**: 854–9.

10. Stocker, R, Neff, T, Stein, S, Ecknauer, E, Trentz, O, Russi, E. Prone positioning and low-volume pressure-limited ventilation improve survival in patients with severe ARDS. *Chest* 1997; **111**: 1008–17.

11. Amato, MB, Barbas, CS, Medeiros, DM, *et al.* Effect of a protective-ventilation strategy on mortality in the acute respiratory distress syndrome. *N Engl J Med* 1998; **338**(6): 347–54.

12. The Acute Respiratory Distress Syndrome Network. Ventilation with lower tidal volumes as compared with traditional tidal volumes for acute lung injury and the acute respiratory distress syndrome. *N Engl J Med* 2000; **342**(18): 1301–8.

13. Ranieri, VM, Suter, PM, Tortorella, C, *et al.* Effect of mechanical ventilation on inflammatory mediators in patients with acute respiratory distress syndrome. *JAMA* 1999; **282**: 54–61.

14. Ranieri, VM, Giunta, F, Suter, PM, Slutsky, AS. Mechanical ventilation as a mediator of multisystem organ failure in acute respiratory distress syndrome. *JAMA* 2000; **284**: 43–4.

15. Slutsky, A. Mechanical ventilation: report of American College of Chest Physicians Consensus Conference. *Chest* 1993; **104**: 1833–59.

16. Gattinoni, L, D'Andrea, L, Pelosi, P Vitale, G, Pesenti, A, Fumagalli, R. Regional effects and mechanism of positive end-expiratory pressure in early adult respiratory distress syndrome. *JAMA* 1993; **269**: 2122–7.

17. Hickling, K. Recruitment greatly alters the pressure volume curve: a mathematical model of ARDS lungs. *Am J Respir Crit Care Med* 1998; **158**: 194–202.

18. Jonson, B, Richard, JC, Straus, C, *et al.* 1999. Pressure–volume curves and compliance in acute lung injury. Evidence of recruitment above the lower inflection point. *Am J Respir Crit Care Med* 1999; **159**: 1172–8.

19. Brimioulle, S, Vachiery, JL, Lejeune, P, *et al.* Acid–base status affects gas exchange in canine oleic-acid pulmonary edema. *Am J Physiol* (*Heart Circ Physiol* 29) 1991; **260**: H1086.

20. Laffey, JG, Tanaka, M, Engelberts, D, *et al.* Therapeutic hypercapnia reduces pulmonary and systemic injury following *in vivo* lung reperfusion. *Am J Respir Crit Care Med* 2000; **162**: 2287–94.

21. Morris, AH, Wallace, CJ, Menlove, RL, *et al.* Randomized clinical trial of pressure-controlled inverse ratio ventilation and extracorporeal CO_2 removal for adult respiratory distress syndrome. *Am J Respir Crit Care Med* 1994; **149**: 295–305.

22. Hirschl, RB, Pranikoff, T, Wise, C, *et al.* Initial experience with partial liquid ventilation in adult patients with the acute respiratory distress syndrome. *JAMA* 1996; **275**: 383–9.

23. Anzueto, A, Baughman, RP, Guntupalli, KK, *et al.* Aerosolized surfactant in adults with sepsis-induced acute respiratory distress syndrome. Exosurf Acute Respiratory Distress Syndrome Sepsis Study Group. *N Engl J Med* 1996; **334**: 1417–21.

24. Dellinger, RP, Zimmerman, JL, Taylor, RW, *et al.* Effects of inhaled nitric oxide in patients with acute respiratory distress syndrome: results of a randomized phase II trial. *Crit Care Med* 1998; **26**: 15–23.

25. Lundin, S, Mang, H, Smithies, M, Stenqvist, O, Frostell, C, for the European Study Group of Inhaled Nitric Oxide. Inhalation of nitric oxide in acute lung injury: results of a European multicentre study. *Intensive Care Med* 1999; **25**: 911–19.

26. Meduri, GU, Headley, AS, Golden, E, *et al*. Effect of prolonged methylprednisolone therapy in unresolving acute respiratory distress syndrome: a randomized controlled trial. *JAMA* 1998; **280**: 159–65.

27. NIH ARDS Network. Ketoconazole for early treatment of acute lung injury and acute respiratory distress syndrome. *JAMA* 2000; **283**: 1995–2002.

28. Abraham, E, Baughman, R, Fletcher, E, *et al*. Liposomal prostaglandin E_1 (YTLC C-53) in acute respiratory distress syndrome: a controlled, randomized, double-blind, multicenter trial. *Crit Care Med* 1999; **27**: 1478–85.

29. Bernard, GR, Wheeler, AP, Russell, JA, *et al*. The effects of ibuprofen on the physiology and survival of patients with sepsis. *N Engl J Med* 1997; **336**: 912–18.

13

Weaning from mechanical ventilation

STEFANO NAVA, MICHELE VITACCA AND ANNALISA CARLUCCI

THE SIZE OF THE PROBLEM

There are a number of problems when considering the concept of 'weaning'. First, the clinician needs to distinguish between liberation from mechanical ventilation, when support is no longer required, and extubation, when there is no longer a need for the endotracheal tube. Accordingly, after a patient has successfully undergone a trial of unassisted breathing, one must decide whether access to the lower respiratory tract is still required. The term 'weaning success' therefore applies only after both conditions have been met.[1] Another problem is the definition of weaned. What is the minimum time that the patient must remain disconnected from a ventilator to be considered to have 'weaned'? This is rarely addressed in published reports. In most, a time interval of 48 hours after extubation or disconnection from support is specified. The assumption is that, after this, failure is likely to be for non-respiratory reasons. However, this may not be the case. How large is the problem of weaning delay or failure? About 80% of patients admitted for mechanical ventilation in the intensive care unit (ICU) resume spontaneous breathing in a few days. In the remaining 20%, often a combination of unresolved primary illness and pre-existing cardiorespiratory or neuromuscular disease renders discontinuation from mechanical ventilation difficult. The length of weaning is, therefore, dependent upon the aetiology of respiratory failure. When the need for ventilation persists for more than 15 days, as occurs in 2–5% of ICU admissions (depending on case-mix), it carries a poor prognosis (>50% mortality). Moreover, failure of extubation increases the risk for death, prolongs ICU stay and may lead to the need for transfer to long-term care or rehabilitation. In a national survey in Spain,[2] it was reported that 41% of the overall ICU time was devoted to weaning, with large differences between different aetiologies necessitating mechanical ventilation. In patients with chronic obstructive pulmonary disease (COPD), cardiac failure or neurological problems, the process of weaning accounted for >50% of ICU stays.[2]

FACTORS DELAYING WEANING

The causes of weaning delay include:

- unresolved primary illness,
- nosocomial infection,
- pre-morbid COPD or heart failure,

- upper airway problems, such as glottic oedema or bulbar disease,
- corticosteroids,
- impaired consciousness,
- electrolyte disturbances,
- haemodynamic instability,
- critical illness neuropathy/myopathy.

Endotracheal intubation may cause complications that increase morbidity and mortality.[3] Furthermore, the need for sedation or paralysis to enable effective mechanical ventilation, particularly in the initial days of critical illness, may lead to a generalized myopathy. The evidence for this is contentious. The association with, for instance, paralytic agents may be explained by confounding factors such as disease severity. The use of prolonged mechanical ventilation may lead to diaphragmatic atrophy. In one report, this developed after 48 hours in a study performed on rats.[4] However, other animal experiments suggest that diaphragm atrophy does not occur if paralysis is partial or intermittent (only a few contractions per day are required to prevent wasting). Impairment in skeletal muscle strength in the ICU may also be a consequence of electrolyte disturbances[5] or a direct effect of hypercapnia, hypoxia, malnutrition, treatment with corticosteroids and a low cardiac output. Nevertheless, critically ill patients with sepsis and multiple organ failure (MOF) are at risk of developing critical illness neuropathy, which is, in most cases, a combination of myopathy and neuropathy.[6] The weakness of the respiratory muscles that follows is probably one of the major determinants of weaning failure in patients recovering from critical illness. In COPD, the altered shape of the diaphragm, with flattening from hyperinflation, will result in a mechanical disadvantage that will impair function. The force generation of the diaphragm is not the only factor involved in weaning delay. The respiratory pump output, in terms of minute ventilation, will be the result of the balance between the load on the pump and its capacity (Fig. 13.1). In many causes of acute respiratory failure, such as COPD, acute respiratory distress syndrome (ARDS), pneumonia and heart failure, the elastic and resistive loads are elevated as much as three to four times.[7] In COPD, in particular, respiratory muscle training has been suggested as a strategy to increase the strength and endurance of the diaphragm. Similowski et al.[8] demonstrated that the diaphragm in COPD is able to generate a normal pressure, in response to bilateral phrenic nerve stimulation,

when corrected for hyperinflation. Their findings argue against the value of inspiratory muscle training (or weaning by intermittent periods of increased load, e.g. T-tube breathing). Similowski concludes that 'the absence of central inhibition or evidence of chronic fatigue cast doubt on the need to treat patients with interventions intended to improve the contractility of the diaphragm'. More recently, Levine and co-workers[9] provided support for this view when they showed, in biopsy specimens taken from the diaphragm in severe COPD, that there is an increase in the slow-twitch fibres, presumably as an adaptive mechanism that will lead to an increase in resistance to fatigue (see Chapter 2).

Infection is an important cause for delay in weaning. The presence of an endotracheal tube for more than 3 days significantly increases the risk of nosocomial pneumonia (>20% at 10 days of invasive mechanical ventilation). Nosocomial pneumonia results in a longer hospital stay as well as an increase in mortality. The endotracheal tube predisposes to pneumonia:

1. by impairing cough and mucociliary clearance,
2. by allowing aspiration of contaminated secretions that accumulate above the cuff, or

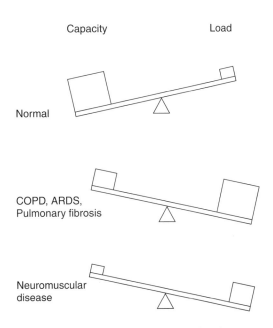

Figure 13.1 *Balance between the loads imposed on the respiratory system and its capacity in normal subjects and in respiratory diseases. COPD, chronic obstructive pulmonary disease; ARDS, acute respiratory distress syndrome.*

3. because bacterial binding to the surface of bronchial epithelium is increased.

The use of non-invasive ventilation reduces the risk of ventilator-associated pneumonia. For this reason, it was recently suggested[10] that the term ventilator-associated pneumonia be replaced by intubation-associated pneumonia. Unfortunately, the use of non-invasive ventilation is not always successful, especially in patients without alveolar hypoventilation, and non-invasive ventilation is currently employed in selected patients with hypercapnic respiratory failure (see Chapter 5). Aspiration of regurgitated stomach contents is a potent cause of ventilator-associated pneumonia, and the risk of this with nasogastric feeding is high. In one study, it occurred in approximately 50% of patients.[11] A semi-recumbent, rather than fully recumbent, body position may reduce regurgitation and thus the frequency of nosocomial pneumonia in patients receiving enteral nutrition.[12]

Cardiac failure is another important cause of delayed weaning. In patients undergoing a trial of spontaneous breathing, a progressive decrease in SvO_2, caused both by a decrease in O_2 transport and an increase in O_2 extraction, increased the failure rate.[13] A protracted ICU stay also leads to complications due to confinement to bed and general de-conditioning, with changes in skeletal muscle composition, altered cardiovascular response to stress, bone demineralization, protein wastage and a decrease in total body water. The central nervous system, endocrine function and blood composition may also alter.[14]

THE WEANING PROCESS

The first step in the weaning process is the *identification* of the patient potentially able to sustain spontaneous breathing. The following requirements are considered necessary.

- Clinical stability, defined as the absence of sepsis, significant bronchospasm, electrolyte imbalance or over-sedation, evidence of profound malnutrition, excessive secretions and/or weak cough or hypotension (systolic <90 mmHg).
- Normal or only mildly disturbed central nervous system function.
- Adequate oxygenation ($PaO_2 > 8.0$ kPa or 60 mmHg) with $FiO_2 < 40\%$ and end-expiratory pressure < 5.0 cmH$_2$O in patients able to trigger the ventilator.

The second step is the choice of the *modality* for liberation from mechanical ventilation. The most common techniques are:

- Pressure support ventilation (PSV): a progressive decrease in pressure support is continued until minimal support is provided, e.g. 8 cmH$_2$O,
- T-piece: a period of spontaneous breathing through the endotracheal tube connected to a T-piece,
- SIMV: the patient can breathe spontaneously between ventilator-delivered breaths.

Pressure support ventilation

PSV is a widely used method of partial mechanical ventilatory support that efficiently reduces the workload of the inspiratory muscles. It can be used during weaning by progressively decreasing the level of assistance. At a pressure support level of 8 cmH$_2$O, the work imposed by the endotracheal tube and demand valve of the ventilator is equivalent to spontaneous breathing, so that extubation will not increase the work of breathing.[15]

T-piece

This is a method of weaning based on the philosophy that the respiratory muscles need retraining, with periods of disconnection from the ventilator for lengthening periods. During these periods, patients receive humidified O_2-enriched gas through a T-piece connected to the endotracheal tube.

Synchronized intermittent mechanical ventilation

In this mode of ventilation, the patient is able to breathe spontaneously between ventilator-delivered breaths. Delay in the timing of machine breaths is referred to as synchronization; a variable 'lock-out' period after machine provided breaths limits breath 'stacking' or hyperventilation. Spontaneous breaths may also be supported – so-called SIMV plus pressure support. The weaning procedure consists of gradually decreasing the number of machine-determined breaths.

Other techniques have also been proposed, e.g. mandatory minute ventilation, volume-assured pressure support and BiPAP. There is no evidence for the routine use of these methods in the clinical practice.

WHAT VENTILATOR MODE SPEEDS WEANING?

Two important multi-centre trials were performed in the mid 1990s by Brochard and co-workers[16] and by Esteban and colleagues.[17] Both compared the following methods: intermittent T-piece breathing, PSV and SIMV. The former study, performed on 456 medical and surgical patients, concluded that the outcome of weaning was influenced by ventilatory strategy and found that the use of PSV (attempted reductions of pressure support by 2–4 cmH_2O twice a day until pressure support was 8 cmH_2O) resulted in significantly faster weaning than the other two techniques. On the other hand, the latter study found that a once-daily trial of spontaneous breathing with a T-piece of gradually increasing duration led to extubation three times more quickly than SIMV and twice as quickly as PSV. In this study, the minimum target pressure support level before extubation was 5 cmH_2O. The explanation for these contrasting results is that the method employed is probably less important than the patient pathology in determining the duration of mechanical ventilation. Confidence and familiarity with the technique adopted are likely to be more important than the chosen method. Certainly, the rate of failure following extubation was similar after T-piece weaning and PSV, which suggests that either approach is acceptable in the liberation from mechanical ventilation. In both studies, weaning trials were performed only in those patients who had first failed a 2-hour T-piece trial. These patients represented about 25% of all patients who had reached the criteria for weaning. Accordingly, the majority of patients judged 'weanable' (75%), according to the above criteria, could be safely extubated after a single brief trial of spontaneous breathing. More recently, it has been shown that successful extubation can be achieved using a shorter trial period (30 min) of spontaneous breathing.[18] Before proceeding to extubation, additional aspects that require consideration are the volume and character of secretions and the ability of the patient to cough effectively. In addition to an adequate cough reflex, patient

co-operation and good bulbar function are necessary. The criteria to judge the outcome of a period of T-piece breathing are:

- subjective comfort,
- physiological stability (no significant increment in heart rate and respiratory rate),
- absence of an acute respiratory acidosis or hypoxemia, defined as $PaO_2 < 8.0$ kPa on 40% inspired O_2.

EXTUBATION CRITERIA

Many parameters have been proposed to predict successful extubation: the Index of Rapid Shallow Breathing (RSB), or Tobin's Index.,[19] has a predictive utility superior to other proposed indices such as vital capacity, maximal inspiratory pressure (Pimax) or tidal volume, and is simpler and less invasive than complex measurements such as neuromuscular drive to breathe $(P_{0.1})$, the Work of Breathing Index, CROP (acronym for compliance, rate, oxygenation and pressure) or other parameters of respiratory mechanics. The RSB Index relates respiratory frequency and tidal volume (RR/Vt) with a threshold of >105 breaths mL^{-1} predicting weaning failure. Despite good sensitivity in predicting success when RSB <105, the index lacks specificity. Thus, some patients with an RR/Vt > 105 may, in fact, succeed, whereas a few with RR/Vt < 105 may fail.[1]

WEANING PROTOCOLS

The concept of using a standardized protocol to wean patients from mechanical ventilation is popular in the USA. Therapist-driven protocols combine extubation criteria with daily care plans, changes in therapy being directed by changes in measurable patient variables. The daily screening of respiratory function by nurses or respiratory therapists, followed by trials of spontaneous breathing and notification to the patients' physicians when the trials are successful, can reduce the duration of ventilation, the cost of intensive care and the rate of complications.[20] Whereas these protocols may be applied in the USA, where respiratory therapists are directly involved in the weaning procedure, they may not be in Europe, where only 22% of respiratory therapists working in

ICUs are directly involved in ventilator management.[21] Therapist-driven protocols are a consensus of medical knowledge and opinion that are summarized into a care plan or algorithm, with changes in therapy directed by changes in objectively measurable patient variables. It is important to stress the specific roles of the respiratory therapists in this procedure. With the institution of therapist-driven protocols, the interaction between the therapist and nurse regarding the indications for arterial blood-gas and maximal inspiratory pressure (MIP) measurements, bronchial secretions management or number of hours of T-tube breathing results in a significant change in the behaviour of nursing and medical staff. The whole therapist-driven protocol team consists of the physician, patient, family, nurse and a respiratory therapist. It addresses the prevention of the deleterious effects of bed rest, communication, emotional support, psychological well-being and function. The initial evaluation includes assessment of the patient and ventilator status and patient–ventilator synchrony. This evaluation is performed routinely every 2 hours and with each ventilator setting change. The use of respiratory therapists is also important during the application of non-invasive ventilation, one of the keys to the success of which is the continuous

monitoring, preparation and nursing of patients. For this reason, in the first phases of treatment, the presence of the respiratory therapist and/or nurse is necessary to ensure correct positioning of the mask, to coach the patient, to aspirate bronchial secretions and to ensure compliance and tolerance. Nursing input is clearly important and may affect success. In one study, a significant inverse correlation was found between the duration of mechanical ventilation and availability of nurses as assessed by a nursing index.

A major limitation to 'accelerated' extubation remains the lack of criteria that guarantee success. However, removing the endotracheal tube does not necessarily mean that respiratory support cannot be provided. Instead of relying upon spontaneous ventilation in the immediate post-extubation period, non-invasive ventilation, with face or nasal mask, can be employed as a 'bridge'. This technique has been validated in a randomized, multi-centre Italian study in patients with COPD.[22] The trial involved patients intubated for acute hypercapnic respiratory failure, either after initial failure of or contraindications to non-invasive ventilation. Patients were initially sedated, and often paralysed, and frequent bronchial toilet was performed in the first 6–12 hours. In the subsequent 24–36 hours, sedation was reduced and mechanical ventilation provided with pressure support. At 48 hours after intubation, a T-piece trial was performed if the patients were haemodynamically stable, had a normal temperature, were alert and had no evidence of pneumonia. Strict criteria, similar to the Brochard et al.[16] extubation requirements, were used to judge failure of the T-piece trial. Patients who failed this trial (50 of the initial 68 patients) were than randomized to either re-institution of full mechanical ventilation and conventional weaning or temporary reconnection to the ventilator, until previous arterial blood-gas levels were reached, and then extubation onto non-invasive ventilation. In both groups, weaning proceeded by daily reductions in the level of pressure support and intermittent spontaneous breathing trials twice a day (Fig. 13.2). The mean durations of ventilatory support and ICU stay and the 60-day mortality were significantly reduced in the non-invasively ventilated group. Importantly, none of the patients weaned non-invasively developed nosocomial pneumonia, whereas 7 (28%) of those who continued with endobronchial ventilation did. Another study, employing non-invasive ventilation a few days after intubation in patients with hypercapnic respiratory

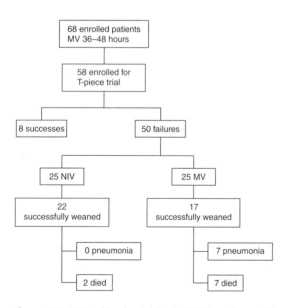

Figure 13.2 *NIV to aid early extubtion in COPD (see reference 22). Distribution of the patients according to treatment and outcomes. MV, mechanical ventilation; NIV, non-invasive ventilation.*

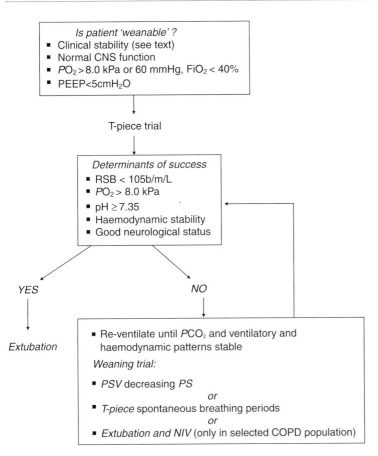

Figure 13.3 *Algorithm for weaning from mechanical ventilation. CNS, central nervous system; PEEP, positive end-expiratory pressure; RSB, Index of Rapid Shallow Breathing; PSV, pressure support ventilation; NIV, non-invasive ventilation; COPD, chronic obstructive pulmonary disease.*

failure due to COPD or restrictive thoracic disease, showed similar results, although the reduction in infectious complications did not achieve statistical significance.[23] Finally, a study using non-invasive ventilation for weaning patients without pre-existing COPD (most following lung transplant procedures) also reported that nosocomial pneumonia can be avoided by using non-invasive PSV and that the duration of mechanical ventilation, the duration of ICU stay and the need for re-itubation can be reduced.[24] These studies therefore suggest that non-invasive ventilation may allow patients to be extubated earlier, more successfully and with fewer complications than conventional weaning procedures.

However, weaning with non-invasive ventilation should be performed with caution. Published studies pertain mostly to patients with hypercapnic respiratory failure (pump failure) due to COPD who had been carefully selected to be haemodynamically stable with PaO_2:FiO_2 ratio ≥ 1.5, no evidence of infection or depressed consciousness and an effective cough. Until large-scale studies have been undertaken, it is difficult to quantify how many intubated COPD patients may be successfully managed this way. Further studies are also needed to assess the feasibility of the technique in other forms of respiratory failure. Keeping in mind these limitations, a practical algorithm for the weaning process is proposed in Figure 13.3.

SELF-EXTUBATION

Unplanned extubation occurs in 8–14% of patients.[25,26] It occurs more frequently with oral intubation, with insufficient sedation, in patients with COPD and when the fixation of the tube is poor. The re-intubation rate varies in different series, but is considerably lower after unplanned extubations that complicate a weaning trial (15–30%) than after those occurring when the patients are receiving full ventilatory support (75–80%). These figures suggest that a considerable proportion of patients could be liberated from mechanical ventilation at an earlier time! An unplanned extubation is not unimportant, because it appears to increase the duration of mechanical ventilation and the length of ICU and hospital stay when compared with patients re-intubated following extubation failure. The mortality rate, interestingly, is not increased. On the other hand, when successful, unplanned extubation clearly reduces the length of mechanical ventilation, but has no other measurable beneficial impact.[26]

POST-EXTUBATION FAILURE

Failure following extubation is a common problem. The incidence ranges from 3.3% to 23.5%.[27] The prognosis in these patients is poor, with a hospital mortality of 30–40%, depending on whether the cause is respiratory or non-respiratory. The time to re-intubation is an independent predictor of outcome. As re-intubation *per se* is an insufficient explanation for the high mortality rate, it has been claimed that clinical deterioration during the period of unsupported ventilation may allow the development of secondary organ failure that then leads to a poor prognosis.[28] The prolonged period of unsupported ventilation may arise because the clinician wishes to avoid re-intubation due to the severity of underlying disease or because of concerns about the well-recognized complications of continued intubation and mechanical ventilation.

Hilbert and co-workers have described the so-called 'sequential use' of non-invasive ventilation, consisting of intermittent periods of non-invasive ventilation for 30 min every 3 hours.[29] During periods of spontaneous unsupported ventilation, patients can be monitored and returned to non-invasive ventilation if SaO_2 falls to <85% or the respiratory rate increases to >30 breaths min^{-1}.[28] This sequential use has been successfully employed in the management of COPD patients and may be applied to all patients identified as at risk of post-extubation failure. The limitation of this study is the use of historical controls. However, the use of sequential non-invasive ventilation significantly reduced the need for endotracheal re-intubation, the mean duration of ventilatory assistance and the length of ICU stay, and the

mortality was (not statistically) three times higher in the group treated conventionally. This study also demonstrated a lower incidence of pneumonia in the group treated non-invasively (7% versus 20%).

Randomized, controlled studies are needed to confirm the utility of non-invasive ventilation in these circumstances (post-extubation hypercapnia), but also in those with hypoxaemic respiratory failure.

WEANING FAILURE

Weaning failure, defined as mechanical ventilation persisting after recovery from the initial critical illness, is commonly due to a pre-existing disease[29] and/or neuromuscular disease. In a subset of COPD patients, weaning may be particularly difficult or even impossible. This may relate to the advanced nature of their disease, with a severe mechanical load being placed upon the respiratory muscles. Advanced age, respiratory muscle weakness (possibly due to treatment with corticosteroids) or co-existent cardiac disease may contribute to difficulties in the weaning process. Once recovered from the acute phase illness, patients may continue to require intensive nursing and/or physiotherapy care for weeks before they can be finally weaned or even be discharged ventilator dependent. In one study, these severely compromised patients, although only representing 3% of the total number of patients admitted to the ICU, consumed almost 40% of the total days of care.[30]

Patients are often judged as having failed weaning if they are still ventilator dependent 14–21 days following recovery from the admission illness. This arbitrary threshold needs clarification, as does the incidence of such patients in the ICU. There may well be considerable differences between hospitals and between countries, reflecting admission criteria and differences in the withdrawal of mechanical ventilation (see Chapter 21). In many European countries, high dependency, step-down or long-term ventilation units may offer the opportunity for continued weaning of such patients. Despite recovery from the acute illness, they may require intensive nursing and physiotherapy care, nutritional and psychological support and a more gradual weaning process before being judged totally ventilator dependent. One study showed that 60% of patients considered 'unweanable' at the time of ICU discharge regained respiratory autonomy after a relatively short (mean 17 days) stay in a specialized respiratory apecial care unit.[31] For those patients discharged to home mechanical ventilation by tracheostomy, the mortality rate at 1 year is considerably higher, at 62–87%, compared to the group successfully weaned (23–54%). Moreover, the former group remained severely disabled and house bound.[32,33]

NUTRITIONAL, PSYCHOLOGICAL AND REHABILITATIVE ASPECTS

Malnutrition and psychological aspects are important reasons for weaning difficulties.[34,35] A decrease in body weight is a recognized feature of advanced COPD and is especially severe in recurrently hospitalized patients. Nutritional state, measured as percentage of ideal body weight, influences mortality independently of the degree of airflow obstruction. It has been suggested that the main contributor to weight loss in COPD is an inadequate dietary intake for energy expenditure. The risk of being hospitalized for an episode of acute respiratory failure is significantly increased in patients with a low body mass index (<20 kg m^{-2}).[36]. Interestingly, in one report, body mass index and serum albumin were independently related to survival in acute respiratory failure. Malnutrition may contribute to respiratory and skeletal muscle weakness and have other metabolic consequences. On the other hand, excessive nutritional supplements will increase CO_2 production and thus the amount of ventilation necessary to maintain normocapnia. Further investigations may be necessary to determine whether nutritional intervention may improve clinical outcome in weaning. Metabolic disorders, such as diabetes, often associated with malnutrition, may lead to a decrease in immunological defences, so that patients are more prone to infections that prolong mechanical ventilation.[37] The correlation between body mass index and impaired respiratory muscle force may explain why malnourished patients are more likely to take longer to wean.

Psychological problems have also been frequently reported in patients in whom weaning is difficult, although the literature is limited. Overall, psychological problems are found in more than 50% of ICU patients, compared to an incidence of <1% in non-ICU hospitalized patients.[38] Sleep disturbance in the ICU is very common and may be implicated in the psychological disturbance of patients. Being mechanically ventilated involves a loss of independence and often ineffective communication, and promotes passivity. Depressive reactions often develop, making the process of weaning more difficult. Some studies have investigated the use of respiratory feedback to reduce anxiety. By using visual and auditory feedback of tidal volume, coupled with a display of the frontalis muscle electromyograph, relaxation was induced. The protocol significantly reduced ventilation time.[39] Although these preliminary results are encouraging, the requirement for trained personnel and sophisticated equipment limits its application. Indeed, there is considerable controversy about whether biofeedback is a useful, or necessary, addition to relaxation techniques. Studies have been often poorly controlled and the results cannot be generalized. Biofeedback may have a place when used in a comprehensive multi-modal treatment plan.

Dyspnoea (and resulting anxiety) is a frequent problem for patients with COPD. In particular, difficulty in gaining independence from the ventilator may relate to paradoxical breathing patterns, excessive respiratory drive and anxiety. A major goal in the rehabilitation process is early mobilization. In addition to avoiding the adverse effects of prolonged inactivity, there are several advantages to getting out of the bed, e.g. improved mechanics of ventilation, the mobilization of secretions and the promotion of self-confidence. It has been shown that COPD patients recovering from acute respiratory failure benefit from early mobilization, compared to patients who received standard medical therapy.[40] Patients treated with such a protocol showed improved effort tolerance, maximal inspiratory effort and dyspnoea score.

VOLUME-REDUCTION SURGERY AND TRANSPLANTATION

No studies have systematically investigated whether lung-volume-reduction surgery (LVRS) or lung transplantion is appropriate in the patient who has failed weaning. Nevertheless, it has been reported that LVRS in selected ventilator-dependent COPD patients can result in improved gas exchange and respiratory mechanics, which enable successful weaning.[41] Inability to walk at least 200 m in 6 min, before or after pulmonary rehabilitation, and the presence of significant hypercapnia are pre-operative predictors of a longer hospital and ICU stay, duration of mechanical ventilation and of the need for chest tube drainage in COPD patients undergoing elective bilateral LVRS.[42] The implication of this in economic terms is that cost was directly related to length of stay in the ICU: the range being 11%–30 % of the total costs of the LVRS programme.[43,44] A thoracoscopic approach, compared to open surgery, for LVRS may offer a shorter ICU stay, fewer days with an endotracheal tube, fewer respiratory complications and a lower mortality rate.[45] For patients with cystic fibrosis, the mean duration on ventilatory support for survivors of bilateral sequential lung transplantation is 3.1 days, with a range of 1–12 days; the mean ICU and hospital stays were 4.7 days (range 1–13 days) and 28 days (range 12–79 days), respectively[46]

CONCLUSION

Although we now have a 'science' of weaning, with evidence on which to base practice, there remains an 'art' to the process. The move to less sedation, more interactive modes of ventilation and greater emphasis on general rehabilitation in the weaning patient must be leading to less morbidity and, it is hoped, mortality.

REFERENCES

1. Manthous, C, Schmidt, GA, Hall, J. Liberation from mechanical ventilation. A decade of progress. *Chest* 1998; **114**: 886–901.
2. Esteban, A, Alia, I, Ibanez, J, Bonito, S, Tobin, MJ. Modes of mechanical ventilation and weaning: a national survey of Spanish hospitals. *Chest* 1994; **106**: 1188–93.
3. Stauffer, JL. Complications of translaryngeal intubation. In *Principles and practice of mechanical ventilation*, ed. M. Tobin. New York, McGraw Hill, 1994; 711–47.
4. Le Bourdelles, G, Vires, N, Bockzowki, J, Seta, N, Pavlovic, D, Aubier, M. Effects of mechanical

ventilation on diaphragmatic contractile properties in rats. *Am J Respir Crit Care Med* 1994; **149**: 1539–44.
5. Agusti, AG, Torres, A, Estopa, R, Agustividal, A. Hypophosphatemia as a cause of failed weaning: the importance of metabolic factors. *Crit Care Med* 1984; **12**: 142–3.
6. Hund, EF, Fogel, W, Kreger, D, *et al*. Critical illness polyneuropathy: clinical findings and outcomes of a frequent cause of neuromuscular weaning failure. *Crit Care Med* 1996; **24**: 1328–33.
7. Broseghini, C, Brandolese, R, Poggi, R, *et al*. Respiratory mechanics during the first day of mechanical ventilation in patients with pulmonary edema and chronic airway obstruction. *Am Rev Respir Dis* 1988; **138**(2): 355–61.
8. Similowski, T, Yan, S, Gauthier, AP, Macklem, PT, Bellemare, F. Contractile properties of the human diaphragm during chronic hyperinflation. *N Engl J Med* 1991; **325**: 917–23.
9. Levine, S, Kaiser, L, Leferovich, J, Tikunov, B. Cellular adaptations in the diaphragm in chronic obstructive pulmonary disease. *N Engl J Med* 1997; **337**: 1799–806.
10. Kramer, B. Ventilator-associated pneumonia in critically ill patients. *Ann Intern Med* 1999; **130**(12): 1027–8.
11. Elpern, EH, Scott, MG, Petro, L, Ries, MH. Pulmonary aspiration in mechanically ventilated patients with tracheostomies. *Chest* 1994; **105**: 563–6.
12. Drakulovic, MB, Torres, A, Bauer, TT, Nicolas, JM, Nogue, S, Ferrer, M. Supine body position as a risk factor for nosocomial pneumonia in mechanically ventilated patients: a randomised trial. *Lancet* 1999; **354**: 1851–8.
13. Jubran, A, Mathru, M, Dries, D, Tobin, MJ. Continuous recordings of mixed venous oxygen saturation during weaning from mechanical ventilation and the ramifications thereof. *Am J Respir Crit Care Med* 1998; **158**: 1763–9.
14. Bortz, WM. Disuse and aging. *JAMA* 1982; **248**: 1203–8.
15. Brochard, L, Rue, F, Lorino, H, Lemaire, F, Harf, A. Inspiratory pressure support compensates for the add-itional work of breathing caused by the endotracheal tube. *Anesthesiology* 1991; **75**: 739–45.
16. Brochard, L, Rauss, A, Benito, S, *et al*. Comparison of three methods of gradual withdrawal from ventilatory support during weaning from mechanical ventilation. *Am J Respir Crit Care Med* 1994; **150**: 896–903.
17. Esteban, A, Frutos, F, Tobin, MJ, *et al*. A comparison of four methods of weaning from mechanical ventilation. Spanish Lung Failure Collaborative Group. *N Engl J Med* 1995; **332**: 345–50.

18. Esteban, A, Alia, I, Tobin, MJ, *et al*. Effect of spontaneous breathing trial duration on outcome of attempts to discontinue mechanical ventilation. Spanish Lung Failure Collaborative Group. *Am J Respir Crit Care Med* 1999; **159**: 512–18.

19. Yang, KL, Tobin, MJ. A prospective study of indexes predicting the outcome of trials of weaning from mechanical ventilation. *N Engl J Med* 1991; **324**: 1445–50.

20. Ely, EW, Baker, A, Dunagan, D, *et al*. Effect of the duration of mechanical ventilation on identifying patients capable of breathing spontaneously. *N Engl J Med* 1996; **335**: 1864–9.

21. Norrenberg, M, Vincent, JL, A profile of European intensive care unit physiotherapists. *Intensive Care Med* 2000; **26**: 988–94.

22. Nava, S, Ambrosino, N, Clini, E, *et al*. Noninvasive mechanical ventilation in the weaning of patients with respiratory failure due to chronic obstructive pulmonary disease. A randomized, controlled trial. *Ann Intern Med* 1998; **128**: 721–8.

23. Girault, C, Daudenthum, I, Chevron, V *et al*. Non-invasive ventilation – a systematic extubation and weaning technique in acute-on-chronic respiratory failure: a prospective, randomized controlled study. *Am J Respir Crit Care Med* 1999; **160**: 86–92.

24. Kilger, E, Briegel, J, Haller, M, *et al*. Effects of noninvasive positive pressure ventilatory support in non-COPD patients with acute respiratory insufficiency after early intubation. *Intensive Care Med* 1999; **25**: 1374–9.

25. Chevron, V, Menard, JF, Richard, JC, Girault, C, Leroy, J, Bonmarchand, G. Unplanned extubation: risk factors of development and predictive criteria for reintubation. *Crit Care Med* 1998; **26**: 1049–53.

26. Epstein, SK, Nevins, ML, Chung, J. Effect of unplanned extubation on outcome of mechanical ventilation. *Am J Respir Crit Care Med* 2000; **161**: 1912–16.

27. Epstein, SK, Ciubataru, RL, Wong, JB. Effect of failed extubation on the outcome of mechanical ventilation. *Chest* 1997; **112**: 186–92.

28. Espstein, SK, Ciubotaru, RL. Independent effects of etiology of failure and time to reintubation on outcome for patients failing extubation. *Am J Respir Crit Care Med* 1998; **158**: 489–93.

29. Hilbert, G, Gruson, D, Gbikpi-Benissan, G, Cardinaud, JP. Sequential use of noninvasive pressure support ventilation for acute exacerbations of COPD. *Intensive Care Med* 1997; **23**: 955–61.

30. Daly, BJ, Rudy, ED, Thompson, KS, *et al*. Development of a special care unit for chronically ill patients. *Heart Lung* 1991; **20**: 45–52.

31. Nava, S, Confalonieri, M, Rampulla, C. Intermediate respiratory intensive care units in Europe: a European perspective. *Thorax* 1998; **53**: 798–802.

32. Menzies, R, Gibbons, W, Goldberg, P. Determinants of weaning and survival among patients with COPD who require mechanical ventilation for acute respiratory failure. *Chest* 1989; **95**: 398–405.

33. Nava, S, Rubini, F, Zanotti, E, *et al*. Survival and prediction of successful ventilator weaning in COPD patients requiring mechanical ventilation for more than 21 days. *Eur Respir J* 1994; **7**: 1645–52.

34. Al-Saady, NM, Blackmore, CM, Bennett, ED. Hight fat, low carbohydrate enteral feeding lowers $PaCO_2$ and reduces the period of ventilation in artificially ventilated patients. *Intensive Care Med* 1989; **15**: 290–5.

35. Holliday, JE, Hyers, TM. The reduction of weaning time from mechanical ventilation using tidal volume and relaxation biofeedback. *Am Rev Respir Dis* 1990; **141**: 1214–20.

36. Kessler, R, Faller, M, Fourgaut, G, Mennecier, B, Weitzenblum, E. Predictive factors of hospitalization for acute exacerbation in a series of 64 patients with chronic obstructive pulmonary disease. *Am J Respir Crit Care Med* 1999; **159**: 158–64.

37. Almirall, J, Bolibar, I, Balanzo, X, *et al*. Risk factors for community-acquired pneumonia in adults: a population-based case-control study. *Eur Respir J* 1999; **13**: 349–55.

38. Criner, GJ, Isaac, L. Psychological problems in the ventilator-dependent patient. In *Principles and practice of mechanical ventilation*, ed. M. Tobin. New York, McGraw-Hill, 1994; 1163–75.

39. Acosta, F. Biofeedback and progressive relaxation in weaning the anxious patient from the ventilator: a brief report. *Heart Lung* 1988; **17**(3): 299–301.

40. Nava, S. Rehabilitation of patients admitted to a Respiratory Intensive Care Unit. *Arch Phys Med Rehabil* 1998; **79**: 849–54.

41. Criner, GJ, O'Brien, G, Furukawa, S, *et al*. Lung volume reduction surgery in ventilator dependent COPD patients. *Chest* 1996; **110**: 877–84.

42. Szekely, LA, Oelberg, DA, Wright, C, *et al*. Preoperative predictors of operative morbidity and mortality in COPD patients undergoing bilateral lung volume reduction surgery. *Chest* 1997; **111**: 550–8.

43. Albert, RK, Lewis, S, Wood, D, Benditt, J. Economic aspects of lung volume reduction surgery. *Chest* 1996; **110**: 1068–71.

44. Elpern, EH, Behner, KG, Klontz, B, Warren, WH, Szidon, P, Kesten, S. Lung volume reduction surgery. An analysis of hopsital costs. *Chest* 1998; **113**: 896–99.

45. Roberts, JR, Bavaria, JE, Wahl, P, Wurster, A, Friedberg, JS, Kaiser, LR. Comparison of open and thoracoscopic bilateral volume reduction surgery: complications analysis. *Ann Thorac Surg* 1998; **66**: 1759–65.

46. Wiebe, K, Wahlers, T, Harringer, W, Hardt, H, Fabel, H, Haverich, A. Lung transplantation for cystic fibrosis: a single center experience over 8 years. *Eur J Cardiothorac Surg* 1998; **14**: 191–6.

14

Community-acquired pneumonia

WEI SHEN LIM AND JOHN T MACFARLANE

BACKGROUND EPIDEMIOLOGY

Community-acquired pneumonia (CAP) is common. In the UK, there are approximately 261 000 general practice consultations for CAP, which annually result in 83 000 hospital admissions. The estimated incidence of CAP is 5–11 per 1000 adult population per year. The elderly carry the burden of the disease, those ≥65 years of age comprising 65% of patients with CAP in the UK.

Most respiratory infection is managed in the community. CAP accounts for about 5–12% of adult lower respiratory tract infection managed by general practitioners (GPs) in the community. It has been estimated that for every 100 cases of CAP seen in primary care, 20 are referred to hospital and, of these, only one to two (10%) will require admission to an intensive care unit (ICU). The proportion of patients admitted to ICU varies in different countries (New Zealand, 1–3%; UK, 5%; USA, 12–18%; Germany, 35%) and is influenced by ICU designation and admission criteria.

Mortality rates range from 6% to 15% in hospitalized patients, increasing to 22–54% in ICU series. Again, this broad range reflects admission criteria and is consequently proportionately related to the rates of mechanical ventilation of patients in ICU, which vary from 50% to 87%.

PATIENT CHARACTERISTICS

Based on cohort studies conducted over the last 20 years, the mean age of patients with CAP admitted to ICUs is around 50 years, ranging from 18 to 89 years. Associated chronic illness is common (70%), with >30% of cases having underlying lung disease. In Spain, high alcohol intake has been noted in many patients.

The time from the onset of symptoms to ICU admission is generally about 4 days. Patients later found to have pneumococcal infection tend to be admitted more quickly compared to patients with *Legionella* or *Mycoplasma* infections. Importantly, half to three-quarters of the admissions to ICUs occur within the first 24 hours of hospital admission. Whether earlier ICU referral would result in a better outcome is unclear. In a cross-sectional study comparing patients admitted to the ICU at one hospital 10 years apart, no change in mortality was noted, despite a reduction in the numbers of unplanned emergency ICU admissions resulting from cardiopulmonary arrest which fell from 25% to 17%.

GETTING ADMITTED TO THE INTENSIVE CARE UNIT

ICU admission is usually a result of acute respiratory failure requiring assisted ventilation. An unstable clinical condition precipitated by septic shock or acute renal failure accounts for other cases admitted. The American Thoracic Society recommended that the presence of either one of two major criteria, or two of three minor criteria (Table 14.1) should prompt ICU care.[2] These admission criteria have been tested, with admission to a specialized tertiary referral ICU as the outcome measure. A high sensitivity (98%) was demonstrated, but there was low specificity (32%).[3] Modifying the criteria to include both major and minor features has been suggested to increase the sensitivity and specificity. However, these recommendations require validation.

The British Thoracic Society has defined severe CAP as the presence of two or more of the following features measured on hospital admission:[4]

- respiratory rate ≥ 30 min^{-1},
- diastolic blood pressure ≤ 60 mmHg,
- urea > 7 mmol L^{-1}.
- mental confusion

This severity prediction rule has been widely validated and has an overall sensitivity of 83% and a specificity of 70% for predicting mortality.[5–7] Its value in predicting the need for ICU admission has not been tested. However, no admission criteria can be ideal, especially as there is no universally accepted definition for severe CAP. These recommendations help inform the decision to refer or admit a patient for ICU care, but cannot replace what is, ultimately, a clinical decision. Access to a high dependency unit (HDU) or monitored respiratory care beds will be an alternative option in some hospitals with such facilities, where the

Table 14.1 *Criteria for severe community-acquired pneumonia according to the 2001 American Thoracic Society recommendations*

Major criteria
  Need for mechanical ventilation
  Septic shock

Minor criteria
  Systolic blood pressure ≥ 90 mm Hg
  PaO_2/FiO_2 ratio < 250
  Multilobar disease

need for assisted ventilation is not deemed immediate. No guidelines for admission to a HDU have been published, but they are likely to be similar to those for ICU admission.

We recommend the following as indications for considering transfer to an ICU:

- severe CAP as judged by the British Thoracic Society severity prediction rule,
- inability to maintain $PaO_2 > 8$ kPa despite maximal O_2 therapy,
- severe acidosis with pH < 7.26,
- the presence of, or worsening, CO_2 retention,
- a depressed level of consciousness or patient exhaustion,
- shock – defined as a ≥ 1-hour decrease in systolic blood pressure of ≥ 40 mmHg from baseline or a systolic blood pressure of < 90 mmHg after adequate volume replacement.

The influence of age and co-morbidity

Advancing age blunts the immune response, both locally and systemically. Older people are therefore at higher risk of developing pneumonia and are more likely to present with atypical symptoms, such as the absence of pyrexia. It has been suggested that, with increasing age, the mortality of CAP also increases. Studies conducted *exclusively* in older patients have yielded conflicting results and suggest that, at least in hospitalized patients, an age ≥ 65 years does not increase mortality.[8–10] Studies of prognostic factors have yielded similar results. In two studies conducted in Europe, patients aged ≥ 65 years admitted to the ICU with CAP did not have a higher ICU mortality.[11,12] However, this could be due to more stringent ICU admission criteria in the elderly. Furthermore, the risk of mortality following discharge from the ICU is not known. Nonetheless, on balance, the evidence does not suggest that age alone should deny ICU admission to the elderly.

IN THE INTENSIVE CARE UNIT

Microbial pathogens

Depending on the range of diagnostic tests employed, a pathogen is identified in 40–82% of cases. The frequency of identification of pathogens in 14 CAP ICU studies is shown in Figure 14.1.

Streptococcus pneumoniae is the most commonly detected pathogen in these studies. In areas where there is a high prevalence of penicillin-resistant *Strep. pneumoniae*, there is as yet no strong evidence to indicate that patients with penicillin-resistant pneumococcal pneumonia (PRPP) have a more severe illness. Currently, most cases display only low to intermediate ($0.1–1$ mg L^{-1}) levels of resistance and remain susceptible to high doses of penicillin. However, as the proportion of high-level resistant (≥ 2 mg L^{-1}) cases increases, the clinical importance and severity of PRPP may alter. Many of these PRPP isolates are also resistant to erythromycin (25% in the USA). In the UK, the prevalence of penicillin-resistant *Strep. pneumoniae* is still relatively low (2–4% in isolates from invasive samples).

The importance of *Legionella* infection in patients admitted to the ICU with CAP was underlined by studies conducted in the 1980s and emerging mainly from the UK and Spain. In the UK, it accounted for 12–30% of cases. More recent studies have not always found *Legionella* infection to be as prominent. In one centre in Spain, the frequency dropped from 14% in 1984 to 2% in 1996. This fall in frequency may, in part, be due to year-to-year variation and to increased use of macrolides in the early treatment of CAP in the community.[13] A knowledge of local epidemiological patterns is therefore important.

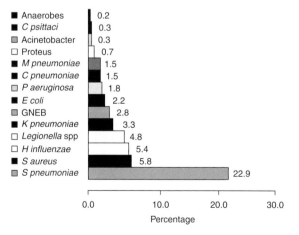

Figure 14.1 *Pathogens identified in patients with CAP admitted to an ICU from 14 studies. GNEB, Gram-negative enteric bacilli. (Figures are under-represented as they do not include studies in which specific pathogens are mentioned, e.g.* Escherichia coli.*)*

Legionella pneumonia is commonly perceived as having a high mortality, probably reflecting both the high proportion of patients with *Legionella* infection who are admitted to the ICU compared to those with other infections and the unusually high publicity this infection has attained.[14] However, *Legionella* is not an independent risk factor for mortality in CAP and does not increase the mortality in those patients who require mechanical ventilation.[15]

Clinical features considered typical for *Legionella* pneumonia include a dry cough, neurological symptoms, such as mental confusion and headache, diarrhoea and a low sodium level. In the UK, over half of all cases are associated with travel abroad in the 10 days prior to onset of illness. Unfortunately, none of these features is specific for *Legionella* infection and none can be relied upon to confidently discriminate infection caused by *Legionella* sp. from other pathogens. Rhabdomyolysis is an uncommon but well-recognized complication. Creatinine kinase levels $>50\,000$ U L^{-1} have been reported, and acute renal failure may be precipitated. Interestingly, the organism has been demonstrated by immunofluorescence in renal biopsy samples in such cases.[16]

In all studies, the other atypical pathogens (*C. pneumoniae*, *C. psittici*, *M. pneumoniae* and *C. burnetti*) are found in only 2–3% of cases. Mortality in these cases tends to be lower, consistent with the generally less severe nature of these infections.

Staphylococcus aureus is well recognized as an important pathogen in severe CAP and carries a high mortality (60–100%). In about 50% of cases, it is associated with recent influenza virus infection. It therefore needs to be considered in the winter months during high influenza activity. In France, it is reported to be a more frequent cause of severe CAP (15%),[11] although the reason for this is not clear. In a typical case, there is a history consistent with influenza followed up by a period of relative recovery, before further deterioration within 2 weeks. Infection may be complicated by lung abscess formation, cavitation and empyema. Pneumatoceles have been described, more commonly in paediatric cases. Methicillin-resistant *Staph. aureus* (MRSA) is an increasing problem, particularly in nosocomial infection in the ICU. Patients at risk for MRSA pneumonia who come from outside of the hospital include the elderly, the immunocompromised and those with recent prolonged hospitalization during which MRSA colonization may have developed. MRSA is a well-recognized pathogen in nosocomial pneumonia, but patients presenting with CAP as a result of MRSA infection are now being reported. Another risk factor may be admission from a nursing home facility. A rise in the importance of community-acquired MRSA infection will have significant implications for the empiric antibiotic therapy of CAP, and the evolution of this situation requires close surveillance.

Some centres, mostly in Spain, have reported a relatively high rate (4–5%) of infection with *Pseudomonas aeruginosa* in CAP associated with a high mortality – up to 100%. Significant co-morbidity, in particular underlying chronic lung disease, may be the explanation, and an independent association of *P. aeruginosa* infection with mortality has not been firmly established. Similarly, infection by Gram-negative enteric bacilli (GNEB), especially the Enterobacteriaceae, has been inconsistently associated with a higher mortality. Patients admitted from a nursing home facility are thought to be at greater risk of acquiring GNEB-related CAP. This association has been mainly described in North America and may not apply in other countries where different healthcare systems exist and where the health of nursing home residents may differ substantially.

The importance of geographical variation in the pattern of pathogens seen is exemplified by the high frequency of *Burkholderia pseudomallei* (7–21%) compared to *Strep. pneumoniae infection (4–5%) in* CAP ICU patients reported in retrospective studies from Singapore.[17] This reflects the endemicity of *B. pseudomallei* in the region that includes Northern Australia and Thailand. In South Africa, *Klebsiella pneumoniae* was the second commonest organism isolated after *Strep. pneumoniae* in a 10-year retrospective survey (19% versus 29%).[18]

A microbial agent cannot be identified in approximately 45% of patients, despite intensive microbiological investigations. In the past, attempts have been made to use clinical, laboratory and radiological features to define the responsible pathogen. There is now good evidence that this approach is unreliable.[19,20] As a result, empiric antibiotic therapy must therefore continue to be directed at the most probable range of pathogens determined by local epidemiological data.

MICROBIOLOGICAL INVESTIGATIONS

The value of diagnostic tests to identify microbial agents in CAP has been questioned, especially as a change in antibiotic therapy as a result does not appear to reduce mortality. The limitations to microbiological investigations include the following.

- A lack of sensitivity and specificity of diagnostic tests available. Prior antibiotic use, in particular, reduces the diagnostic rate. In hospital studies of CAP, about 35% of patients report receiving antibiotics prior to hospital admission. Apart from patients transferred immediately to the ICU upon presentation to hospital, almost all patients will have received at least one dose of antibiotic.
- Time delay in obtaining results. Results will not generally be quickly available (except Gram staining of sputum), whereas antibiotic administration needs to be prompt. Serological tests that rely on a rise in antibody titres yield results only 2–3 weeks later.
- The presence of mixed infections. The importance of co-pathogens in regard to diagnostic testing and antibiotic choice is a difficult issue. Mixed infections have been reported in up to 30% of patients hospitalized with CAP. The identification of a single pathogen, therefore, does not rule out the presence of a second. Most co-infections involve an atypical pathogen or virus with a bacterial pathogen, usually *Strep. pneumoniae*. Whether specific treatment for the atypical pathogen in such circumstances is necessary is unclear. Certainly, where *C. pneumoniae* has been found together with *Strep. pneumoniae*, recovery is reported despite antibiotic therapy directed only against *Strep. pneumoniae*.[21–23]

On the other hand, the early identification of a pathogen can be useful through confirmation of the diagnosis and choice of antibiotic regimen. A more focused antibiotic regimen favourably affects the development of adverse drug reactions, complications and antibiotic resistance. The introduction of rapid detection methods, such as antigen detection and polymerase chain reactions, is therefore welcomed. These diagnostic tools are less affected by prior antibiotic use (though not immune to it) and, in theory, can offer a result within hours of the appropriate sample being taken. Commercial kits for the detection in urine of *Legionella* and pneumococcal antigen are now available and may prove to be valuable as part of a diagnostic package. It is our practice to perform the diagnostic tests detailed in Table 14.2 in all cases of CAP admitted to the ICU.

Percutaneous needle biopsy for the bacteriologic diagnosis of pneumonia has regained interest recently. A positive microbiological culture result is possible in 33–80% of cases. The specificity is felt to be good as there is less contamination by oropharyngeal flora, although this has not been evaluated carefully. The most common complication is pneumothorax (up to 30% of procedures), although most are small and do not require drainage. Haemoptysis occurs in 1–5%. Fatal air embolism is a rare but recognized complication. Contraindications to the procedure include:

- poor pulmonary reserve,
- bleeding diathesis,
- lack of patient co-operation,
- mechanical ventilation.

Table 14.2 *Suggested microbiological investigations in patients with severe community-acquired pneumonia*

Gram stain and culture of sputum and respiratory samples
Pneumococcal antigen tests on sputum, respiratory samples and/or urine
Urine for *Legionella* antigen
Sputum or other respiratory sample for *Legionella* culture and direct immunofluorescence to *Legionella* sp., *Chlamydia* sp., influenza A and B, parainfluenza 1–3, adenovirus, respiratory syncytial virus and *Pneumocystis carinii* (if at risk)
Initial and follow up viral and atypical pathogen (including *Legionella*) serology with the initial sample being tested without waiting for the follow-up sample
Collection of lower respiratory tract samples by more invasive techniques, such as bronchoscopy, and deep tracheal sampling by catheter should be considered. Percutaneous fine-needle aspiration may be useful in patients who are not on positive pressure ventilation[37]

The risk of pneumothorax is important in patients who are receiving assisted positive pressure ventilation, and consequently the technique has limited use for patients with severe CAP, except when performed by a very skilled and experienced operator. Therefore, we feel that, currently, percutaneous lung biopsy is not recommended as a routine diagnostic test in CAP. Its role in selected patients, such as the severely ill, remains to be evaluated.

Prognosis

Studies conducted to identify prognostic factors in patients admitted to the ICU differ from other hospital studies of severity assessment in CAP, especially in the use of mortality as the outcome measure. The most consistently independently associated prognostic factors are the presence of either septic shock or progression of chest radiography changes during the ICU stay. (Septic shock has been defined in various ways. A common definition is a ≥ 1-hour decrease in systolic blood pressure of ≥ 40 mmHg from baseline or a resultant systolic blood pressure of <90 mmHg after adequate volume replacement.) Other risk factors are detailed in Table 14.3.

A large, French, multi-centre study over a 10-year period, and involving 472 patients, identified nine important variables from which a prediction model was constructed.[4] Patients were initially stratified into three groups, based on six risk factors assessable on ICU admission. Mortality risk estimates were subsequently adjusted according to the development of three other prognostic factors (Table 14.4). This model appears promising, but, in its current form, is complicated and remains to be tested in different settings. The initial stratification of patients into three risk groups, if subsequently validated, may prove to be a useful prognostic tool.

Table 14.3 *Factors independently associated with death in the ICU*

Anticipated death within 4–5 years
Simplified Acute Physiology Score (SAPS) >12
Acute renal failure
Bacteraemia
Infection with *Strep. pneumoniae*
Infection with Gram-negative enteric bacilli
Non-pneumonia-related complications

Table 14.4 *A prognostic model for predicting ICU mortality*

Risk factors on ICU admission	Points	Risk factors during ICU stay	Points
Age ≥40 years	1	Sepsis-type complication (ARDS, shock, multi-organ failure)	4
Anticipated death ≤5 years (based on co-morbid index)	1	Hospital-acquired lower respiratory tract infection	1
Non-aspiration pneumonia	1	Non-specific complications (deep venous thrombosis, pulmonary embolism, gastrointestinal bleed)	2
Multilobar (>1) lobe involvement	1		
Acute respiratory failure requiring MV <12 hours	1		
Septic shock ≥1 hour (decrease in SBP of ≥40 mmHg from baseline or resultant SBP <90 mmHg after volume replacement)	3		

Initial points	Class	Initial risk of mortality (%)		Adjusted risk of mortality (%) Additional points (during ICU stay)		
				0	1–2	>2
0–2	I	4	♦	1	1	50
3–5	II	25		2	39	86
6–8	III	60		49	49	93

Adapted from reference 4. ICU, intensive care unit; MV, mechanical ventilation; SBP, systolic blood pressure; ARDS, acute respiratory distress syndrome.

MANAGEMENT STRATEGIES

Antibiotics

The early institution of appropriate antibiotics has been shown to improve outcome.[24] The administration of antibiotics should not be postponed. This is especially pertinent in the early admission period, when multiple tasks may need to be performed simultaneously. The choice of antibiotic is crucially determined by the local epidemiological pattern of likely pathogens. In the UK, where pneumococcal and *Legionella* infection predominate, a combination of a β-lactamase-stable antibiotic and a macrolide ± rifampicin is recommended as empirical therapy (Table 14.5). A rise in liver enzymes can be expected with rifampicin given at a dose of 600 mg intravenously twice daily. This is usually harmless and resolves once the drug is stopped. The authors' practice is to reduce the intravenous dose after 3 days to 600 mg once daily and to stop the drug after a total of 7 days if the patient is responding adequately. Whether the addition of rifampicin to a macrolides

is more effective in proven *Legionella* infection is untested. Similarly, although the quinolones have been found to be more active than macrolides in animal studies, there are no controlled trials demonstrating their superiority. As there is extensive clinical experience with the macrolides in the treatment of *Legionella* infection, and no evidence of emerging resistance, it seems reasonable to continue using them as first-line therapy, with the quinolones being employed as second-line agents in the event of drug intolerance, allergy or failure.

Flucloxacillin should be added when *Staph. aureus* infection is suspected. It is worth noting that the third-generation cephalosporins are less active than the first-generation and second-generation against *Staph. aureus*. For MRSA infection, vancomycin remains the antibiotic of choice. Extra coverage for Gram-negative enteric bacilli (e.g. with an aminoglycoside) and pseudomonal infection (e.g. with ceftazidime) is not routinely required in the UK in view of the low frequency (2–3%) of these pathogens. Where these infections are more common, different recommendations may apply. The European Respiratory Society and Italian guidelines for the

Table 14.5 *Recommended empirical antibiotics for severe community-acquired pneumonia of unknown cause*

Preferred
Amoxicillin/clavulanate 1.2 g t.d.s. i.v.
or
Cefuroxime 1.5 g t.d.s. i.v.
or
Cefotaxime 1 g t.d.s. i.v.
or
Ceftriaxone 2 g o.d. i.v.
plus
Erythromycin 500 mg q.d.s. i.v.
or
Clarithromycin 500 mg b.d. i.v.
with or without
Rifampicin 600 mg o.d. or b.d. i.v.

Alternative
For those intolerant of preferred regimen, or where there are
    local concerns over *Clostridium difficile*-associated diar-
    rhoea related to β-lactam use Levofloxacin 500 mg b.d. i.v.
plus
Benzylpenicillin 1–2 g 6-hourly i.v.

---

management of CAP do not recommend the use of anti-pseudomonal agents, whereas in the Netherlands, they are recommended for patients with severe chronic obstructive airways disease or structural lung disease.[25–27] Anaerobic infection is uncommon. The need for adding anaerobic cover should therefore be assessed individually and take into account known risk factors such as poor dentition and the likelihood of aspiration. The Infectious Diseases Society of America has published recommendations for the empirical antibiotic treatment of severe CAP.[28]

Non-antibiotic therapy

NON-INVASIVE VENTILATION

Failure to maintain adequate oxygenation (PaO_2 >8 kPa or SaO_2 >90%), despite high-flow O_2 supplementation, may indicate the need for assisted ventilation. Continuous positive airways pressure (CPAP), by recruiting under-ventilated alveoli and allowing an increase in fractional FiO_2, may correct hypoxaemia and avoid the need for intubation (see Chapter 5). It has been shown to be effective in

hypoxia resulting from CAP as well as in viral and *Pneumocystis carinii* pneumonia, although there are no randomised, controlled trials. Non-invasive ventilation (see Chapter 5) may be employed when CO_2 retention develops. Confalonieri *et al.* have reported a randomized, controlled trial of 56 patients with CAP in which the intubation rate was significantly reduced by non-invasive ventilation.[29] A rapid and sustained reduction in respiratory rate was evident in patients treated with non-invasive ventilation and the need for mechanical ventilation was reduced by half (21% in patients treated with non-invasive ventilation compared to 50% in controls). The intensity of nursing care workload, duration of hospitalization and hospital mortality remained unchanged. Patients treated with non-invasive ventilation need to be closely monitored, particularly for evidence of retention of respiratory secretions. Review of clinical response is important and criteria for endotracheal intubation should be unambiguous. In all instances, the availability of non-invasive ventilation should not result in inappropriate delay in the initiation of mechanical ventilation when necessary. Centres experienced in non-invasive ventilation are likely to report the best results.

SPECIAL VENTILATORY APPROACHES

In pneumonia, hypoxia is mediated primarily by perfusion of units of low or no ventilation. Hypoxic pulmonary vasoconstriction, which attempts to improve VQ matching through the release of prostaglandins, may be abnormal in pneumonia and be partly responsible.

Positioning

Positioning the patient with unilateral consolidation with the involved side up may increase perfusion to the dependent, uninvolved lung by gravity. Ventilation perfusion matching is thereby improved, with improvement in hypoxaemia.[30]

Differential lung ventilation

Ventilatory requirements may differ substantially between the two lungs in patients with unilateral involvement. By using a double-lumen tube, ventilation to each lung can, theoretically, be individually optimized. For instance, higher levels of positive end-expiratory pressure (PEEP) may be applied to the less compliant pneumonic lung. In practice, double ventilation is very difficult and rarely effective.

Extra-corporeal membrane oxygenation

Extra-corporeal membrane oxygenation (ECMO) has been used in adults with respiratory failure due to CAP who have failed to maintain adequate levels of oxygenation despite aggressive ventilation techniques. However, as yet, there are only isolated case reports and better evidence is required before such experimental approaches can be justified.

Pharmacological manipulation

Anti-inflammatory Drugs Theoretically, cyclo-oxygenase inhibitors, such as aspirin and indomethacin, should reduce prostaglandin-induced loss of hypoxic vasoconstriction. However, in exploratory studies, although improvement in intrapulmonary shunts has been demonstrated, commensurate improvements in oxygenation did not occur.[31]

Prostacyclin and Nitric Oxide Local selective vasodilatation in better ventilated lung areas by aerosolized prostacyclin or inhaled nitric oxide decreases intrapulmonary shunt. An improvement in oxygenation is therefore possible. Although studied most in adult respiratory distress syndrome (ARDS), these drugs may be helpful in patients with pneumonia.[32]

ADJUVANT AGENTS
Steroids

In the past, steroids have been used in septic shock complicating infection, but without success. A preliminary study of intravenous hydrocortisone in CAP suggests that inflammatory markers, including tumour necrosis factor-α (TNF-α), interleukin (IL)-1β, IL-6 and CRP, are reduced.[33] Further work to delineate clinical benefit is awaited.

Granulocyte colony-stimulating factor

Granulocyte colony-stimulating factor (G-CSF) increases the production and function of neutrophils. It is widely used in treating neutropenia in patients receiving chemotherapy. There is evidence that in non-neutropenic patients with CAP, it reduces complications (empyema, ARDS, disseminated intravascular coagulation) and/or length of hospitalization. A phase I trial has shown that, given subcutaneously for 10 days (at doses of 75–650 μg

day^{-1}) in combination with appropriate antimicrobial therapy, it is safe. There has, as yet, been no evidence of increased tissue damage as a result of enhanced neutrophil activation.[34]

PATIENT NOT IMPROVING

Patients who do not respond to initial treatment have a higher mortality. Early re-assessment and appropriate intervention are therefore required. Possibilities to consider include:

- incorrect or additional unrecognized diagnosis, e.g.
  1. pulmonary embolism
  2. foreign-body inhalation
  3. proximal obstructing endobronchial tumour
  4. bronchiolitis obliterans organizing pneumonia
  5. hospital-acquired infection

- a pathogen resistant to initial antimicrobial therapy
  1. natural resistance, e.g.
     (a) fungus: aspergillus, coccidiomycosis
     (b) *Mycobacteria: M. tuberculosis*
     (c) virus: chicken pox
     (d) parasite: *Pneumocystis carinii*
     (e) bacteria: *P. aeruginosa*

  2. acquired resistance, e.g.
     (a) penicillin-resistant *Strep. pneumoniae*
     (b) methicillin-resistant *Staph. aureus*

- drug non-compliance, hypersensitivity or drug-related complications, e.g.
  1. inadequate dose
  2. *Clostridium difficile*-associated diarrhoea
  3. phlebitis at intravenous cannula site

- defective host immune response, e.g.
  1. undiagnosed immunocompromised state, e.g. human immunodeficiency virus (HIV) infection, uncontrolled diabetes mellitus
  2. underlying cancer
  3. cystic fibrosis

- complication of infection, e.g.
  1. lung abscess
  2. empyema
  3. metastatic infection
  4. ARDS

Para-pneumonic effusions are a common complication, occurring in 20–60% of patients with CAP. The majority are small and resolve in step with the main site of pulmonary infection with antibiotics. However, 5–10% of para-pneumonic effusions progress to become empyemas unless adequately drained. In deciding to drain a para-pneumonic effusion, clinical factors, radiological findings and pleural fluid characteristics need to be taken into consideration. Persistent fever, features suggestive of anaerobic infection (aspiration, alcoholism), infection with *Staph. aureus*, *Staph. pyogenes* or *K. pneumoniae* and larger effusions are the most important features that indicate the need for further evaluation. Ultrasound and computerized tomography (CT) scanning are both useful investigations (see Chapter 7). Whenever possible, the effusion should be tapped and pleural fluid sent for determination of pH, Gram stain and culture. (Pleural fluid pH is tested anaerobically using a heparinized syringe through a standard blood-gas machine.) The presence of frank pus or the growth of micro-organisms is diagnostic of an empyema, and a pH of <7.2 is highly suggestive.[35] In these circumstances, and when loculations are demonstrated radiologically by ultrasound or CT, early drainage is indicated. A small to moderate-sized catheter (8–16 French gauge) is adequate in most instances, but requires irrigation with saline one to four times per day to maintain patency. The instillation of intrapleural thrombolytics is useful in promoting drainage and preventing the development of loculations within the pleural cavity.[36] Streptokinase and urokinase have both been tested. Different doses and methods of instillation have been reported. One 'protocol' is detailed in Table 14.6. Where frank pus is present, the insertion of a large-bore chest drain (size 22–34 French gauge) is the traditional approach and early consultation with a thoracic surgical colleague is recommended. Pleural decortication, or open drainage with rib resection, is sometimes still required in difficult cases.

Complete evaluation of the patient who does not appear to be responding to treatment begins with a reappraisal of the history of illness, with collaborating information obtained from relatives, friends or witnesses. It may also involve repeating laboratory investigations, including blood cultures, assessing HIV status and performing CT scans, ultrasound

Table 14.6 *Protocol for instillation of intrapleural streptokinase*

1. Position a size 12–14 French catheter in the most dependent portion of the pleural collection
2. Connect to an underwater seal and keep on continuous suction (− 20 cmH$_2$0)
3. Flush catheter with 20 mL saline every 6 hours
4. Instill 250 000 IU streptokinase in 20 mL saline in place of one of the saline flushes 12 hourly
5. Close off the catheter for 2 hours after instilling streptokinase; return to suction thereafter

Doses of streptokinase may be given for 3–5 days, depending on the clinical situation and response

assessment of pleural and abdominal cavities and echocardiography. Bronchoscopy is indicated to exclude post-obstructive pneumonia or lung abscess. It can be performed on patients supported by non-invasive ventilation see Chapter 5). Lung biopsy is only necessary in a tiny proportion of patients in whom the diagnosis remains unclear despite less invasive investigations. The differential diagnosis includes:

- bronchiolitis obliterans organizing pneumonia,
- malignancy, e.g. primary lymphoma, broncho-alveolar cell carcinoma,
- hypersensitivity pneumonitis,
- eosinophilic pneumonitis,
- drug-induced pneumonitis,
- pulmonary vasculitis, e.g. Wegener's granulomatosis,
- granulomatous disorders, e.g. sarcoidosis, berylliosis,
- pulmonary alveolar proteinosis.

SUMMARY

CAP is common and is severe in some patients. Although there are no randomised, controlled trials, for some patients, prompt and appropriate management in an ICU probably reduces mortality. Admission criteria and the likely pathogens encountered are strongly influenced by geography, healthcare resources and population characteristics. The review offered here may therefore need tailoring to the different situations encountered in day-to-day clinical practice.

REFERENCES

1. Hirani, NA, Macfarlane, JT. Impact of management guidelines on the outcome of severe community acquired pneumonia. *Thorax* 1997; **52**: 17–21.

2. Niederman, MS, Mandell, LA, Anzueto, A, *et al.* Guidelines for the management of adults with CAP. *ABRCCM* 2001; **163**: 1730–54.

3. Ewig, S, Ruiz, M, Mensa, J, *et al.* Severe community-acquired pneumonia. Assessment of severity criteria. *Am J Respir Crit Care Med* 1998; **158**: 1102–8.

4. The British Thoracic Society, BTS guidelines for the management of CAP. *Thorax* 2001; **56**: Supplement IV.

5. Anonymous. Community-acquired pneumonia in adults in British hospitals in 1982–1983: a survey of aetiology, mortality, prognostic factors and outcome. The British Thoracic Society and the Public Health Laboratory Service. *Q J Med* 1987; **62**: 195–220.

6. Lim, WS, Macfarlane, JI, Boswell, TC, *et al.* SCAPA: Study of CAP aetiology in adults admitted to hospital: implications for management guidelines. *Thorax* 2001; **56**: 296–301.

7. Neill, AM, Martin, IR, Weir, R, *et al.* Community acquired pneumonia: aetiology and usefulness of severity criteria on admission. *Thorax* 1996; **51**: 1010–16.

8. Riquelme, R, Torres, A, El-Ebiary, M, *et al.* Community-acquired pneumonia in the elderly: a multivariate analysis of risk and prognostic factors. *Am J Respir Crit Care Med* 1996; **154**: 1450–5.

9. Janssens, JP, Gauthey, L, Herrmann, F, Tkatch, L, Michel, JP. Community-acquired pneumonia in older patients. *J Am Geriatr Soc* 1996; **44**: 539–44.

10. Venkatesan, P, Gladman, J, Macfarlane, JT, *et al.* A hospital study of community acquired pneumonia in the elderly. *Thorax* 1990; **45**: 254–8.

11. Leroy, O, Bosquet, C, Vandenbussche, C, *et al.* Community-acquired pneumonia in the intensive care unit: epidemiological and prognosis data in older people. *J Am Geriatr Soc* 1999; **47**: 539–46.

12. Rello, J, Rodriguez, R, Jubert, P, Alvarez, B. Severe community-acquired pneumonia in the elderly: epidemiology and prognosis. *Clin Infect Dis* 1996; **23**: 723–8.

13. Ruiz, M, Ewig, S, Torres, A, *et al.* Severe community-acquired pneumonia. Risk factors and follow-up epidemiology. *Am J Respir Crit Care Med* 1999; **160**: 923–9.

14. Woodhead, MA, Macfarlane, JT, Rodgers, FG, Laverick, A, Pilkington, R, Macrae, AD. Aetiology and outcome of severe community-acquired pneumonia. *J Infect* 1985; **10**: 204–10.

15. Woodhead, MA, Macfarlane, JT. Legionnaires' disease: a review of 79 community acquired cases in Nottingham. *Thorax* 1986; **41**: 635–40.

16. Shah, A, Check, F, Baskin, S, Reyman, T, Menard, R. Legionnaires' disease and acute renal failure: case report and review. *Clin Infect Dis* 1992; **14**: 204–7.

17. Tan, YK, Khoo, KL, Chin, SP, Ong, YY. Aetiology and outcome of severe community-acquired pneumonia in Singapore. *Eur Respir J* 1998; **12**: 113–15.

18. Feldman, C, Ross, S, Mahomed, AG, Omar, J, Smith, C. The aetiology of severe community-acquired pneumonia and its impact on initial, empiric, antimicrobial chemotherapy. *Respir Med* 1995; **89**: 187–92.

19. Farr, BM, Kaiser, DL, Harrison, BD, Connolly, CK. Prediction of microbial aetiology at admission to hospital for pneumonia from the presenting clinical features. British Thoracic Society Pneumonia Research Subcommittee. *Thorax* 1989; **44**: 1031–5.

20. Fang, GD, Fine, M, Orloff, J, *et al.* New and emerging etiologies for community-acquired pneumonia with implications for therapy. A prospective multicenter study of 359 cases. *Medicine* 1990; **69**: 307–16.

21. Torres, A, El Ebiary, M. Relevance of *Chlamydia pneumoniae* in community-acquired respiratory infections [editorial]. *Eur Respir J* 1993; **6**: 7–8.

22. Kauppinen, MT, Saikku, P, Kujala, P, Herva, E, Syrjala, H. Clinical picture of community-acquired *Chlamydia pneumoniae* pneumonia requiring hospital treatment: a comparison between chlamydial and pneumococcal pneumonia [see comments]. *Thorax* 1996; **51**: 185–9.

23. Lieberman, D, Schlaeffer, F, Boldur, I, *et al.* Multiple pathogens in adult patients admitted with community-acquired pneumonia: a one year prospective study of 346 consecutive patients. *Thorax* 1996; **51**: 179–84.

24. Meehan, TP, Fine, MJ, Krumholz, HM, *et al.* Quality of care, process, and outcomes in elderly patients with pneumonia. *JAMA* 1997; **278**: 2080–4.

25. Vegelin, AL, Bissumbhar, P, Joore, JC, Lammers, JW, Hoepelman, IM. Guidelines for severe community-acquired pneumonia in the western world. *Neth J Med* 1999; **55**: 110–17.

26. Gialdroni, GG, Bianchi, L. Guidelines for the management of community-acquired pneumonia in adults. Italian Society of Pneumology. Italian

Society of Respiratory Medicine. Italian Society of Chemotherapy. *Monaldi Arch Chest Dis* 1995; **50**: 21–7.

27. ERS Task Force Report. Guidelines for management of adult community-acquired lower respiratory tract infections. European Respiratory Society. *Eur Respir J* 1998; **11**: 986–91.

28. Bartlett, JG, Breiman, RF, Mandell, LA, File, TM Jr. Community-acquired pneumonia in adults: guidelines for management. The Infectious Diseases Society of America. *Clin Infect Dis* 1998; **26**: 811–38.

29. Confalonieri, M, Potena, A, Carbone, G, *et al*. Acute respiratory failure in patients with severe community-acquired pneumonia. A prospective randomized evaluation of noninvasive ventilation. *Am J Respir Crit Care Med* 1999; **160**: 1585–91.

30. Dreyfuss, D, Djedaini, K, Lanore, JJ, Mier, L, Froidevaux, R, Coste, F. A comparative study of the effects of almitrine bismesylate and lateral position during unilateral bacterial pneumonia with severe hypoxemia. *Am Rev Respir Dis* 1992; **146**: 295–9.

31. Ferrer, M, Torres, A, Baer, R, Hernandez, C, Roca, J, Rodriguez-Roisin, R. Effect of acetylsalicylic acid on pulmonary gas exchange in patients with severe pneumonia: a pilot study. *Chest* 1997; **111**: 1094–100.

32. Walmrath, D, Schneider, T, Pilch, J, Schermuly, R, Grimminger, F, Seeger, W. Effects of aerosolized prostacyclin in severe pneumonia: impact of fibrosis. *Am J Respir Crit Care Med* 1995; **151**: 724–30.

33. Monton, C, Ewig, S, Torres, A, *et al*. Role of glucocorticoids on inflammatory response in nonimmunosuppressed patients with pneumonia: a pilot study. *Eur Respir J* 1999; **14**: 218–20.

34. DeBoisblanc, BP, Mason, CM, Andresen, J, *et al*. Phase 1 safety trial of Filgrastim (r-metHuG-CSF) in non-neutropenic patients with severe community-acquired pneumonia. *Respir Med* 1997; **91**: 387–94.

35. Heffner, JE, Brown, LK, Barbieri, C, DeLeo, JM. Pleural fluid chemical analysis in parapneumonic effusions. A meta-analysis. [Published erratum appears in *Am J Respir Crit Care Med* 1995; **152**(2): 823.] *Am J Respir Crit Care Med* 1995; **151**: 1700–8.

36. Davies, RJ, Traill, ZC, Gleeson, FV. Randomised controlled trial of intrapleural streptokinase in community acquired pleural infection. *Thorax* 1997; **52**: 416–21.

37. Ruiz-Gonzalez, A, Falguera, M, Nogues, A, RubioCaballero, M. Is *Streptococcus pneumoniae* the leading cause of pneumonia of unknown etiology? A microbiologic study of lung aspirates in consecutive patients with community-acquired pneumonia. *Am J Med* 1999; **106**: 385–90.

15

Nosocomial pneumonia

JEAN-LOUIS VINCENT, BAUDOUIN BYL AND DALIANA PERES BOTA

INTRODUCTION

Derived from the Latin word for hospital (*noso-comium*), a nosocomial infection is an infection acquired in hospital as opposed to in the community. The critically ill patient is particularly at risk of developing nosocomial infection. In a large, single-day point prevalence study of nosocomial infection in intensive care units (ICUs) across Europe (the EPIC study), 45% of the 10038 patients occupying an ICU bed had a nosocomial infection.[1] The most common type of infection was nosocomial pneumonia, reported in 47% of infected patients (Fig. 15.1). Nosocomial pneumonia is therefore common on the ICU and is not only associated with increased morbidity and mortality, but also with prolonged ICU stay and costs.[2] Awareness of the associated risk factors facilitates early diagnosis and treatment, and specific preventive strategies may help limit the development of this complication. This chapter discusses basic definitions and epidemiology, diagnosis, potential risk factors, prevention and therapy.

DEFINITIONS AND EPIDEMIOLOGY

ICU nosocomial pneumonia may be broadly defined as a pneumonia that develops while on the ICU but that was not present on ICU admission. However, within this broad definition, varying time intervals and other criteria have been specified by different authors. Most agree that ICU-acquired pneumonia refers to any infection occurring 48 hours or more after ICU admission. Many investigators also separately classify ventilator-acquired pneumonia (VAP) as an infection that occurs more than 24 or 48 hours after the patient has been intubated and mechanically ventilated. The quoted incidence of nosocomial pneumonia on the ICU ranges from 9% to 47%, with the variation relating to the ICU case-mix and differences in the definitions and diagnostic techniques used.[3–6] Specific groups of ICU patients such as trauma patients have a higher incidence of nosocomial infection.[3,7]

Mortality associated with the development of nosocomial pneumonia varies considerably, with some studies reporting a crude mortality ranging from 40% to 70%,[4,6,8,9] while other studies have attempted to identify the increased mortality specifically attributable to its development (27–45%).[10,11] Nosocomial pneumonia may itself cause increased mortality, but it could also be that it is the sicker patients with inherently higher mortality who develop nosocomial pneumonia and the pneumonia itself is only a marker of the higher mortality seen in such patients.

The most commonly identified organisms are *Pseudomonas aeruginosa* and *Staphylococcus aureus*,

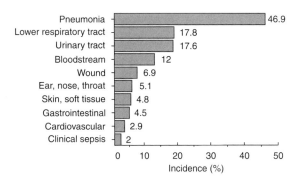

Figure 15.1 *Incidence of ICU-acquired infection in the EPIC study[1] by site of origin, showing pneumonia as the most common nosocomial infection.*

with other causative organisms including *Klebsiella*, *Enterobacter*, *Escherichia coli* and *Acinetobacter* species.[5] The pattern of causative organisms varies among units according to patient case-mix, antibiotic protocols, infection control practices, etc.[12] Mortality seems to be particularly high in patients infected with *Pseudomonas* or *Acinetobacter* species.[10]

PATHOGENESIS

For pneumonia to develop, one or more of the following conditions must exist: impaired host defences; the presence of a sufficient number of organisms in the patient's lower respiratory tract to overcome host defence; or the presence of a particularly virulent organism. Host defences are frequently already reduced in the critically ill population, due to concurrent disease processes. Immunosuppression in the critically ill is primarily due to the release of interleukin-10 (IL-10) and other anti-inflammatory mediators, such as IL-1 receptor antagonist (IL-1Ra) and tumour necrosis factor (TNF) receptors, and produces a state of 'immunoparalysis'. Patients who have been treated with immunosuppressive drugs represent a particularly high-risk group.[13]

The inoculation of infectious organisms into the lower airways can occur in various ways, but (micro)aspiration of colonized oropharyngeal secretions is probably the most important. Whereas micro-aspiration of oropharyngeal secretions is a common event in all individuals, the critically ill,

particularly those receiving mechanical ventilation, have a higher incidence of upper airway colonization with potentially pathogenic organisms and figures as high as 80% have been reported.[14,15] Aspiration of gastric contents is more likely to occur in patients with a reduced level of consciousness, during insertion of nasogastric or endotracheal tubes and if there is co-existing oesophageal disease. Alternative routes of entry for infectious organisms to the lower airways include aerosol spread, perhaps more commonly associated with viruses, *Legionella* species and *Mycobacterium tuberculosis*, and haematogenous spread, more common in postoperative patients and in those with long-term intravenous or urinary catheters. Tracheal intubation impairs certain host defence mechanisms, such as cough and mucociliary clearance, putting such patients at greater risk of developing pneumonia. Secretions may collect around the endotracheal cuff and these are not easily removed by suctioning and are prone to colonization. Changes in airway size during swallowing or breathing can allow leakage of these secretions into the lower airways. In addition, respiratory equipment can harbour pathogenic organisms, permitting direct inoculation of the lower airways.

DIAGNOSIS

The diagnosis of nosocomial pneumonia in the ICU may be difficult because the typical features of infection, such as fever, tachycardia, tachypnoea and raised white blood cell counts, are non-specific indicators of an inflammatory response. Patchy alveolar infiltrates on chest X-ray may represent pneumonia, but could also be due to pulmonary oedema, infarction or atelectasis. Non-pathogenic colonization of the upper airways is common in the ICU patient, rendering positive cultures from tracheal aspirates relatively insensitive. Other techniques, including culture of samples obtained by bronchoalveolar lavage (BAL) or by protected specimen brush (PSB), have been suggested to improve diagnostic sensitivity. Although the value of these invasive methods is still debated, a recent randomized trial suggested that, in patients managed according to results from specimens obtained by BAL or PSB, survival improved, antibiotic use was reduced and organ dysfunction resolved earlier than in patients who were managed using non-invasive clinical assessment and microscopic evaluation of endotracheal aspirates.[16]

Bronchoalveolar lavage

BAL specimens are generally obtained by wedging the tip of a bronchoscope in the medium-sized bronchus relevant to the area of alveolar infiltrate identified on the chest X-ray. The lung segment is lavaged with 20–30 mL of sterile isotonic saline and, after 5–10 s, a sample of 5–10 mL is obtained using gentle suction. A culture of $>10^4$ colony-forming units (cfu) mL^{-1} is generally considered to be indicative of pneumonia.[12,17] Non-bronchoscopic BAL (nBAL) specimens may also be obtained using a flexible catheter inserted blindly into the airways, but the source of the secretions obtained will be unknown and diluted by bronchial secretions. This may lead to a false-positive result in a heavily colonized patient or a patient with bronchitis and also to problems related to the threshold value used to diagnose significant infection.

Protected specimen brush

The PSB is a double-lumen brush system that avoids upper airway contamination of the sample. The brush is introduced, either blindly or via fibreoptic bronchoscopy, into the bronchus of a lung segment, with infiltrates seen on chest X-ray. The inner cannula is then advanced further and a specimen obtained. Generally, a culture of $>10^3$ cfu mL^{-1} is considered diagnostic of pneumonia. Problems with PSB include the fact that only a small lung segment is sampled, potentially leading to false-negative results, and, despite the double-lumen system, contamination can still occur. In addition, in patients already receiving antibiotics, PSB sampling has a very low sensitivity.[17]

Direct comparison of BAL with PSB has produced conflicting results, with no general agreement on which has the greater sensitivity or specificity. A recent meta-analysis concluded that both were equally accurate in diagnosing pneumonia, although, in patients already on antibiotics at the time of sampling, BAL is more sensitive.[17]

BAL and PSB techniques are dependent, to a degree, on operator skills and training. Blind non-bronchoscopic sampling may help reduce costs and has been evaluated for both techniques, yielding results similar to those of bronchoscopic sampling.[18,19] Early treatment is important in the outcome from nosocomial pneumonia and concerns have been raised about delays in initiating treatment while culture results from these techniques are awaited. Empiric therapy, based on likely pathogens and local resistance patterns, should be started as soon as the diagnosis is suspected, and adapted as results from such tests become available.

RISK FACTORS

Many risk factors have been reported as being associated with the development of nosocomial neumonia in the critically ill population (Table 15.1). Certain patient groups are at greater risk due to the nature of current or pre-existing disease processes, such as those with trauma, chronic respiratory or cardiac disease, and those who are in a coma. Patients with acute respiratory distress syndrome (ARDS) carry a twofold increase in risk compared to other critically ill patients.[20] Recent studies have shown that there is a reduced risk of nosocomial pneumonia in patients nursed in the semi-recumbent rather than the supine position.[21] The use of antibiotics is more controversial, with some studies suggesting an increased incidence of pneumonia in patients previously treated with antibiotics and others showing a reduced risk. However, prolonged and inappropriate antibiotic therapy may be expected to favour colonization, and hence infection, with resistant organisms.[22]

PREVENTION

With the high associated morbidity and mortality, prevention of nosocomial pneumonia must be seen as an important part of routine ICU patient care. Based on knowledge of the patient groups at risk and other specific aetiological factors, various preventive strategies have been proposed (Table 15.2).

Table 15.1 *Risk factors for the development of nosocomial pneumonia*

Patient-related factors
Trauma, burns
Pre-existing disease: chronic obstructive airways disease, diabetes mellitus, central nervous system disease, liver failure, alcoholism
Malnutrition
Severity of illness
Older age
Smoking habits

Intervention-related factors
Duration of mechanical ventilation
Presence of indwelling catheters: urinary catheters, central venous lines, arterial lines
Use of nasogastric tubes
Prolonged surgery
Excessive use of sedative agents
Inappropriate and prolonged use of antibiotics
Use of antacids/H2 antagonists
Parenteral nutrition
Nasal intubation
Supine positioning

Environment-related factors
Inadequate infection-control procedures
Prolonged ICU stay
Contaminated respiratory equipment

Table 15.2 *Suggested strategies to prevent nosocomial pneumonia*

Adequate infection control policies: hand washing, equipment sterilization, etc.
Semi-recumbent positioning
Subglottic drainage
Selective digestive decontamination
Maintenance of low gastric pH by avoidance of antacids and H2 antagonists
Oral intubation versus nasal intubation
Jejunal versus nasogastric tube
Early enteral feeding (particularly with immune supplemented feeds)
Avoidance of excessive sedation

Adequate infection control and equipment management

Thorough hand washing is the most effective means of limiting the spread of infection, but it is frequently forgotten or inadequate, involving only a cursory holding of the hands under the tap. Some studies have shown that less than 50% of hospital personnel comply with hand-washing protocols,[23,24] and patients' relatives are often better at washing their hands than ICU staff. The use of hand disinfection rather than washing more efficiently reduces the hand carriage of potentially pathogenic organisms and achieves better compliance, probably because it is both quicker and more convenient.[24] The use of disposable gloves and gowns may also help limit the transmission of bacteria between staff and patients, but the evidence for this is less compelling.[25,26] Transport of patients outside the ICU, for whatever reason, is associated with an increased risk of develop-

ing nosocomial pneumonia and should therefore be restricted as far as possible.[27]

Increasing the frequency of ventilator circuit changes does not appear to be beneficial, although the use of heat and moisture exchangers (HMEs) may decrease the incidence of nosocomial pneumonia, perhaps by minimizing the amount of condensate in the circuit. Further research is necessary in this area because existing information is scanty and conflicting and some HMEs may be associated with difficulty in weaning.[28,29] Oral intubation is preferable to nasal intubation and is associated with lower rates of nosocomial sinusitis. Non-invasive ventilation has been associated with reduced rates of infection and should be considered in appropriate patients.[30]

Patient positioning

A recent randomised, controlled trial evaluated the association of nosocomial pneumonia with patient positioning in mechanically ventilated patients.[21] The study was interrupted after a preliminary analysis showed a significant reduction in nosocomial pneumonia in those patients nursed in the semi-recumbent compared to the supine position; this difference was particularly significant in patients receiving enteral nutrition and in those with a reduced Glasgow Coma Score. Other studies have shown similar results, the benefit presumably being due to a reduced incidence of aspiration in this position. Kinetic beds may also be associated with a reduced incidence of nosocomial respiratory infection,[31] but this therapy is expensive.

Subglottal drainage of secretions

The aspiration of secretions that pool above the endotracheal cuff in mechanically ventilated patients may be another factor implicated in the development of nosocomial pneumonia. Special endotracheal tubes are now available with a separate lumen that allows continuous subglottal suctioning of these secretions, but it is not yet clear whether the benefit justifies the additional cost.

Selective digestive decontamination (SDD)

Selective decontamination of the digestive tract (SDD) is designed to prevent infection by eradicating and preventing the carriage of potentially pathogenic aerobic micro-organisms from theoropharynx, stomach and gut. SDD consists of non-absorbable antibiotics (usually polymyxin, tobramycin and amphotericin B) applied topically to the oropharynx and through a nasogastric tube, plus the use of a systemic antibiotic, most commonly cefotaxime. Several studies, although not all, have shown this technique to reduce the incidence of nosocomial pneumonia, particularly in trauma patients, and meta-analyses have confirmed that SDD using a combination of topical and systemic antibiotics can reduce respiratory infection[32] and may have a beneficial effect on mortality.[33] However, SDD is not routinely used in most ICUs because concerns remain regarding the cost and the risk of increasing bacterial resistance and drug toxicity with this approach.

Maintenance of low gastric pH

Antacids and H2-blockers are often used in the ICU population to prevent the development of stress ulcers and gastrointestinal bleeding. However, these agents can increase gastric pH and encourage colonization, and several publications have suggested an increased incidence of pneumonia with these treatments.[34,35] Sucralfate has been proposed as an alternative agent that may be less likely to increase the risk of pneumonia, but it appears to be less effective than H2-blockers in preventing gastrointestinal haemorrhage.[36] On the available evidence, H2-antagonists have superior anti-ulcer activity and minimal, if any, excess risk for pneumonia.

Nutritional support

Malnutrition is a risk factor for nosocomial pneumonia, and achieving adequate nutritional support is an important preventative strategy. However, when administered via a nasogastric tube, enteral nutrition has itself been associated with increased infection rates, possibly because it raises gastric pH, thereby encouraging bacterial colonization. The use of jejunal feeding tubes has been shown both to reduce the incidence of pneumonia and to improve nutritional status. The use of various immune-enhanced feeds including conditionally essential amino acids such as glutamine and arginine, nucleotides and omega-3 fatty acids has been associated with fewer acquired infections than standard feeding solutions, but further studies are needed to define the most beneficial combination of nutrients, to identify the most appropriate target populations and to justify the increased costs.

Avoiding excessive sedation

A reduced conscious level is associated with an increased risk of respiratory complications, and sedative agents should therefore be titrated to the minimal level required to keep each individual patient comfortable and co-operative. Sedation scores may be useful in assessing and adjusting sedation.[37]

TREATMENT

Antibiotic therapy

The treatment of nosocomial pneumonia represents a considerable challenge due to the range of organisms encountered, the frequent polymicrobial nature of these infections and the high incidence of resistant organisms. Maintaining a high index of suspicion and the prompt initiation of therapy are important aspects of management. Appropriate antibiotic selection is essential (Fig. 15.2) because inadequate antibiotic therapy is associated with increased mortality rates.[38] Guidelines for empiric therapy have been drawn up by several groups, and a consensus statement by the American Thoracic Society suggests that treatment should be based on the subdivision of patients into groups according to the severity of their disease and the presence of associated risk factors.[12]

- Group 1 patients are those with mild to moderate infection and without significant risk factors, or with severe but early-onset infection. Monotherapy is considered adequate.
- Group 2 patients are those with both mild to moderate infection and risk factors. These patients are more likely to have infection with more virulent pathogens, including *Pseudomonas aeruginosa*, and need additional coverage. Monotherapy may not be adequate.
- Group 3 patients are those with severe infection and risk factors. These patients are at greatest risk of infection with highly virulent pathogens and many, especially those with late-onset pneumonia, will require combination antibiotic therapy.

Figure 15.2 shows suggested antibiotic regimens for patients with nosocomial pneumonia, but the precise choice of antibiotic will depend on various factors (Table 15.3).

Importantly, once an organism has been isolated and antibiotic sensitivity determined, the antibiotic prescription should be modified accordingly to prevent unnecessary treatment, which increases both the costs and the risk of inducing bacterial resistance. The duration of therapy needs to be assessed on an individual patient basis according to clinical response, but antibiotics are often given for at least 7 days. In cases of Gram-negative pneumonia associated

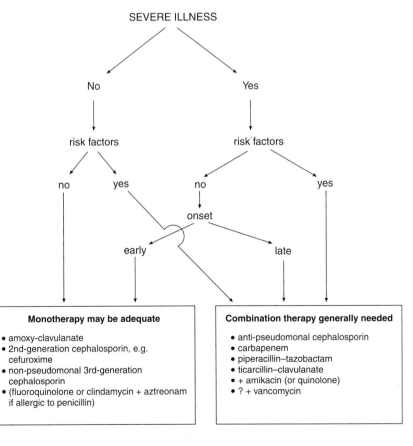

Figure 15.2 *Suggested flowchart to direct antibiotic therapy in patients with nosocomial pneumonia.*

Table 15.3 *Factors influencing the choice of antibiotic in the therapy of nosocomial pneumonia*

Bacteriological information
Epidemiolgic data (literature plus local)
Length of hospitalization
Previous antibiotic therapy
Severity of infection – presence of septic shock
Degree of immunosuppression
Side effects of antibiotics
Costs

with tissue necrosis and cavitation, treatment may need to be prolonged (14–21 days).

Immunomodulating therapies

The suppression of host defence mechanisms is a key factor in the development of nosocomial pneumonia, and therapies aimed at stimulating host defence may therefore be beneficial. Clinical trials have focused on two main agents: interferon-gamma (IFN-γ) and granulocyte-colony stimulating factor (G-CSF).

IFN-γ has been shown to restore monocyte function *in vivo*, but clinical trials using prophylactic IFN-γ in patients with severe trauma or burns have been inconclusive, with no sustained improvement in infection rates.[39]

G-CSF has shown promising results in animal experiments, but, in clinical trials, the results have been less convincing, with no apparent effects of prophylactic use on the incidence of nosocomial pneumonia.[40]

Immunomodulation is an interesting area of ongoing research, but remains experimental at present.

CONCLUSION

The high incidence and associated increase in morbidity and costs associated with nosocomial pneumonia demand that the critical care clinician remains alert to the risk factors and early features of this condition. Prevention should play a key role in limiting the development of nosocomial pneumonia. Simple techniques such as hand washing and disinfection, and placing the patient in the semi-recumbent rather than the prone position must be promoted, and excessive sedation avoided. Other strategies have given less consistent results, and the cost–benefit assessment of these approaches needs to be determined before they can be routinely recommended. Early diagnosis and effective antibiotic treatment can improve prognosis, and immunomodulatory therapies (unproven as yet) may become an important therapeutic adjunct.

REFERENCES

1. Vincent, JL, Bihari, D, Suter, PM, *et al.*, Members of the EPIC International Advisory Group. The prevalence of nosocomial infection in intensive care units in Europe – the results of the EPIC study. *JAMA* 1995; **274**: 639–44.
2. Kappstein, I, Schulgen, G, Beyer, U, Geiger, K, Schumacher, M, Daschner, FD. Prolongation of hospital stay and extra costs due to ventilator-associated pneumonia in an intensive care unit. *Eur J Clin Microbiol Infect Dis* 1992; **11**: 504–8.
3. Chevret, S, Hemmer, M, Carlet, J, Langer, M, European Cooperative Group on Nosocomial Pneumonia. Incidence and risk factors of pneumonia acquired in intensive care units. *Intensive Care Med* 1993; **19**: 256–64.
4. Fagon, JY, Chastre, J, Vuagnat, A, Trouillet, JL, Novara, A, Gibert, C. Nosocomial pneumonia and mortality among patients in intensive care units. *JAMA* 1996; **275**: 866–9.
5. Richards, MJ, Edwards, JR, Culver, DH, Gaynes, RP. Nosocomial infections in combined medical–surgical intensive care units in the United States. *Infect Control Hosp Epidemiol* 2000; **21**: 510–15.
6. Tejada Artigas, A, Bello Dronda, S, Chacon Valles, E, *et al.* Risk factors for nosocomial pneumonia in critically ill trauma patients. *Crit Care Med* 2001; **29**: 304–9.
7. Wallace, WC, Cinat, M, Gornick, WB, Lekawa, ME, Wilson, SE. Nosocomial infections in the surgical intensive care unit: a difference between trauma and surgical patients. *Am Surg* 1999; **65**: 987–90.
8. Kollef, MH. Ventilator-associated pneumonia. A multivariate analysis. *JAMA* 1993; **270**: 1965–70.
9. Torres, A, Aznar, R, Gatell, JM, *et al.* Incidence, risk, and prognosis factors of nosocomial pneumonia in mechanically ventilated patients. *Am Rev Respir Dis* 1990; **142**: 523–8.
10. Fagon, JY, Chastre, J, Hance, AJ, Montravers, P, Novara, A, Gibert, C. Nosocomial pneumonia in ventilated patients: a cohort study evaluating attributable mortality and hospital stay. *Am J Med* 1993; **94**: 281–8.

11. Heyland, DK, Cook, DJ, Griffith, L, Keenan, SP, Brun-Buisson, C. The attributable morbidity and mortality of ventilator-associated pneumonia in the critically ill patient. The Canadian Critical Trials Group. *Am J Respir Crit Care Med* 1999; **159**: 1249–56.

12. American Thoracic Society. Hospital-acquired pneumonia in adults: Diagnosis, assessment of severity, initial antimicrobial therapy and preventative strategies. *Am J Respir Crit Care Med* 1995; **153**: 1711–25.

13. Fayon, MJ, Tucci, M, Lacroix, J, *et al*. Nosocomial pneumonia and tracheitis in a pediatric intensive care unit: a prospective study. *Am J Respir Crit Care Med* 1997; **155**: 162–9.

14. Ewig, S, Torres, A, El-Ebiary, M, *et al*. Bacterial colonization patterns in mechanically-ventilated patients with traumatic and medical head injury. Incidence, risk factors, and association with ventilator-associated pneumonia. *Am J Respir Crit Care Med* 1999; **159**: 188–98.

15. Cardenosa Cendrero, JA, Sole-Violan, J, Bordes Benitez, A, *et al*. Role of different routes of tracheal colonization in the development of pneumonia in patients receiving mechanical ventilation. *Chest* 1999; **116**: 462–70.

16. Fagon, JY, Chastre, J, Wolff, M, *et al*., for the VAP Trial Group. Invasive and noninvasive strategies for management of suspected ventilator-associated pneumonia. *Ann Intern Med* 2000; **132**: 621–30.

17. de Jaeger, A, Litalien, C, Lacroix, J, Guertin, MC, Infante-Rivard, C. Protected brush specimen or bronchoalveolar lavage to diagnose bacterial nosocomial pneumonia in ventilated adults: a metaanalysis. *Crit Care Med* 1999; **27**: 2548–60.

18. Bello, S, Tajada, A, Chacon, E, *et al*. 'Blind' protected specimen brushing versus bronchoscopic techniques in the aetiological diagnosis of ventilator-associated pneumonia. *Eur Respir J* 1996; **9**: 1494–9.

19. Wearden, PD, Chendrasekhar, A, Timberlake, GA. Comparison of nonbronchoscopic techniques with bronchoscopic brushing in the diagnosis of ventilator-associated pneumonia. *J Trauma* 1996; **41**: 703–7.

20. Chastre, J, Trouillet, JL, Vuagnat, A, *et al*. Nosocomial pneumonia in patients with acute respiratory distress syndrome. *Am J Respir Crit Care Med* 1998; **157**: 1165–72.

21. Drakulovic, MB, Torres, A, Bauer, TT, Nicolas, JM, Nogue, S, Ferrer, M. Supine body position as a risk factor for nosocomial pneumonia in mechanically ventilated patients: a randomised trial. *Lancet* 1999; **354**: 1851–8.

22. Fagon, JY, Chastre, J, Domart, Y, *et al*. Nosocomial pneumonia in patients receiving continuous mechanical ventilation. Prospective analysis of 52 episodes with use of a protected specimen brush and quantitative culture techniques. *Am Rev Respir Dis* 1989; **139**: 877–84.

23. Doebbeling, BN, Stanley, GL, Sheetz, CT, *et al*. Comparative efficacy of alternative hand-washing agents in reducing nosocomial infections in intensive care units. *N Engl J Med* 1992; **327**: 88–93.

24. Bischoff, WE, Reynolds, TM, Sessler, CN, Edmond, MB, Wenzel, RP. Handwashing compliance by health care workers: the impact of introducing an accessible, alcohol-based hand antiseptic. *Arch Intern Med* 2000; **160**: 1017–21.

25. Crowe, M, Towner, KJ, Humphreys, H. Clinical and epidemiological features of an outbreak of *Acinetobacter* infection in an intensive therapy unit. *J Med Microbiol* 1995; **43**: 55–62.

26. Eveillard, M, Eb, F, Tramier, B, *et al*. Evaluation of the contribution of isolation precautions in prevention and control of multi-resistant bacteria in a teaching hospital. *J Hosp Infect* 2001; **47**: 116–24.

27. Kollef, MH, Von Harz, B, Prentice, D, *et al*. Patient transport from intensive care increases the risk of developing ventilator-associated pneumonia. *Chest* 1997; **112**: 765–73.

28. Manthous, CA, Schmidt, GA. Resistive pressure of a condenser humidifier in mechanically ventilated patients. *Crit Care Med* 1994; **22**: 1792–5.

29. Le Bourdelles, G, Mier, L, Fiquet, B, *et al*. Comparison of the effects of heat and moisture exchangers and heated humidifiers on ventilation and gas exchange during weaning trials from mechanical ventilation. *Chest* 1996; **110**: 1294–8.

30. Nourdine, K, Combes, P, Carton, MJ, Beuret, P, Cannamela, A, Ducreux, JC. Does noninvasive ventilation reduce the ICU nosocomial infection risk? A prospective clinical survey. *Intensive Care Med* 1999; **25**: 553–5.

31. Nelson, LD, Choi, SC. Kinetic therapy in critically ill trauma patients. *Clin Intensive Care* 1992; **3**: 248–52.

32. Vandenbroucke-Grauls, CM, Vandenbroucke, JP. Effect of selective decontamination of the digestive tract on respiratory tract infections and mortality in the intensive care unit. *Lancet* 1991; **338**: 859–62.

33. Liberati, A, D'Amico, R, Pifferi, S, *et al*. Antibiotics for preventing respiratory tract infections in adults receiving intensive care. *Cochrane Database Syst Rev* 2000; **2**: CD000022.

34. Cook, DJ, Reeve, BK, Guyatt, GH, *et al*. Stress ulcer prophylaxis in critically ill patients. Resolving discordant meta-analyses. *JAMA* 1996; **275**: 308–14.

35. Messori, A, Trippoli, S, Vaiani, M, Gorini, M, Corrado, A. Bleeding and pneumonia in intensive care patients given ranitidine and sucralfate for prevention of stress ulcer: meta-analysis of randomised controlled trials. *Br Med J* 2000; **321**: 1103–6.

36. Cook, D, Guyatt, G, Marshall, J, *et al*. A comparison of sucralfate and ranitidine for the prevention of upper gastrointestinal bleeding in patients requiring mechanical ventilation. *N Engl J Med* 1998; **338**: 791–7.

37. Detriche, O, Berré, J, Massaut, J, Vincent, JL. The Brussels Sedation Score: the use of a simple clinical sedation scale can avoid excessive sedation in mechanically ventilated patients in the intensive care unit (ICU). *Br J Anaesth* 1999; **83** 698–701.

38. Kollef, MH, Ward, S. The influence of mini-BAL cultures on patient outcomes: implications for the antibiotic management of ventilator-associated pneumonia. *Chest* 1998; **113**: 412–20.

39. Wasserman, D, Ioannovich, JD, Hinzmann, RD, Deichsel, G, Steinmann, GG. Interferon-gamma in the prevention of severe burn-related infections: a European phase III multicenter trial. *Crit Care Med* 1998; **26**: 434–9.

40. Heard, SO, Fink, MP, Gamelli, RL, *et al*. Effect of prophylactic administration of recombinant human granulocyte colony-stimulating factor (filgrastim) on the frequency of nosocomial infections in patients with acute traumatic brain injury or cerebral hemorrhage. *Crit Care Med* 1998; **26**: 748–54.

16

Infection in the immunocompromised patient

DAVID GHEZ, JEAN-FRANÇOIS TIMSIT AND JEAN CARLET

INTRODUCTION

Although at one time limited to rare constitutional diseases or haematological malignancies, immune deficiency has become progressively more prevalent in recent years. Acquired immunodeficiency syndrome (AIDS) accounts for a large proportion of this increase in cases, but the more powerful and effective immunosuppressive drug regimens now used have also increased both the incidence and the variety of clinical patterns of acquired immune deficiency encountered. Consequently, many more immunocompromised patients require intensive care unit (ICU) admission with serious infections caused by both common and opportunistic pathogens.

The occurrence of a pneumonia in an immunocompromised host is a daunting challenge because it may rapidly become life threatening, diagnosis is often difficult, and patient survival depends greatly on the speed with which the diagnosis is made and the appropriate treatment instituted. Clinical presentation is often atypical and a wide range of microorganisms may be responsible. In addition, other non-infectious causes of pulmonary infiltrates, such as intra-alveolar haemorrhage, may present a remarkably similar clinical picture and, although less frequent, should also be considered.

PATHOPHYSIOLOGY: TYPES OF IMMUNE DEFICIENCY AND THEIR RELATIONSHIP TO INFECTIONS

The nature and magnitude of the immune deficiency and its impact on specific host defence mechanisms are relevant to the clinician, because they largely determine which pathogens will be involved (Table 16.1). The aetiology of the immune deficiency may be complex. It can be related to the underlying disease itself, to the immunosuppressive therapy and, frequently, to both. The nature of the immunosuppressive therapy – type, duration, cumulative dose – is particularly important. The temporal sequence of the administration of the different elements of the immunosuppressive regimen is also relevant, particularly after transplantation.

Table 16.1 *Major causes of immunodeficiency and associated pulmonary pathogens (HIV infection excluded)*

Type of immunodeficiency	Underlying diseases	Pulmonary pathogens

Neutropenia	Chemotherapy induced
	Agranulocytosis
	Leukaemias
	Connective tissue diseases:
	    Systemic lupus erythematosus
	    Rheumatoid arthritis
	    (Felty'syndrome)
	Common variable immunodeficiency
		Enterobacteriaceae,
		Pseudomonas aeruginosa
		Gram-positive bacteria
		Aspergillus spp.

Cell-mediated immunity	Corticosteroid treatment
	Haematological malignancies:
	    Hodgkin's disease
	    Lymphomas
	    Angioimmunoblastic lymphadenopathy
	Connective tissue diseases:
	    Systemic lupus erythematosus
	    Wegener's granulomatosis
	Sarcoidosis
	BMT
	Organ transplantation
	Constitutional immunodeficiencies:
	    Hyper-IgM syndrome
		Viruses:
		    CMV, HSV, VZV, RSV,
		    adenovirus, rhinovirus, influenza,
		    parainfluenza virus, enteroviruses,
		    HSV6 (BMT)
		Protozoans:
		    Toxoplasma gondii
		Fungi:
		    Aspergillus spp
		    Pneumocystis carinii
		    Cryptococcus neoformans
		    Coccidioides immitis[a]
		Bacteria:
		    Legionella pneumophila
		    Mycobacterium tuberculosis
		    Atypical mycobacteria
		    Nocardia asteroides
		    Strongyloides stercoralis[a]

Humoral immunity	Multiple myeloma
	Splenectomy
	BMT
	Constitutional immunodeficiencies:
	    Common variable immunodeficiency
	    Agammaglobulinaemia
		Encapsulated bacteria:
		    Streptococcus
		    pneumoniae
		    Haemophilus influenzae
		    Salmonella sp.

[a]In areas of endemicity.
HIV, human immunodeficiency virus; CMV, cytomegalovirus; HSV, herpes simplex virus; VZV, varicella-zoster virus; RSV, respiratory syncytial virus; BMT, bone marrow transplantation.

Other factors include:

- alterations of natural barriers,
- uraemia,
- malnutrition,
- concomitant infection with immunomodulating viruses such as Epstein–Barr virus (EBV), cytomegalovirus (CMV) and hepatitis viruses.

The spectrum of potential pathogens in the immunocompromised host is particularly broad. Although there is no rule, the nature of the organisms most likely to cause an infection depends mostly on the type and duration of the immune defect (Tables 16.1 and 16.2). Infection with human immunodeficiency virus (HIV) produces quantitative and functional defects in cell-mediated immunity. When antiretroviral therapy fails or is not taken, HIV-infected people experience a progressive decline in the number of circulating CD4 lymphocytes and are increasingly at risk of opportunistic infections. Functional defects in macrophage function associated with an impairment of some cytokine production diminish the host response to intracellular pathogens. Infection with pyogenic bacteria is

Table 16.2 *Probable causative organisms according to time course and pattern of immunosuppression*

Condition	Type of infection
Neutropenia	<2 weeks: Gram-negative bacilli, Gram-positive cocci >2 weeks: increased risk of invasive pulmonary aspergillosis (less frequently *Candida* spp)
Transplantation Bone marrow 　Early infections	Before engraftment: 　Identical to that of neutropenic patients After engraftment: 　Nosocomial bacterial pneumonia (also consider *Legionella*) 　*Aspergillus* (bimodal: day 20 and 80), other fungi (*Blastomycosis, Coccidioïdomycosis*) in areas of endemicity 　CMV (recipient + or donor + , especially between day 30 and 60)
Late infections	HSV, HSV6 　Toxoplasmosis (*Pneumocystis carinii*) Community-acquired bacteria (encapsulated bacteria: *Strep. pneumoniae, Haemophilus influenzae*) Respiratory viruses, VZV Aspergillosis (less frequent after day 100) *Pneumocystis carinii, Cryptococcus neoformans* Mycobacteria, *Nocardia asteroides*
Solid organ 　Early infections	Nosocomial bacterial pneumonia: Gram-negative bacilli, *Staphylococcus aureus, Legionella* sp (*Pseudomonas* if cystic fibrosis) CMV (donor + /recipient −) Aspergillosis (especially in lung transplant recipients) *Mycobacterium tuberculosis* (increased risk in renal transplant recipients) *Pneumocystis carinii* *Toxoplasmosis* (donor + /recipient −)
Late infections	Community-acquired bacteria (encapsulated bacteria: *Strep. pneumoniae, H. influenzae*) Respiratory viruses, CMV *Pneumocystis carinii, Cryptococcus neoformans* Mycobacteria, *Nocardia asteroides*
HIV-infected patients CD4 >800–1000 10^6/litre	Bacterial pneumonia: *Strep. pneumoniae, Staph. aureus, H. influenzae, Legionella* Aspiration pneumonia
Early decline CD4 250–800 10^6/litre	As for HIV-infected patients plus: *Mycobacterium tuberculosis* If non-infectious infiltrates: non-specific interstitial pneumonitis, lymphoid interstitial pneumonitis, Kaposi's sarcoma, non-Hodgkin lymphoma) consider opportunistic infection
CD4 < 200 10^6/litre	*Pneumocystis carinii* Cryptococcosis (in USA and Africa), histoplasmosis, aspergillosis, toxoplasmosis (in France) CMV infection, *Mycobacterium avium intracellulare* Pseudomonal pneumonia

CMV, cytomegalovirus; HSV, herpes simplex virus.

increased by other immunological defects, which include the spontaneous activation of B-lymphocytes accompanied by decreased responsiveness to neoantigens, a reduced level of type-specific antibodies and impaired chemotaxis, phagocytosis and bacterial killing of neutrophils.

EPIDEMIOLOGY OF SEVERE PNEUMONIA IN IMMUNOCOMPROMISED HOSTS

Outcome predictors and prognosis

Approximately 4–5% of hospitalized HIV-infected patients are admitted to the ICU, half of them with respiratory failure.[1] Several studies in the mid-1980s showed an extremely high mortality (86–100%) for AIDS patients requiring mechanical ventilation for respiratory failure. The prognosis of *Pneumocystis carinii* pneumonia (PCP) in AIDS patients gradually improved and, in the 1990s, reports of improved survival were noted in AIDS patients requiring mechanical ventilation, with a mortality of 40–70%. This improved survival is probably related to a combination of factors, including patient selection, earlier diagnosis, antiretroviral therapy, anti-*Pneumocystis* prophylaxis and corticosteroid therapy.[2] Similar reasons might be advanced to explain the improved survival of cancer patients, whose overall mortality in the ICU is now 40–50 %.[3] General severity scores, although strongly associated with prognosis, nonetheless underestimate the risk of death in this population. The outcome for cancer patients admitted to the ICU is adversely affected by respiratory insufficiency, the need for mechanical ventilation and the development of septic shock, but neutropenia *per se* is not an independent predictor of death in recent studies.[4] Allogenic bone marrow transplantation (BMT) has the highest mortality: 18% ICU survival and 5 % 6-month survival in patients requiring mechanical ventilation.[5] Autologous BMT has a better outcome from ICU admission.

In general, the ICU outcome of immunocompromised patients is related to the number of organs that fail and particularly to the use of mechanical ventilation. The increasing use of non-invasive ventilation in this setting has improved the prognosis of BMT patients.[6] Non-invasive ventilation was also shown to improve morbidity and hospital mortality (13/26 versus 20/26, $p = 0.02$) of other immunocompromised patients with acute respiratory failure in a recent randomized study.[7]

Causes of pulmonary infiltrates according to the immune status: epidemiology and preventive strategies

Infections are responsible for more than 60% of pulmonary infiltrates in immunocompromised patients.[8] A thorough analysis of the underlying conditions and their treatments, and their influence on the immune system, is required to define empirically the spectrum of possible pathogens (Table 16.2). Some settings are particularly frequent and should therefore be detailed.

NEUTROPENIA

Neutropenia (neutrophil count < 1500 mm^{-3}) is more frequently encountered with the increasing use of cytotoxic drugs to treat malignancies and inflammatory diseases. The vulnerability to infections is not identical in every neutropenic patients as it depends on several cofactors, including the degree of the neutropenia, its duration and the alterations of the natural barriers. An absolute neutrophil count $< 500 \times 10^9$ L^{-1} and a rapidly falling granulocyte count are major risk factors for infections, whereas they are less frequent above 500×10^9 L^{-1}. Defects in neutrophil function caused by chemotherapy increase the susceptibility to infections, and changes in the gastrointestinal tract related to the chemotherapy facilitate invasion of the bacteria flora both from the mouth and via the bowel.

Bacterial pneumonia

Fever has an infectious origin in more than 60% of neutropenic patients and is often due to a primary bacteraemia. However, lung infections represent the principal cause of admission to the ICU of neutropenic patients. The majority of bacteria are acquired by the patient after hospital admission. Enterobacteriaceae, *Pseudomonas* spp. and nosocomial multi-resistant Gram-negative bacteria are the classical pathogens, but Gram-positive organisms are being isolated with an increasing frequency related to the presence of indwelling catheters (*Staphylococcus* species), prophylactic antibiotic therapy with fluoroquinolones and lesions of the oral mucosa (*Streptococcus viridans*). They now account for more than 60% of the isolated organisms in blood cultures.[9] Nosocomial outbreaks of *Legionella* species pneumonia have also been reported.

Aspergillosis

Neutropenia lasting for more than 2 weeks is associated with a high risk of pulmonary aspergillosis.[10] Because the post-therapeutic aplasia may last between 30 and 40 days, patients receiving induction chemotherapy for acute leukaemia are therefore particularly at risk. Early antifungal treatment and bone marrow recovery may allow the control of the infection. In patients who remain deeply neutropenic, survival beyond 3 weeks is uncommon because dissemination to other organs, especially the brain, often occurs.

Other pneumonias

Pulmonary infections caused by common respiratory viruses have been described mostly in patients suffering from haematological malignancies. Fungi, including *Candida*, *Fusarium* and *Trichosporon* species, may cause lung infiltrates, usually in the setting of a disseminated haematogenous infection.

ALLOGENEIC BONE MARROW TRANSPLANTATION

Allogeneic BMT combines neutropenia and major alterations of monocyte/macrophage functions in the early phase post-transplantation with a profound and long-lasting impairment of cell-mediated and humoral immunity. Pulmonary diseases represent 40–60% of complications and the estimated mortality exceeds 30%. Diffuse alveolar haemorrhage is a frequent complication in patients with pulmonary infections who require mechanical ventilation.[5] The different pathogens affect the recipient at different times in the post-transplantation course, although there are some overlaps (Table 16.2). One-half of the infections occur in the first 4–6 weeks following bone marrow grafting.[11] Additional risk factors for infectious complications include engraftment failure (resulting in prolonged neutropenia), HLA mismatch, volunteer-unrelated donor, use of T-depleted bone marrow, acute graft-versus-host disease (GVHD; with subsequent use of high-dose steroids and anti-lymphocyte globulins) and chronic GVHD.

The risk periods for certain infections are changing in relation to:

- the reduction in the length of the neutropenic period with the use of granulocyte colony stimulating factor (G-CSF) and peripheral blood stem cells,
- the increasing shift of viral (especially CMV) and fungal infections to the late period (after day 100) as effective early preventive strategies have been developed, such as ganciclovir prophylaxis for the prevention of CMV reactivation in seropositive recipients, and fluconazole prophylaxis for candidiasis.

Early infections (< 3-months-post-transplantation)

Bacterial Pneumonia Bacterial pneumonias occurring before engraftment, i.e. during the neutropenic phase, are clinically and bacteriologically similar to chemotherapy-induced neutropenia. It affects up to 20% of patients.[11] In addition to common respiratory tract pathogens, the high toxicity of pre-transplant therapy (especially total-body irradiation) on the digestive tract and the occurrence of digestive acute GVHD facilitates the translocation of enteric organisms. Legionellosis is rare because of the systematic decontamination of the water supply.

Fungal Pneumonia Invasive pulmonary aspergillosis, whose overall incidence varies from 4% to 10%,[10] remains one of the most feared complications following allogeneic BMT. The risk factors are:

- prolonged neutropenia before BMT,
- time to engraftment,
- previous history of *Aspergillus* colonization or infection,
- use of immunosuppressive drugs to treat an acute GVHD.

It has a bimodal distribution, with peaks at day 20 and day 80. Its mortality remains as high as 95%, despite early diagnosis and therapy.

Systemic candidiasis frequently occurs after BMT, but the diagnosis of primary pulmonary candidiasis is controversial, with many authorities believing that it arises secondary to hematogeneous dissemination.

The systematic use of prophylaxis has considerably decreased the incidence of PCP in BMT recipients, which is less than 10%, usually in patients who cannot take pentamidine or cotrimoxazole prophylaxis.[11]

Viral Pneumonia CMV infections remain one of the most important causes of morbidity and mortality after allogeneic BMT. CMV active infection occurs preferentially between day 30 and 60 after BMT, by reactivation of a latent endogenous virus in CMV-seropositive BMT recipients. CMV pneumonia reflects a severe disseminated infection, which, once declared, has a 30–70% mortality, despite the use of antiviral agents and immunoglobulins.[11] Preventive approaches, such as the systematic administration of ganciclovir to high-risk patients, have proven effective, but drug-induced neutropenia occurs in up to 30% of patients treated. Early pre-emptive antiviral therapy using repeated monitoring of pp65 antigenaemia and surveillance bronchoalveolar lavage (BAL) is preferable.

Herpes simplex virus (HSV) has become uncommon with the prophylactic use of aciclovir during the first month after transplantation. HSV-6 may cause an interstitial pneumonia.

Parasitic Pneumonia In the first 2 months post-BMT, the reactivation of a latent *Toxoplasma gondii* infection may cause pulmonary infiltrates, in the setting of a disseminated disease. The incidence of *T. gondii* is only 0.9%, but it has a mortality rate over 95%. Serologic tests have no diagnostic value, but may serve to identify the group of patients at risk. The diagnosis is difficult and often only made at autopsy; it relies on the visualization of tachyzoites in the BAL and, more recently, polymerase chain reaction (PCR).

Late infections
(>3 months post-transplantation)

Bacterial Pneumonia Because of the long-lasting defect in humoral immunity and the functional asplenia induced by total body irradiation, *Streptococcus pneumoniae* and *Haemophilus influenzae* are the main pathogens responsible for late bacterial pneumonia. Legionellosis remains a risk in these patients. Pulmonary infections caused by *Nocardia* species or *Mycobacterium* spp are rare.

Viral Pneumonia Common viruses such as adenovirus, respiratory syncytial virus (RSV), rhinoviruses, enteroviruses, influenza and parainfluenza viruses can cause devastating disease in severely immunocompromised hosts, especially after BMT, and are frequently associated with bacterial superinfection. The incidence has increased in recent years, probably due to improved methods of detection. The prognosis is poor in patients with pneumonia and the mortality rate in patients with respiratory failure requiring mechanical ventilation has been reported to be over 90%. Adenovirus infection can present as a disseminated disease responsible for severe hepatitis, gastroenteritis and encephalitis.

CMV pneumonia is less common more than 3 months after transplantation, but may occur in association with intense immunosuppression, particularly associated with the use of T-cell-depleted grafts and chronic GVHD. In one study, the incidence of CMV infection after day 100 was 4.8%, with a mortality rate of 70%.[11]. Interestingly, late-onset CMV infection has been reported in patients given prophylactic or early ganciclovir therapy, probably due to an inability completely to restore their immune response to CMV.

Most cases of varicella-zoster virus (VZV) infections represent reactivation of a pre-existing infection and occur in up to 50% of patients. Visceral dissemination, which may involve the lungs, has been described in 5% of patients.

Fungal Pneumonia It is likely that aspergillosis also plays a significant role in fatal infections during the late period, but its frequency has not been defined precisely.

AUTOLOGOUS BONE MARROW TRANSPLANTATION

Intensification of the therapeutic regimen followed by autologous BMT is now routinely used to treat haematological malignancies and is increasingly performed in solid tumours. Although the procedure yields a considerably lower mortality than allogeneic BMT (around 5–10%), the neutropenic period is often complicated by infections, the incidence of bacterial pneumonia being around 3%.[12] Because the neutropenia usually lasts less than 2 weeks, invasive aspergillosis has an incidence of 2%.[10] CMV and other opportunistic infections are rare. The use of G-CSF seems to decrease the risk of severe infectious complications and mortality. The use of peripheral blood stem cells also shortens the neutropenic phase, but the benefits are debated.

ORGAN TRANSPLANTATION

Although organ transplantation has achieved a 1-year survival rate exceeding 80%, it can be followed by life-threatening complications, amongst which pulmonary diseases are most prominent. Infections are the cause of approximately two-thirds of pulmonary infiltrates.[13] In recent years, the incidence of infectious complications has decreased with the use of cyclosporin and tacrolimus. Pulmonary infections have different presentations and causes, according to the timing post-transplantation. Early infections, which occur when the immunosuppression is maximal, are more frequent and have a higher mortality. Because these patients receive a maintenance immunosuppression to avoid graft rejection, they remain particularly susceptible to opportunistic pathogens.

Bacterial pneumonia

Approximately 5% of solid-organ transplant recipients develop bacterial pneumonia, more frequently in the first 3 months. The incidence of bacterial pneumonia depends on the tranplantation site: it is highest in recipients of heart and/or lung (around 20%) and less common in liver or renal transplant patients. Identified risk factors are the occurrence of primary CMV infection, splenectomy, graft rejection and anti-rejection therapy. The global mortality of bacterial pneumonia in solid-organ transplantation is above 40% and that of early pneumonia exceeds 60%.

Gram-negative bacilli, *Staphylococcus aureus* and *Legionella* species predominate in the first 3 months. Lung allograft recipients are at greater risk for pneumonia than other organ transplant recipients, because:

- the lung is directly exposed to the environment,
- the transplanted lung is denervated, with impaired mucociliary function and cough reflex,
- patients typically require a higher level of immunosuppression to prevent rejection.

Patients transplanted for end-stage disease secondary to cystic fibrosis are often colonized by *Pseudomonas* spp and *Burkholderia cepacia* and require particularly close surveillance. Empirical therapy must include agents against the *Pseudomonas* strains that are prevalent in the institution. Empyema and lung abscess require aggressive therapy, with immediate drainage of potentially infected collections. Late-onset bacterial pneumonia is less frequent, primarily caused by community-acquired bacteria, e.g. *Strep. pneumoniae* and *H. influenzae*, and has a much better prognosis.

Mycobacterium tuberculosis infections, either primary or reactivation, occur in approximately 1% of solid-organ transplant recipients. *M. tuberculosis* pneumonia only rarely develops early after transplantation. It occurs mostly in recipients of kidney transplants, because the prevalence of tuberculosis is high in patients undergoing chronic haemodialysis. Tuberculosis is often disseminated and may be particularly severe.

The incidence of *Nocardia asteroides* infections varies between transplant centres (0–20%, mean 3%). *Nocardia* infection presents with pneumonia in 90% of cases, but also with brain abscess (30%), and occasionally involves the skin, eye or joints. The clinical signs are often non-specific and subacute. Chest radiograph findings include nodular, segmental or multilobar infiltrates. Cavitation and pleural effusion are frequent. Even with appropriate antimicrobial therapy, the mortality appraches 50%. The infected patients should receive cotrimoxazole indefinitely as relapse can occur even after prolonged treatment.

Viral pneunonia

CMV infections are frequent in organ transplant recipients and present at a similar time to that described for BMT recipents. However, unlike BMT, the donor's seropositivity represents the highest risk factor for the development of symptomatic CMV disease. Reactivation of latent virus is often less severe than primary infection following transplantation. Interestingly, CMV manifestations depend on the organ transplanted. Recipients of lung or heart–lung transplants are at higher risk of CMV pneumonitis and bronchiolitis obliterans. Prophylactic ganciclovir therapy appears to reduce the incidence and severity of disease following renal transplantation and delays the disease in lung transplant recipients.

HSV pneumonitis has become a rare event with the implementation of oral aciclovir prophylaxis, with an incidence of 1–10%, the highest-risk group being heart and lung transplant recipients. As in BMT, EBV, VZV and common respiratory viruses can cause a severe, diffuse, interstitial pneumonia.

Parasitic pneumonia

Pulmonary toxoplasmosis occurs primarily in seronegative patients who receive an allograft from a seropositive donor. Because of the predilection of the parasite for muscle tissue, it is more frequent after heart transplantation. In one study of *T. gondii*-seronegative recipients of allografts from *T. gondii*-seropositive donors, 57% of heart, 20% of liver and < 1% of kidney transplant recipients acquired primary *T. gondii* infection. It is usually a fulminant disseminated disease with a mortality that exceeds 90%.[14,15]

Strongyloides stercoralis has been called the 'Trojan horse' because it possesses an autoinfection cycle that can cause a chronic asymptomatic infestation for decades after an exposure in endemic areas. Depression of the cell-mediated immunity may result in the so-called hyperinfestation syndrome associated with haemorrhagic pulmonary consolidation, diffuse bilateral alveolar opacities leading to acute respiratory distress syndrome (ARDS) and gastrointestinal symptoms. An associated bacteraemia and/or meningitis caused by enteric bacteria occur in 50% of cases. There is often no hypereosinophilia. The parasite is recovered on direct examination of sputum, BAL or stool. When the diagnosis is suspected, immediate treatment must be instituted. Prophylactic treatment before transplantation is needed in endemic areas. The prognosis is poor.

Fungal pneumonia

As in BMT recipients, the implementation of prophylaxis against PCP has dramatically decreased the risk of this infection.

Pulmonary aspergillosis pneumonia occurs within the first 2 months following tranplantation, but, with the exception of lung or heart–lung transplant recipients, it has a low incidence (<5%) compared to BMT. Disseminated disease occurs in 50% of these patients and is almost invariably fatal.

Other causes of fungal pneumonia include *Cryptococcus neoformans*, *Coccidioides immitis* and *Histoplasma capsulatum*.

HUMAN IMMUNODEFICIENCY VIRUS INFECTION

The number of HIV-infected patients admitted to the ICU has decreased following highly active antiretroviral therapy. However, the absolute rate of opportunistic infections remains high, e.g. PCP had an incidence of 46 per 1000 patient-years in 1997,[16] and some patients are still admitted with undiagnosed HIV disease. The CD4 count remains the best surrogate marker of host immune response in HIV-infected patients (see Table 16.2). Patients with a CD4 count >500 mm^{-3} are mainly at risk of common bacterial pneumonia. As CD4 falls lower, infections caused by relatively virulent pathogens such as *M. tuberculosis* may appear. Opportunistic infections, especially PCP, occur when the CD4 count falls below 200 mm^{-3}. Under 100 mm^{-3}, cryptococcosis, *M. avium* complex and toxoplasmosis may cause disseminated infections and pneumonias.

Bacterial pneumonia

Bacterial pneumonia is a frequent cause of ICU admission for HIV-infected patients, caused by *Strep. pneumoniae* (penicillin-resistant strains are frequent), *Pseudomonas aeruginosa* and *Staph. aureus*.[17] Pneumococcal pneumonia is frequently associated with positive blood cultures. Pseudomonal pneumonia is becoming a common complication, especially in patients with low leucocyte and CD4 counts. Chest radiographs are often atypical, mimicking PCP in half the cases. Intrapulmonary cavitations, abscesses and empyema are frequent.

Despite the widespread introduction of effective primary and secondary prophylaxis, *P. carinii* remains the cause in 50–90% of HIV-infected patients admitted to the ICU with pneumonia. Primary and secondary prophylaxis by cotrimoxazole, dapsone or aerosolized pentamidine is recommended when the CD4 count falls below 200 mm^{-3}.[18] The clinical presentation is typically insidious, with mild symptoms that progress over weeks or months. There may be surprisingly little clinical distress despite severe hypoxaemia (*Pa*O$_2$ often <50 mmHg on room air). The usual appearance is bilateral perihilar interstitial infiltrates, which, in severe forms, can progress to diffuse confluent alveolar shadowing. Hilar or mediastinal adenopathies are rare and suggest an alternative or concomitant process. Cotrimoxazole for 3 weeks in association with steroids remains the treatment of choice. The ICU mortality is under 20%.[19] The adverse prognostic factors of PCP in ICU are: the need for mechanical ventilation after 3 days of ICU stay and/or for more than 5 days, the occurrence of nosocomial infections and pneumothorax.

Tuberculosis

Tuberculosis may occur at any stage in HIV disease and is less frequently responsible for admission to the ICU. Positive tuberculin tests or contact with a person with active tuberculosis should lead to preventive treatment.[18] In the early stage of HIV disease, its clinical presentation resembles adult post-primary disease. Later, the presentation is often atypical, cavitation is rare but hilar and mediastinal lymph-adenopathy, diffuse and miliary shadowing or pleural effusion are frequent. A high proportion of patients have an extrapulmonary disease involving the bone marrow, liver, pericardium and meninges.[17] Disseminated tuberculosis is responsible for septic shock and multi-system organ failure. The suspicion of tuberculosis warrants immediate conventional anti-tuberculous therapy. Steroids are frequently used for severe miliary tuberculosis and may be life saving.

Pulmonary infection with *C. neoformans* usually occurs as part of disseminated infection with meningoencephalitis. This disease is common in France, the USA and Africa and rarer in other European countries such as the UK. The presenting symptoms and chest radiographic appearance are non-specific. Serum, BAL and cerebrospinal fluid cryptococcal antigen are always positive. The diagnosis is established by the culture of BAL fluid or a transbronchial biopsy specimen or, in disseminated disease, by the culture of blood or cerebrospinal fluid.

OTHER IMMUNODEFICIENT STATES

Humoral defiency and hyposplenism

Splenectomy or functional hyposplenism (e.g to sickle-cell disease, SLE) renders patients particularly sensitive to encapsulated bacteria such as *Strep. pneumoniae*, H. influenzae or non-typhi salmonella, which can take a fulminant course. Patients with hypogammaglobulinaemia (common variable immunodeficiency, lymphoproliferative disorders, especially multiple myeloma) that entails an opsonization defect, have a similar risk.

Collagen tissue diseases

Various alterations in cell-mediated immunity have been described in patients suffering from collagen tissue diseases, particularly SLE, rheumatoid arthritis and Wegener's granulomatosis. Whereas these defects alone appear rarely to be responsible for severe opportunistic infections, the immunodeficiency is frequently exacerbated by treatment (steroids, cyclophosphamide, methotrexate, cyclosporin). Community-acquired bacteria are

the main causes of infectious pneumonia, but a wide range of opportunistic pathogens should always be considered, amongst which mycobacteria and *P. carinii* are the most common. *Aspergillus* is a rare cause of pulmonary infiltrates and occurs in patients receiving prolonged corticosteroid therapy. The aggressive treatment with high-dose steroids and cyclophosphamide used in Wegener's granulomatosis increases the risk of opportunistic infection, particularly PCP, which was a significant cause of mortality before the systematic use of prophylaxis.

Haematological malignancies

Lymphoproliferative diseases may cause various defects in cellular and humoral immunity that increase the susceptibility to opportunistic pathogens (particularly *P. carinii*). Mycobacterial infections are increased in hairy-cell leukaemia. Infectious complications occurring in acute leukaemias are usually related to the neutropenia, but other pathogens have occasionally been reported to cause pulmonary infections. Some treatments (especially steroids and 2-chloro-deoxyadenosine) deeply depress cellular immunity, which favours the development of opportunistic infections.

Trauma patients, severe sepsis and other ICU patients with severe prolonged organ dysfunction

Critical illness is associated with profound cellular and humoral immune dysfunction, probably related to excess production of pro-inflammatory and anti-inflammatory mediators. Hormonal, nutritional and genetic factors, as well as the increasing use of corticosteroïds in septic patients, contribute to the impairment of immune function. Consequently, the severely ill ICU patient may develop infections with low-grade pathogens such as *Staphylococcus epidermidis*, *Aspergillus fumigatus* or cytomegalovirus.

NON-INFECTIOUS CAUSES

Non-infectious causes of pulmonary infiltrates are found in more than 30% of immunocompromised hosts and should be systematically eliminated (Table 16.3). A detailed description of their characteristics is beyond the scope of this chapter. Because they can

Table 16.3 *Non-infectious causes of pulmonary infiltrates*

Pulmonary oedema
  Cardiogenic
  Non-cardiogenic
      Conditioning regimen
      Veno-occlusive disease
      Graft-versus-host disease
Alveolar haemorrhage
Pulmonary embolism
Bronchiolitis obliterans
Toxic: irradiation
Immunoallergic
  Methotrexate
  Bleomycin
Idiopathic interstitial pneumonia
Leukaemic relapse
Leukostasis (acute leukaemias)
Retinoic acid syndrome
Capillary leak syndrome
Alveolar proteinosis
Pulmonary lymphoma
EBV post-transplant lymphoproliferative disease
Kaposi's sarcoma

EBV, Epstein–Barr virus.

present with a wide variety of pulmonary complications whose specific treatment relies on an increase of the immunosuppressive therapy, collagen vascular disease may cause difficult diagnostic and therapeutic problems. In patients with haematological malignancies, the aetiologies are dominated by pulmonary haemorrhage, pulmonary oedema, leukaemic relapse and transfusion reactions.

DIAGNOSTIC STRATEGY

The diagnostic approach to the evaluation of pneumonia in the immunocompromised is based on the medical history.[20] The understanding of the expected 'timetable of infections' depending on the particular programme of immunosuppression plays a major role in the differential diagnosis (see Table 16.2). Knowledge of the modes of onset and progression of the pneumonia process is also useful. An acute or fulminant onset suggests conventional pyogenic bacterial infections (and, for non-infectious causes, pulmonary embolism, pulmonary oedema, leukoagglutinin reaction or pulmonary haemorrhage). A subacute onset suggests viral,

Legionella, *Mycoplasma*, *Pneumocystis*, *Aspergillus* or *Nocardia* infection. A more protracted course, over several weeks, suggests fungal or tuberculous infections.

Prior prophylaxis must also be reviewed. For example, compliance with cotrimoxazole prophylaxis practically rules out the diagnosis of PCP.

Clinical features

Even if the main symptom at admission is pneumonia, a careful physical examination is needed. The clinical presentation of these pneumonias may overlap considerably. Moreover, some processes are occasionally caused by mixed infection or can reflect infections superimposed on another non-infectious process. Clinical features specific to particular aetiologies have already been discussed. In neutropaenic patients, the clinical presentation is either pneumonia or ARDS due to sepsis caused by bacterial or fungal infections.

The initial examination should include a chest radiograph, standard laboratory tests, two peripheral blood cultures and blood gases.

Radiological findings

Although no particular chest X-ray pattern is specific for a given pathologic process, particularly in the immunosuppressed patient, some patterns are more characteristic. The distribution and location of chest-imaging abnormalities might help in the differential diagnosis (Table 16.4). Neutropenia may greatly modify or delay the appearance of pulmonary lesions. Atelectasis may be the only radiological clue to the presence of a clinically important bacterial pneumonia.

Computerized tomography (CT) scanning provides more information, which may aid diagnosis, and it is also the best method for predicting whether bronchoscopy will be helpful. It also enables a CT-guided biopsy to be performed, if necessary to make the diagnosis, and allows for transparietal needle biopsy of pulmonary nodules.

Pulmonary samples

Immunocompromised patients with pulmonary dysfunction should have a sputum Gram stain. If

Table 16.4 *Diagnosis according to chest radiograph appearances in pneumonia of acute and subacute onset*

Chest radiograph abnormality	Acute onset of symptoms	Subacute or chronic onset of symptoms
Consolidation	Pyogenic bacteria[a] Legionnaires'disease Intra-alveolar haemorrhage Pulmonary oedema (cardiogenic or not)	Fungal Nocardial Tuberculosis

Peri-bronchovascular/interstitial	Pulmonary oedema
	Leukoagglutinin reaction
		Viral
		Pneumocystis (diffuse alveolar in severe
		  forms)
		Radiation (adjoin the edges of the
		  radiation field)
		Drug induced

Nodular infiltrate	(Right-sided endocarditis)	Tumours Kaposi's sarcoma Aspergillosis Toxoplasmosis *Nocardia* (macronodules) Tuberculosis (miliary)
Cavitation	Gram-negative bacilli *Staphylococcus aureus*	Necrotic tumours Tuberculosis *Nocardia* Aspergillosis (*Pneumocystis*: atypical cysts)
Hilar and mediastinal lymph nodes		Tumours ++ Mycobacteria +++ Fungus
Pleural effusion	Cardiogenic pulmonary oedema (bilateral) Bacteria	Mycobacteria Fungus (except *P. carinii*) Tumours

[a]Bacterial pneumonia frequently leads to discrete infiltrates in neutropenic patients.

pleural fluid is present, it should be sampled and examined for infection and malignancy. Sputum stain and culture for mycobacteria should also be routine. Blood cultures should be taken and serum cryptococcal antigen requested. Induced sputum can be useful in diagnosing pneumocystosis in HIV-infected patients, but these tests have little value in other immunocompromised patients.

In neutropenia, bronchoscopy with BAL is of limited value in the diagnosis of pulmonary infection, particularly fungal infection, because of a high rate of false-positive bacterial isolates caused by contamination from the upper airway and a poor yield in the diagnosis of fungal infection.

Usually, in non-neutropenic patients, fibreoptic bronchoscopy is needed to make the diagnosis.[11,20] However, if patients are still breathing spontaneously, bronchoscopy can precipitate the need for mechanical ventilation. In this case, empirical antimicrobial treatment should be given. Bronchoscopy should be delayed to confirm the diagnosis after the initial improvement of the patient or performed if the patient deteriorates and requires mechanical ventilation. Nevertheless, an aggressive approach to diagnosis limits drug toxicity and interactions and the risk of potentially lethal superinfection without exposing the patient to potentially inadequate therapy.

BAL has become the procedure of choice in the evaluation of diffuse pulmonary infiltrates because it has a high diagnostic yield, especially with viruses, *P. carinii* and *M. tuberculosis*. In order to maximize the sensitivity, bacterial, fungal and viral culture of BAL fluid should be performed in addition to shell vial centrifugation culture and staining for viral antigens. Cytological evaluation should be performed by an experienced pathologist to look for viral inclusion bodies and fungal elements using specific stains. It can also confirm a non-infectious process such as alveolar haemorrhage. Non-diagnostic findings from BAL are common, especially in the evaluation of nodular lesions. In such a situation, a diagnosis should be pursued with transbronchial biopsy, which has a higher sensitivity, but there is an increased risk of pneumothorax and haemorrhage and it cannot be performed in patients with thrombocytopaenia or severe ARDS. Transthoracic needle aspiration for peripheral lesions has a low yield, with significant risks of pneumothorax (5–10%) and haemoptysis (3–5%). Open-lung biopsy will provide a diagnosis in the majority of cases and should be considered both when the empirical treatment is toxic or interacts with another medication and, particularly, if the patient has a reasonable prognosis from the underlying disease.

Because obtaining lung tissue is potentially hazardous, other possible sites from which diagnostic tissue could be obtained should be sought. This applies especially to moulds that invade the bloodstream because the organism can often be identified in more easily accessible sites such as the skin, sinuses and bone marrow. Diagnostic tests according to specific pathogens are summarized in Table 16.5.

TREATMENT

Treatment of respiratory insufficiency

Mechanical ventilation is associated with an increased risk of death in immunocompromised patients,[5] because of the very high risk of nosocomial infections. CPAP and non-invasive ventilation[6,7] should be tried, before intubation and mechanical ventilation, when O_2 therapy via facemask has failed. These techniques are also useful during and after bronchoscopy with BAL in patients with severe hypoxaemia.

Empirical antimicrobial treatment

The sudden onset of symptoms and an often fulminant course of the disease are characteristic of infections in immunocompromised patients, particularly the neutropenic patient. Therefore, the antimicrobial therapy has to be instituted as early as possible and usually before microbiological results are available.

NEUTROPENIA

The majority of pathogens associated with new episodes of acute pneumonia are bacteria. Because of the absence of neutrophils, clinical and radiological data are frequently absent or not specific. Consequently, the first-choice antibacterial treatment must be broad spectrum and adapted to the bacterial species and their antibiotic susceptibility prevalent in the institution. A combination of an aminoglycoside and an extended-spectrum β-lactamin is recommended for initial therapy.[9] Vancomycin is appropriate in institutions where methicillin-resistant staphylococci are frequent or when the direct stain of the sputum examination shows Gram-positive cocci. During prolonged neutropenia, amphotericin B should be added when *Aspergillus* or *Candida* spp infection is suspected.

The use of G-CSF has been shown to shorten the duration of neutropenia after low-risk chemotherapy. However, the results of several randomized trials have shown that G-CSF was ineffective in reducing either the incidence of infectious complications or the overall mortality. However, G-CSF or GM-CSF might be useful in cases of severe sepsis or septic shock or pneumonia.[21] G-CSF may be responsible for the development of ARDS.[22].

INFECTIONS IN NON-NEUTROPENIC PATIENTS

In non-neutropenic patients with haematological malignancy, the causes of pulmonary infection are similar to those in immunocompetent patients. In the case of acute onset, common pyogenic bacterias and *Legionella* spp should be the targets of the initial treatment.

When the onset of symptoms is delayed in patients receiving immunosuppressive therapy, *P. carinii* infection and tuberculosis should be considered, especially in cases of bilateral diffuse infiltrates. On the basis of AIDS experience, prednisolone should be added when PCP is suspected.

Table 16.5 *Value of diagnostic tests for different pathogens*

Pathogens	Diagnostic tests	Comments
Pyogenic bacteria	Sputum Bronchoscopy with tracheal aspirate and BAL Blood cultures	Oropharyngeal contamination If possible according to severity of respiratory symptoms
Legionnaires' disease	Direct imunofluorescence (sputum) Urinary antigen + + Culture (BCYE)	Poor sensitivity Culture: 5–21 days to grow the organism
Nocardia asteroides	Sputum or bronchoscopy: Gram-positive beaded filaments (Gram stain) and culture (Ziehl–Nielsen or Kinyoun stain)	
Tuberculosis	Sputum tracheal aspirate or BAL Tissue biopsy Ziehl–Nielsen staining or immunofluorescence Culture (Lowenstein)	Direct examination is often negative in immunocompromised hosts
Fungi		
P. carinii	BAL: cyst or trophozoites (immunofluorescence or) toluene blue	90% sensitivity, especially in AIDS patients; PCR is a very specific method
Aspergillus spp.	Definite diagnosis: septated non-pigmented hyphae in tissue biopsy (Gomory methamine silver or acid Schiff stains) and positive culture BAL: smear, culture and antigen detection	Isolation of *Aspergillus* spp. from the respiratory specimen: positive predictive value of invasive *Aspergillus* infection of 72% in patient with haematological malignancy, and 82% in BMT recipients Aspergillus antigen (EIA, ELISA or immunoblot) serially, probably valuable in BMT PCR assays
Cryptococcus neoformans	BAL: direct examination and culture Positive serum cryptococcal antigen	
Parasites		
T. gondii	BAL: tachyzoites (eosine/methylene blue or Giemsa staining) PCR methods, Culture on MRC5 cells	The absence of serum *T. gondii* IgG makes the diagnosis unlikely, especially in AIDS
Strongyloides stercoralis	Direct stool (concentration) Sputum BAL	Repeat tests + + +
Viruses		
RSV	Nasopharynx, tracheal aspirate or BAL: culture (gold standard) or rapid antigen detection	
CMV	BAL: shell vial assay, antigen, cytopathogenic effect Biopsies	

RSV, respiratory syncytial virus; CMV, cytomegalovirus; BAL, bronchoalveolar lavage; BCYE, buffered charcoal yeast extract; PCR, polymerase chain reaction; MRC5 cells, AIDS, autoimmune deficiency syndrome; BMT, bone marrow transplantation; EIA, enzyme immune assay; ELISA, enzyme linked immunoadsorbent assay.

Table 16.6 *Suggested initial treatment of severe pneumonia according to suspected pathogens*

Pathogen	Antimicrobial treatment	Additional comments
Pyogenic bacteria		Broad-spectrum antimicrobials if neutropenia
Legionnaires' disease		Imipenem + amikacin or ceftriaxone + imipenem are alternative treatments
Nocardia asteroides	Erythromicin 4 g day^{-1} i.v. and rifampicin 20 mg kg^{-1} day^{-1} for 21 days Cotrimoxazole + amikacin	Consider ethambutol (15 mg kg^{-1} day^{-1}) if risk of drug resistance Prednisone 1–2 mg kg^{-1} day^{-1} in miliary tuberculosis
Mycobacterium tuberculosis	Isoniazid (5 mg kg^{-1} day^{-1}) + rifampicin(10 mg kg^{-1} day^{-1}) + pyrazinamide (15 mg kg^{-1} day^{-1})	
Pneumocystis carinii	Cotrimoxazole (sulphamethoxazole 100 mg kg^{-1} day^{-1}, trimethoprim 20 mg kg^{-1} day^{-1}) for 21 days (second choice: pentamidine i.v. 4 mg kg^{-1} day^{-1}) and prednisone 40 mg b.d. for 5 days, 20 mg b.d. for 5 days, 20 mg o.d. for 11 days	Fever and impairment of respiratory function may occur when steroids are decreased
Aspergillus fumigatus	Amphotericin B 1.5 mg kg^{-1} day^{-1} (and 5-flucytosine 100–150 mg kg^{-1} day^{-1}, dosage + +) If creatinine clearance < 30%: amphotericin B lipid complex 5 mg kg^{-1} day^{-1} or amphotericin B colloidal dispersion 5 mg kg^{-1} day^{-1} or liposomal amphotericin 3–5 mg kg^{-1} day^{-1}	G-CSF therapy has to be discussed in neutropenic patients Amphotericin continued until 3 g or for 2 weeks after resolution of all clinical signs and symptoms. Consolidation therapy for the entire period of immunosuppression: itraconazole 400–800 mg day^{-1} (dosage + + +) Consider surgical resection of aspergilloma
Cryptococcus neoformans	Amphotericin 0.7–1 mg kg^{-1} day^{-1} plus flucytosine 100 mg kg^{-1} day^{-1} for 2 weeks, then fluconazole 400 mg day^{-1} or fluconazole 400–800 mg day^{-1}	In HIV-infected patients, consolidation treatment must be continued for at least 10 weeks
Histoplasma capsulatum	Amphotericin B 0.7 mg kg^{-1} day^{-1} (or one of the lipid preparations at 3 mg kg^{-1} day^{-1} for patients with renal impairement) Then itraconazole 200 mg day^{-1} or fluconazole 800 mg day^{-1}	Consider prednisone 60 mg day^{-1} for 2 weeks
Respiratory syncytial virus	Ribavirin (aerosolized) 6 g in 300 mL of water continuous nebulization 18–24 hours daily for 3–7 days and i.v. immunoglobulin	Use closed system to prevent exposure to hospital personnel (teratogenicity)
CMV	Ganciclovir 5 mg kg^{-1} day^{-1} b.d. plus polyvalent immunoglobulin	
VZV	Aciclovir 10 mg kg^{-1} 8 h^{-1} for 7 days	
Toxoplasma gondii	Pyrismethamine 50 mg day^{-1} + (sulphadiazine 4 g day^{-1} or clindamycin 2.4 g day^{-1})	

| Strongyloides stercoralis | Thiabendazole 25 mg kg^{-1} for 7–10 days or ivermectine 200 μg kg^{-1} day 1, 2, 15, 16 +++ | Associated bacteraemia or bacterial meningitis is frequent Thiabendazole 25 mg kg^{-1} for 3 days must be given before immunosuppressive therapy in areas of endemicity |

CMV, cytomegalovirus; VZV, varicella-zoster virus; HIV, human immunodeficiency virus; G-CSF, granulocyte colony stimulating factor; i.v., intravenous; b.d., twice daily; o.d., once daily.

In AIDS patients with a CD4 count > 200 mm^{-3}, bacterial pneumonia is the most common cause of respiratory infection leading to admission to the ICU. In the case of diffuse alveolar infiltrates with miliary lesions, hilar or mediastinal lymph nodes or cavitation, an anti-tuberculous treatment should be empirically started. For diffuse lesions and subacute onset of symptoms, PCP should be treated. Macrolides should be added if atypical pneumonia is suspected.

Other specific treatments of pathogens should be chosen according to previous anti-infective prophylaxis, clinical history and results of specific tests and are summarized in Table 16.6. These are often toxic and should be carefully chosen on the results of diagnostic tests.

CONCLUSION

Pulmonary infections in the immunocompromised host are an increasing problem for intensive care clinicians. In the neutropenic patient, the prognosis is related to the promptness of a broad-spectrum antibacterial treatment. In the non-neutropenic host, treatment should be given that covers the common respiratory pathogens. Diagnostic tests, particularly bronchoscopy and BAL, remain the key investigations in making the diagnosis and avoiding potentially toxic empirical therapy. If possible, respiratory support should be provided non-invasively and tracheal intubation avoided.

REFERENCES

1. Casalino, E, Mendoza-Sassi, G, Wolff, M, et al. Predictors of short- and long-term survival in HIV-infected patients admitted to the ICU. Chest 1998; 113: 421–9.
2. Sprung, C, Eidelman, LA. Triage decisions for intensive care in terminally ill patients. Intensive Care Med 1997; 23: 1011–14.
3. Kress, JP, Christenson, J, Pohlman, AS, Linkin, DR, Hall, JB. Outcomes of critically ill cancer patients in a university hospital setting. Am J Respir Crit Care Med 1999; 160: 1957–61.
4. Staudinger, T, Stoiser, B, Mullner, M, et al. Outcome and prognostic factors in critically ill cancer patients admitted to the intensive care unit. Crit Care Med 2000; 28: 1322–8.
5. Huaringa, AJ, Leyva, FJ, Giralt, SA, et al. Outcome of bone marrow transplantation patients requiring mechanical ventilation. Crit Care Med 2000; 28: 1014–17.
6. Antonelli, M, Conti, G, Bufi, M, et al. Noninvasive ventilation for treatment of acute respiratory failure in patients undergoing solid organ transplantation: a randomized trial. JAMA 2000; 283: 235–41.
7. Hilbert, G, Gruson, D, Vargas, F, et al. Non invasive ventilation in immunosuppressed patients with pulmonary infiltrates, fever, and acute respiratory failure. N Engl J Med 2001; 244: 481–7.
8. Rubin, HR, Greene, R. Clinical approach of the compromised host with fever and pulmonary infiltrates. In Clinical approach to infection in the compromised host, ed. RH Rubin, LS Young. New York: Plenum Medical Book Company, 1994; 121–62.
9. Pizzo, PA. Management of fever in patients with cancer and treatment induced neutropenia. N Engl J Med 1993; 328: 1323–32.
10. Stevens, DA, Kan, VL, Judson, MA, et al. Practice guidelines for diseases caused by Aspergillus. Clin Infect Dis 2000; 30: 696–709.
11. Soubani, AO, Miller, KB, Hassoun, PM. Pulmonary complications of bone marrow transplantation. Chest 1996; 109: 1066–77.
12. Nosanchuk, JD, Sepkowitz, KA, Pearse, RN, White, MH, Nimer, SD, Armstrong, D. Infectious complications of autologous bone marrow and peripheral stem cell transplantation for refractory leukemia and lymphoma. Bone Marrow Transplant 1996; 18: 355–9.
13. Fishman, JA, Rubin, RH. Infection in organ transplant recipients. N Engl J Med 1998; 338: 1741–51.

14. Speirs, GE, Hakim, M, Wreghitt, TG. Relative risk of donor-transmitted *Toxoplasma gondii* infection in heart, liver and kidney transplant recipients. *Clin. Transplant* 1988; **2**: 257.

15. Gallino, A, Maggiorini, M, Kiowski, W, *et al.* Toxoplasmosis in heart transplant recipients. *Eur J Clin Microbiol Infect Dis* 1996; **15**: 389.

16. Kovacs, JA, Masur, H. Prophylaxis against opportunistic infections in patients with human immunodeficiency virus infection. *N Engl J Med* 2000; **342**: 1416–29.

17. Miller, R. HIV-associated respiratory diseases. *Lancet* 1996; **348**: 307–12.

18. 1999 USPHS/IDSA guidelines for the prevention of opportunistic infections in persons infected with human immunodeficiency virus. *Clin Infect Dis* 2000; **30**: S29–65.

19. Bedos, JP, Dumoulin, JL, Gachot, B, *et al. P. carinii* pneumonia requiring intensive care management: survival and prognostic study in 110 patients with human immunodeficiency virus. *Crit Care Med* 1999; **6**: 1109–15.

20. Mayaud, C, Cadranel, J. A persistent challenge: the diagnosis of respiratory disease in the non-AIDS immunocompromised host. *Thorax* 2000; **55**: 511–17.

21. Ozer, H, Armitage, JO, Bennett, CL, *et al.* 2000 update of recommendations for the use of hematopoietic colony-stimulating factors: evidence-based, clinical practice guidelines. *J Clin Oncol* 2000; **18**: 3558–85.

22. Schilero, GJ, Oropello, J, Benjamin, E. Impairment in gas exchange after granulocyte colony stimulating factor (G-CSF) in a patient with the adult respiratory distress syndrome. *Chest* 1995; **107**(1): 276–8.

17

Pleural disease

WOLFGANG FRANK AND ROBERT LODDENKEMPER

INTRODUCTION

The pleura is a delicate, double-layer structure that is physiologically characterized by a regulated fluid turnover that maintains a low-protein pool of less than 30 mL at a production rate of 0.3 mL kg^{-1} day^{-1}. The mechanisms for fluid transport (ultrafiltration and active clearance) also provide the energy supply for the creation of the ventilation-modulated and gravity-modulated negative pleural pressure. The gliding function of the fluid film results in mechanical coupling with the chest wall to ensure lung expansion in any physiological condition. Whereas the pleural cleft does not appear to be of vital importance for respiratory function, it is responsible for its vulnerability to a variety of local and distant disease processes that may interfere with lung expansion. Fluid accumulation due to inflammatory or non-inflammatory causes and lung collapse from traumatic or spontaneous pneumothorax are the most important. Empyema and bronchopleural fistula may complicate these conditions. Significant pleural problems occur in 30% of all general intensive care patients, mainly in the form of effusion (20%). The incidence of empyema and para-pneumonic effusion is around 5% and pneumothorax and bronchopleural fistula account for roughly 10%, with some overlap between these figures.[1]

PLEURAL EFFUSION

Effusion is the most common manifestation of pleural disease, and the biochemical profile of pleural fluid provides the basis for the classical distinction between a transudate and an exudate. The clinical importance of this distinction relates to the aetiological causes and consequent therapeutic implications. Low-protein-containing transudates, representing a plasma ultrafiltrate, usually result from extrapleural disease interfering with hydrostatic–oncotic fluid balance. Protein-rich exudates indicate direct inflammatory or neoplastic pleural involvement. Increased vascular permeability and vascular injury are the basic mechanisms, but impaired lymph drainage may be a contributory factor in both transudates and exudates. In the non-critically ill patient, approximately 40% of effusions are transudates, so that the odds for a patho-anatomic pleural cause in an undefined effusion are 0.6 or less. Taking into account the high prevalence of cardiac dysfunction in intensive care, the ratio is probably less in this setting. Indeed, the majority of exudates in surgical cases (e.g. post-thoracotomy) may still have cardiac dysfunction and/or excessive fluid administration as the principal cause. When assessing the clinical relevance of pleural effusion in the medical patient, however, it is important to realize that even small fluid collections indicate severe impairment of regulatory mechanisms, because the pleural drainage system may accommodate a 20-fold increase (=700 mL) of the low normal fluid influx.

Causes of pleural effusion

TRANSUDATIVE EFFUSION

Extrapleural or systemic diseases associated with transudative effusions are listed in Table 17.1. Congestive cardiac failure (CCF) is the most important cause. Approximately half of all patients with CCF will develop transudative effusion, which will be bilateral in 88% of cases. Unilateral effusion is more common on the right side. Left heart (mainly diastolic) dysfunction is the essential pathophysiological mechanism, as indicated by a correlation with pulmonary venous pressure and reflected by pulmonary capillary wedge pressure. In CCF, elevation of systemic venous pressure may be contributory by increasing systemic capillary filtration. Another mechanism appears to be elevated 'back pressure' at the lymphatic–venous junction (thoracic duct–jugular vein), with a consequent decrease in lymphatic clearance. Both these mechanisms are believed to explain a transudate in constrictive pericarditis due to diastolic dysfunction of the right ventricle. Isolated right ventricular systolic dysfunction, for example due to increased after-load in pul-

monary hypertension, does not cause pleural effusion, even when severe (PAP $\geqslant$50 mmHg). The occurrence of pleural effusion in right heart failure therefore suggests either associated left heart dysfunction or pericardial constriction. In acute left ventricular failure with pulmonary oedema, over 90% of patients will have radiologically obvious, or concealed, effusions.

In hepatic dysfunction complicating cirrhosis, about 8% of patients will have an effusion, with a striking 90% right-sided predominance. Hypoalbuminaemia is an important pathogenic mechanism, but a fluid shift from peritoneum to pleura contributes – a condition referred to as 'porous diaphragm syndrome'. The right-sided preference is so characteristic as to require exclusion of a peritoneal cause in recurrent or therapeutically unresponsive right-sided transudates. The same mechanism applies in chronic pleural effusions seen in continuous ambulant peritoneal dialysis (CAPD).

Other causes of transudates, usually bilateral, include nephrotic syndrome and renal failure. Both hypoproteinaemia and fluid overload result in gross ascites, pleural effusions and generalized peripheral oedema. Transudative effusion may occur in pleural inflammation such as pneumonia, thromboembolic disease or malignancy, but is unusual. Interestingly, long-standing transudates may undergo partial resorption and appear as exudates (so-called pseudo-exudates), especially with diuretic therapy.

Table 17.1 *Causes of transudative effusions*

Disease/condition	Approximate relative frequency (%)	Comments/causes
Congestive heart failure	80	Elevated hydrostatic pressure, hypoproteinaemia
Hepatic cirrhosis	8	and pleuro-peritoneal communication
Nephrotic syndrome	4	Hypoproteinaemia, systemic fluid overload
Other (total)	8	
Continuous ambulant peritoneal dialysis		Pleuro-peritoneal communication
Hypoalbuminaemia		Hypoproteinaemia,
Urinothorax		Obstructive uropathy
Atelectasis[a]		Effusion 'e vacuo'
Constrictive pericarditis		Increased central venous pressure
Trapped lung[a]		Adjacent inflammation
Superior vena cava obstruction		Venous hypertension and lymphatic obstruction
Sarcoidosis[a]		Inflammation
Pulmonary embolism[a]		Elevated hydrostatic pressure ± inflammation

[a]Also exudative effusion possible.

EXUDATIVE EFFUSION

Exudative effusion results from inflammation of the pleura, with leakage of blood constituents (in particular protein) from damaged pleural capillaries caused by systemic (mostly inflammatory or neoplastic) disorders, adjacent organ disease (pulmonary, mediastinal, abdominal) or primary pleural pathology. Differential diagnosis is therefore difficult, as indicated in Table 17.2. With respect to critical care, the important causes are more restricted:

- infection accounts for about 50% of cases,
- malignant disease for 25.5%,
- thromboembolic disease for 19%,
- gastrointestinal disease for 4%,
- autoimmune disease, tuberculosis and others for 1.5%.[1]

Malignant effusion ('pleuritis carcinomatosa') is common, with carcinoma of the lung (22%), breast (20%) and gastrointestinal tract (17%) predominating and accounting together for about 60% of malignant causes.[7] Effusions with no detectable tumour seeding are termed *para-neoplastic*; occasionally, they may have transudative characteristics or result from secondary problems such as atelectasis, pneumonia, impaired lymph drainage or systemic factors. Tuberculous pleurisy should be suspected when

there is a predominance of lymphocytes, multiloculation on imaging and a positive PPD test, although this may be falsely negative in 30% of cases.

Pulmonary embolism is an important, and often overlooked, cause of pleural (mainly exudative) effusion, with a reported incidence of up to 18% of all non-cardiac pleural effusions.[1] The possibility of pulmonary embolism should be considered in any non-attributable effusion, a situation not infrequently encountered in the respiratory critical care patient.

Chylothorax is a rare, but serious, mostly right-sided, specific cause of exudative effusion. Its clinical significance is related to the specific problem of controlling the spilling of chyle into the pleural cavity. The most common cause is injury to the thoracic duct by malignancy (in particular lymphoma), and trauma is the second most common cause, with inflammation (e.g. tuberculosis, sarcoidosis) and even benign lymphatic disease or central venous thrombosis as rare aetiologies. Chylothorax is easily diagnosed by its characteristic milky appearance and the diagnosis is confirmed by chemical analysis with triglyceride levels >110 mg dL^{-1} or lipid electrophoresis in ambiguous cases. In pseudo-chylothorax, also referred to as 'cholesterol pleurisy' – pathophysiologically an entirely different condition – the turbidity

Table 17.2 *Causes of exudative effusion*

Infectious	*Gastrointestinal disease*	*Connective tissue disease*
Bacterial pneumonia	Pancreatitis	Lupus pleuritis
Atypical pneumonias	Pancreatic pseudocyst	Rheumatoid pleurisy
Parasites	Subphrenic abscess	Mixed connective tissue disease
Nocardiosis	Hepatic, splenic abscess	Sjögren syndrome
Fungal disease	Hepatitis	Churg–Strauss syndrome
Tuberculosis	Chylous ascites	Wegener's granulomatosis
AIDS	Oesophageal rupture	Familial Mediterranean fever
Post-transplant		
	Malignancy	*Iatrogenic and traumatic*
Other inflammatory conditions	Carcinoma	Misplaced CVP catheter
Pulmonary embolism	Sarcoma	Perforated oesophagus
Radiation therapy	Lymphoma/leukaemia	Haemothorax
Asbestos pleuritis	Mesothelioma	
Sarcoidosis	Chylothorax	*Miscellaneous*
ARDS	AIDS	Meigs syndrome
Post-thoracotomy syndrome		Leiomyomatosis
Uraemic pleurisy		Yellow nail syndrome
Post-transplant		Cholesterol effusion
		Chylothorax
		Hypothyroidism

AIDS, autoimmune deficiency syndrome; ARDS, acute respiratory distress syndrome is due to a high and diagnostic cholesterol content (>200 mg dL^{-1}). The condition may develop in long-standing pleural collections, usually non-bacterial, such as post-traumatic effusion, rheumatic or tuberculous pleurisy. Haemothorax is considered to be present when the fluid approximates to blood. Because sanguinous effusion with haematocrit values as low as 5% may appear to be blood, the diagnosis of haemothorax requires laboratory proof by a defining haematocrit $> 50\%$ of circulating blood. Blunt or penetrating chest trauma is the main cause, but malignancy, pulmonary infarction, (iatrogenic) bleeding disorders and spontaneous pneumothorax may be causative.

Clinical findings

Clinical signs and symptoms are closely related to the amount of intrathoracic volume displacement and will cause varying degrees of dyspnoea. With large effusions, respiratory failure type I is common, often associated with hyperventilation. Respiratory failure type II, unless in compressive effusion, is unusual and would suggest co-existing obstructive airway disease. Major distress (orthopnoea) will require several litres of fluid, resulting in lung compression or mediastinal shift and possibly even causing central venous congestion and a low cardiac output secondary to constriction. The sensitivity of physical examination in small effusions is limited (300–400 mL) and loculated collections may escape detection.

Imaging

Conventional **chest radiography** (CXR) and **ultrasonography** are the basic imaging techniques. Blunting of the costo-phrenic angle is the first evidence, requiring >175 mL for detection. In the supine position of debilitated patients, the classical laterally ascending contour sign is lost and at least 500 mL is necessary to produce a diffuse, ground-glass opacity on supine CXR. Ultrasound is more sensitive than CXR and will detect effusions as small as 50–100 mL. It is particularly useful in evaluating multilocular and encapsulated effusions. Echogeneity to high-frequency (5–10 MHz) ultrasound has been shown to correlate with pleural fluid density and may have some predictive value in the distinction between

transudates and exudates.[2] In addition, extended technical capabilities using convex or sector scanners and additional probing windows (suprasternal, parasternal, infraclavicular, subcostal) have expanded the investigational range to a depth of 26 cm, therefore reaching more central areas of the diaphragm and major portions of the mediastinum. Thus, it allows evaluation of diaphragm motility in the spontaneously breathing patient, although, in controlled mechanical ventilation, paralysis may be missed. Ultrasonography is also valuable for the distinction between a subdiaphragmatic and a pleural cause of suspected effusion. However, the posterior mediastinum, hilum, paravertebral area and subscapular region still remain blind areas.

Therefore, the advantages of ultrasonography are:

- precise bedside visualization and localization of effusion,
- guidance for diagnostic and therapeutic interventions,
- detection of loculations, adhesions and septae,
- it may give clues as to the effusion profile,
- it allows evaluation of diaphragm motility and exclusion of subdiaphragmatic processes,
- it is safe and repeatable,
- it is easy to perform and inexpensive.

Computed tomography (CT) clearly offers greater imaging information and is:

- often necessary to assess the relative contributions of pleural or lung pathology in complex situations, such as multiple air–fluid levels that may result from pleural or intrapulmonary infection,
- essential for investigating mediastinal involvement.

It also provides an image that is more accessible to the non-radiologist and interpretation is less operator dependent than ultrasonography. However, its value is limited by the fact that it is only usually available outside of the intensive care unit/high dependency unit (ICU/HDU), with attendant risks when transporting the critically ill.

Portable CT facilities are now available in larger ICU settings. CT is unreliable in assessing the presence of septal loculations, for which ultrasonography is superior. Technical developments, such as high resolution (HRCT) or helical scanning, allow multiplanar or three-dimensional reconstruction, and intravenous contrast enhancement will increase the information yield. The ability to scan rapidly, e.g. during a breath hold, has revolutionized image quality. The overall accuracy of HRCT in diffuse pleural thickening was 97% in a recent study.[3] The sensitivity of CT for malignant infiltration of the chest wall remains limited. Three-dimensional techniques have been used successfully to study pleural surface infiltration, identifying visceral pleural involvement in 92%, compared to 17% of patients with two-dimensional CT imaging.[3]

Magnetic resonance imaging (MRI) is now the gold standard for imaging infiltrative chest-wall processes. Its better soft-tissue assessment compared to CT, improved spatial resolution and imaging versatility make it the best option for detecting disruption, invasion or thickening of the pleural membranes. In one study, T1-weighted, contrast-enhanced MRI sequences correctly identified 15/18 cases of malignant and 16/18 cases of benign chest-wall disease.[4] The problems of access, however, make this rarely a realistic possibility in the critically ill.

Diagnostic procedures

THORACOCENTESIS

Once clinical or imaging findings have established the presence of fluid, thoracentesis is the next diagnostic step. If there is reasonable evidence for a condition associated with transudates, thoracentesis is only required should it fail to respond to medical therapy. With large effusions, thoracentesis can be percussion guided; with small effusions, ultrasound guidance provides increased safety and efficacy. For diagnostic purposes, 10–20 mL should be aspirated into an optionally anticoagulant-conditioned (e.g. sodium citrate) syringe and appearance, smell and specific gravity should be noted, as well as requesting basic biochemical, cytological and microbiologic studies. PF may be serous (clear or turbid), suppurative, sanguinous, chylous or frankly haemorrhagic. Light's criteria, based upon the protein and lactate contents and their ratio compared to serum, have been traditionally employed to differentiate transudates from exudates and have 98% sensitivity, 77% specificity and an overall accuracy of 95%.[5] More recently, consideration of cholesterol has shown additional value, increasing specificity (91%) but reducing sensitivity (81%).[5] Therefore, their combined use is advised.

The following are the cut-off values for discriminating between exudates and transudates (with the pleural:plasma ratio in parentheses):

- protein $</>$3 g dL^{-1} (0.5)
- LDH $</>$200 IU ($</>$0.6)
- cholesterol $</>$60 mg dL^{-1} ($</>$0.3).

Glucose and pH values are also helpful parameters. Low values of both are characteristic of empyema, tuberculosis, rheumatic effusion and malignancy, and reflect enhanced local anaerobic metabolism. The analysis of cellular components helps in the differentiation of inflammatory and neoplastic aetiologies. An exclusive neutrophil leucocytosis characterizes empyema and para-pneumonic effusion, a relative lymphocytosis or eosinophilia suggest various inflammatory and non-inflammatory conditions, as listed up in Table 17.3.[6]

Cytological analysis requires considerable experience to reliably discriminate inflammation from malignancy. The diagnostic yield of conventional cytology is generally reported to be 40–70%, but 87% sensitivity has been reported.[1,6,7] The yield with advanced cytological analysis (immunocytology, immunocytometry, flow cytometry) is 70–80%, with up to 91% sensitivity and 100% specificity being reported. A panel of commercially available markers – mostly monoclonal antibodies (MAb) – is now often used to detect and identify tumour cells.

Immunological parameters such as rheumatoid factor, anti-nuclear antibodies, anti-neutrophil cytoplasmatic antibodies (c-ANCA) and components of the complement cascade (C3, C4) may confirm a systemic clinical condition as causative, but their sensitivity is limited. Measurement of interleukin and other cytokines, e.g. interferon-gamma (IFN-γ and tumour necrosis factor-alpha (TNF-α) may prove helpful in the diagnosis of tuberculous or rheumatic effusions. Adenosine deaminase (ADA) has been suggested as useful in suspected tuberculosis, with reported 100% sensitivity and 87.5% specificity; however, its accuracy appears largely modified by epidemiological factors (age and regional tuberculosis prevalence).[8] Initial enthusiasm concerning the potency of polymerase chain reaction (PCR) and nucleic acid amplification techniques (NAAT) in general for the diagnosis of tuberculous pleurisy has been dampened by a reported limited overall sensitivity of 47–87%, in both pleural fluid

Table 17.3 *Conditions associated with lymphocytosis (>80%) and eosinophilia (>10%) in the pleural fluid*

Disease/condition	Comment
Pleural lymphocytosis	
Tuberculosis	Most frequent cause (90–95% lymphocytes)
Lymphoma	~100 %, in particular non-Hodgkin
Chylothorax	
Rheumatic effusion	Associated with trapped lung
Sarcoidosis	Very rare (>90% lymphocytes)
Malignancy	In about 50%, but <70% lymphocytes
Yellow nail syndrome	Very rare
Pleural eosinophilia	
Pneumothorax	Most common cause, up to 50% eosinophilia
Haemothorax	Delayed occurrence
Previous thoracentesis	Pneumothorax and bleeding related
Pulmonary embolism	May be haemorrhagic
Benign asbestos pleuritis	Up to 50% eosinophilia, presumably often underlying 'idiopatic' pleural effusion
Parasitic disease	Various parasites
Fungal disease	Histoplasmosis, coccidioidomycosis
Allergic and immunological conditions	Drugs, Wegener's granulomatosis
Lymphoma	M. Hodgkin
Carcinoma	Uncommon, even with blood-stained effusion

According to Sahn.[15]

samples and paraffin-embedded tissue specimens, particularly in cultural negative (pauci-bacillary) pleurisy.[9] Carcino-embryonic antigen (CEA) is the only tumour marker of value in malignant effusion, its presence distinguishing adenocarcinoma from mesothelioma.

PLEURAL BIOPSY AND ENDOSCOPY (THORACOSCOPY)

When there is clinical suspicion of pleural pathology, but imaging techniques and thoracentesis provide inconclusive or conflicting results, blind pleural biopsy or thoracoscopy will be required for diagnosis. A recommended scheme is depicted in Figure 17.1.[7,10] Bacterial pleurisy may progress from benign para-pneumonic effusion to empyema.

Blind needle biopsy is useful in suspected tuberculous or malignant effusion. The Tru-cut needle may be preferable to the older Abraham's needle. It should be diagnostic in 74% of malignant causes and, combined with microbiology, in 60% of cases of tuberculosis.[1,6,7,10] However, the ability to biopsy suspicious pleural areas at thoracoscopy, when technically feasible, provides a significantly higher diagnostic yield.

Video-assisted thoracoscopy is a technical expansion of the original direct vision, single-entry technique, which has also led to the development of video-assisted thoracic surgery (VATS). Unlike traditional thoracoscopy, which can be performed with local anaesthesia in the endoscopy unit, VATS requires double-lumen intubation and a general anaesthetic. Whereas medical thoracoscopy may be basically incorporated in an ICU setting, this is probably only exceptionally a realistic option for VATS. Relative contraindications include coagulation disorders, severe cardiac dysfunction and respiratory failure (unless the patient is intubated and ventilated). Apart from the advantage of direct visualization, adhesions and loculations can be broken down, placement of drains optimized and air leaks evaluated in pneumothorax.

The value of medical thoracoscopy may thus be summarized as follows:[10]

- >90% diagnostic ability in exudative effusion,
- staging of mesothelioma or bronchial carcinoma,
- provision of optimum pleurodesis,
- breaking down of loculations and debridement in tuberculosis and empyema,
- assessment of pleural leaks in pneumothorax.

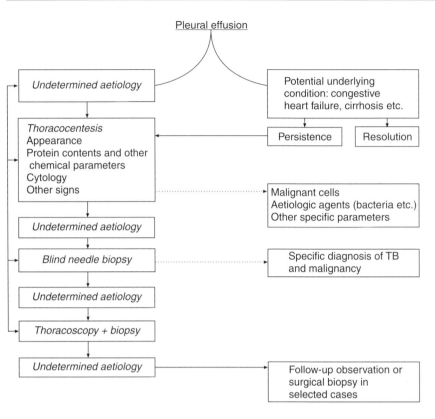

Figure 17.1 *General algorithm for the clinical diagnosis of pleural effusion* [7] *TB, tuberculosis.*

Management of large pleural effusions

In high dependency or intensive care medicine, the management of large effusions is aimed at the urgent restoration of lung expansion to improve gas exchange and allow restoration of venous return in the presence of cardiac embarrassment. Interventions can be divided into systemic and local approaches and also into acute palliative and elective control strategies.

ACUTE PALLIATION

Transudates will respond to therapy aimed at treating the primary cause, for example improving myocardial contractility or correcting fluid overload. Diuretics, and albumin replacement in the case of severe hypoproteinaemic states, are effective, although thoracocentesis may be required initially in respiratory distress or failure. Correction of marked hypoproteinaemia with intravenous albumin should be implemented in a prolonged fashion to avoid detrimental over-expansion of the intravascular fluid compartment. Frusemide infusions are more effective than bolus therapy, but potassium and

magnesium depletion should be avoided. Spironolactone is indicated in hypoproteinaemic states. In view of the evidence favouring its long-term use in CCF, it should now be used in most conditions with generalized oedema unless there is severe impairment of renal function. In the case of a large exudate, tube drainage is the first management strategy. The insertion of a chest drain is conventionally performed in the lateral decubitus position, especially in the ventilated patient. In severe respiratory distress in the spontaneously breathing individual (who may be orthopnoeic), it should be carried out with the patient sitting upright and supported. As vago-vagal syncope may occur, pre-medication with atropine is a wise precaution if this approach is being adopted. Local anaesthesia should be generously infiltrated into the relevant rib interspace (avoiding potential damage to the subcostal neurovascular bundle), with blunt dissection and separation of muscle planes down to the pleura. Alternatively, thoracoscopy-derived trocar systems using a 9-mm external diameter sleeve and a sharp obturator are in common use.

It is important to avoid damage to underlying lung, and drains should not be inserted using force. If there is any doubt as to the presence of loculations and adhesions, ultrasonography should be used to guide placement, although the infiltrating needle will often give warning if the effusion is unexpectedly shallow. Particular attention needs to be paid to fixing the drain after insertion, although purse-string sutures are no longer recommended. Kinking at the skin is a common cause of subsequent failure, and blockage of the tube will increase the risk of surgical emphysema. We favour the use of large-bore, transparent silicone or PVC tubes ($\geqslant$24 F), which provide excellent suppleness with optimum patient tolerance and resistance to kinking and also allow visual patency control. The angle of the drain should be acute, with the skin incision being over the rib immediately below the relevant rib space. A transparent dressing is preferable to allow inspection of the drain site. Immediate relief will usually result from relatively small (500 mL) drainage. Pulmonary re-expansion oedema is unlike to occur, even after the evacuation of large effusions, except in the case of long-standing compressive collections, when the lung has developed complete atelectasis with significant surfactant depletion. However, in order also to avoid hypotensive circulatory effects, drainage should not exceed 1 L hour^{-1} and the suction level should be low (10 cmH$_2$O). Cough provoked by re-expansion is common and may be distressing. Pre-medication with an opiate may therefore be useful if there are no contraindications. However, these aspects are rarely an issue in the ventilated patient.

Long-term control

The majority of effusions that require definitive action for long-term control are caused by malignancy. After initial tube drainage and confirmation of the malignant cause, instillation of pleural irritants to produce a pleurodesis will usually be necessary. The value of large-bore drains ($\geqslant$24 F) in pleurodesis is to optimize instillation and reduce the risk of tube obstruction by viscous, fibrinous exudates or blood. Should this occur, as indicated by the absence of fluctuations that reflect pleural pressure swings in the water column of the drainage bottle, mechanical manipulation to mobilize fibrin deposits or clots can be performed ('milking': Fig. 17.2). Disposable commercial systems that combine fluid collection and suction control systems (including a high-pressure safety valve) are available (Fig. 17.3).

Mechanical wall suction, using a central pressurized air supply, is still in common use and may be combined with a variety of collection systems. One advantage of the venturi-operated system is an (almost) infinite suction reserve with a range in pressure up to 100 cmH$_2$O. For safety reasons, a low-pressure 'thoracic' device is preferred and the routine use of suction levels of 10–20 cmH$_2$O suffices.

Thoracoscopy, as described above, provides optimum placement of chest tubes and helps in predicting likely lung re-expansion. The recognition of the degree of lung encasement by thickened visceral pleura or complicating adhesions is helpful as lung re-expansion is critical for successful pleurodesis. Pleurodesis may be achieved by the instillation of talc powder ('poudrage') with a hand-bulb operated device (intra-thoracoscopic pleurodesis), ensuring widespread powder distribution (Fig. 17.4). Doses up to 8 g have been evaluated as safe. Talc poudrage has been evaluated in controlled, prospective trials and has been shown to provide >90% long-term control in malignant pleurisy.[10,11] Alternatively, agents such as tetracycline or doxycycline can be instilled via the chest tube, with reported success rates between 54% and 96%. A figure around 70% is realistic.[11] The instillation of talc as a slurry, in equivalent doses to poudrage, may be both more effective and better tolerated than tetracycline. Topical analgesia (200–250 mg lidocaine intrapleurally) is useful with additional opiate systemic analgesia when performing pleurodesis. The reported complication rate is around 5%.[7] The clinical course is characterized by an exponential fall in drainage over 3–5 days. When drainage is below 100 mL day^{-1}, the chest tube can be removed. Pleurodesis may also be used in chronic transudative effusion of hepatic origin. However, the presence of ascites carries a lower success rate. The response rate is around 85% in the absence of ascites, but falls to 40% in patients with ascites.[7]

In otherwise refractory chronic transudative and exudative effusions, a pleuro-peritoneal Denver shunt can be useful. This may be inserted using local anaesthesia without important complications. Indications are failure of pleurodesis, particularly in the presence of so-called 'trapped lung' and chylothorax. The device consists of a double-valved pump with an afferent (pleural) and efferent (peritoneal) tube. The pump is implanted subcutaneously and operated by the patient or an assistant two to three times a day. Although peritoneal seeding by

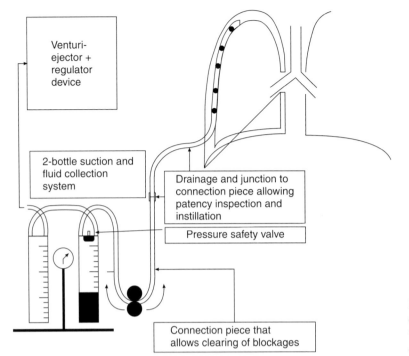

Figure 17.2 *Schematic representation of optimum drainage position and venturi-ejector-operated, two-bottle suction and fluid collection system.*

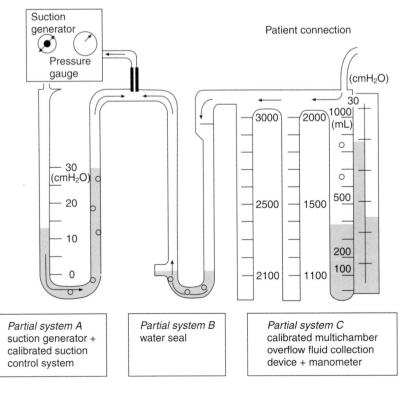

Figure 17.3 *Schematic representation of an integrated three-bottle suction and fluid-collection system. The arrows and bubbles indicate airflow direction, both from the ambient air (suction control system) and from the pleural cavity. If no suction is applied, the system operates as a two-bottle, gravity-dependent, combined water seal and fluid-collection system. The integrated manometer in the fluid-collection system (C) allows monitoring of the actual suction level applied on the patient (= primary suction control gradient delivered by system A (cmH$_2$O) minus height of the water seal column); it also acts as a safety valve to positive pressure.*

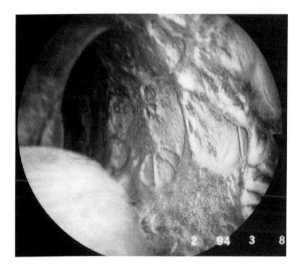

Figure 17.4 *Endoscopic view of thoracoscopic talc poudrage. Note the homogeneous distribution of talc powder across the entire left parietal pleura, adhering lung upper lobe on the left upper margin, free lower lobe at the left lower margin. (See also Plate 7.)*

tumour cells occurs, the benefit of controlling the pleural collection offsets this risk in the short-term palliation of symptoms.

EMPYEMA

Definition, pathogenesis and clinical features

Empyema is defined as a suppurative effusion due to bacterial infection. The most frequent cause is underlying pneumonia. The recovery of obvious pus from the pleural cavity establishes the diagnosis. Serous or turbid effusions that are sterile are termed para-pneumonic effusions. They may, however, pre-date the later development of empyema. Infection accounts for 20% of all pleural effusions, with bacterial pleuritis complicating pneumonia in 20–57%. In 23% of cases, empyema is the result of surgery, and trauma accounts for about 6%. Other causes include oesophageal perforation (5%) pneumothorax (2%) and other miscellaneous causes. Empyema has a peak incidence in the middle-aged and elderly population. Predisposing morbidity has been reported in up to 82% of patients, with alcohol abuse as the leading

risk factor in between 29% and 40% of patients, depending on case-mix. It is clinically important to distinguish:

- the *early exudative stage*, corresponding to a pauci-cellular sterile effusion of 1 to several days duration,
- the *fibrino-purulent stage*, representing classical empyema with abundant leucocytes and bacteria, which progresses to the formation of fibrinous membranes and loculations between 3 days and 3 weeks,
- *chronic empyema*, characterized by organizing adherent peels encapsulating the lung and eventually leading to rupture transcutaneously (empyema necessitans).

Empyema can take a highly variable course, from a well-preserved general status (silent empyema) to severe septic shock, depending on pre-morbidity, antibiotic treatment, immune status, age and aetiology.

Empyema should be suspected if there is:

- persisting or unexplained fever after adequately treated pneumonia,
- persisting elevation of inflammatory markers (CRP, WBC, ESR),
- relevant pre-conditions, such as thoracic or oesophageal surgery or aspiration,
- suggestive faeculent sputum production (broncho-pleural fistula),
- imaging suggesting multi-loculations.

Diagnosis

IMAGING TECHNIQUES

The features distinguishing a simple effusion from empyema are a multi-locular collection, membrane formation indicating thickening of the visceral and parietal pleura and fibrin strands, but empyema may also be monolocular in about 16% of cases. Multi-loculation is not a specific indicator because it may also occur with rheumatic and tuberculous pleurisy. Conventional X-ray may show a convex rather than the typical concave crescent of a free effusion and air within the pleural space, which suggests a bronchopleural fistula. Both ultrasonography and CT have limited sensitivities but high specificity (around 96%) for the detection of parietal and visceral pleural thickening suggestive of bacterial pleuritis. Contrast-enhanced CT is also important in helping to distinguish empyema from lung abscess (which will not require thoracostomy) by the following criteria:

Empyema:

- signs of lung compression,
- smooth margins of membranes,
- dissection of the thickened visceral and parietal pleura ('split-pleura' sign),
- blunt angle with the chest wall,

Lung abscess:

- spherical shape with irregular thick-wall structures,
- absence of lung compression,
- sharp angle with the chest wall,
- visible airway connection,
- demonstration of vasculature around abscess (definite proof).

Bronchoscopy can provide important contributions to the diagnosis of empyema by:

- adding to the microbiological yield in patients with underlying pneumonia,
- allowing definite proof and localization of a bronchopleural communication,

- detecting potential causative conditions such as foreign-body aspirate, tumour or an oesophago-tracheobronchial communication.

Likewise, bronchoscopy may be indicated therapeutically for clearing the airways of secretions or aspirate.

Pleural fluid analysis

Although clinical features may suggest empyema, thoracentesis establishes the diagnosis. Thoracentesis may need to be performed at different locations because, in loculated empyema and para-pneumonic effusion, sterile fluid and pus may be found in different compartments. Pus is instantly recognizable by its appearance and/or the characteristically offensive smell suggesting anaerobic infection. Confusion with chyle or pseudo-chyle may occur when aspiration reveals odourless, whitish-turbid fluid. The parameters in Table 17.4 (referred to as Light's criteria) unequivocally establish the diagnosis and define the stages of bacterial pleuritis from

- uncomplicated para-pneumonic effusion,
- complicated empyema,
- frank empyema.[1,12]

The determination of amylase ($\pm$isoenzymes) may be useful in oesophageal rupture or pancreatitis. Empyema and a complicated para-pneumonic effu-

Table 17.4 *Pleural fluid analysis in para-pneumonic effusion and empyema: indications for tube drainage*

Empyema and complicated para-pneumonic effusion	Indeterminate effusion	Uncomplicated para-pneumonic effusion
Absolute indication for drainage	*Relative indication for drainage*	*No indication for chest drainage*
Frank empyema	Turbid effusion $\pm$ bacterial culture (stain)	Serous – clear effusion
Positive bacterial culture (stain)	Large fluid amounts (>2000 mL)	Negative bacterial culture (stain)
		Fluid amounts (< 2000 mL)
$\pm$Loculations	Loculations	No loculations
Biochemical characteristics:	Biochemical characteristics:	Biochemical characteristics:
(Light's criteria)	glucose 40–60 mg dL^{-1}	glucose > 60 mg dL^{-1}
glucose <40 mg dL^{-1}	LDH < 1000 IU L^{-1}	LDH < 1000 IU L^{-1}
LDH >1000 IUL^{-1}	pH 7.00–7.20	pH < 7.3 ↓ 0
pH < 7.00	WBC 10–15 nL^{-1}	WBC < 10 nL^{-1}
WBC > 15 nL^{-1}		
Bronchopleural fistula		Serial determination
	Serial determination + clinical follow-up	
Drainage	← ⌐ →	*Resolution*

sion are characterized by low pH ($<$7.0) and glucose ($<$40 mg dL^{-1}), a raised LDH ($>$1000 IU L^{-1}) and neutrophil count ($>$15 nL^{-1}), whereas bacterial culture will usually be positive. The clinical significance of subdividing bacterial pleurisy (Table 17.4) is in management: in uncomplicated para-pneumonic effusion, a conservative approach is justified, whereas in empyema and complicated para-pneumonic effusion, drainage is required. Serial determination of Light's criteria is an adjunct to clinical observation in ambiguous cases (indeterminate effusion).

Microbiologic investigation should extend to cultures of blood, sputum and bronchoalveolar lavage (BAL). A wide range of bacterial isolates has been reported (24–94%), obviously due to different rates and intensity of antibiotic pre-treatment and to different methods of sample collection and isolate cultivation (which is particularly true for anaerobes). Importantly, the causative aetiology is changing, with an increasing contribution of Gram-negative micro-organisms, anaerobic isolates and multiple infectious agents. In one series, comprising more than 400 isolates from 336 patients, 56% were mono-infections and 44% multiple (up to four pathogens): 46% Gram positive, 23% Gram negative and 21% anaerobes.[13]

Treatment options

The management of empyema involves both antibiotics and drainage; surgical intervention may be required. Parenteral antimicrobial therapy will need to take account of clinical features such as faeculent fluid or pre-treatment. An empiric scheme is shown in Table 17.5. Therapy should be adjusted by microbiologic isolation as soon as possible.

Tube drainage is indicated:

- with severe sepsis,
- with large quantities of effusion ($>$2 L),
- in the presence of air in the pleural space (indicating bronchopleural fistula),
- following Light's criteria-based fluid assessment (see Table 17.4).

We favour the use of double-lumen catheters (Fig 17.5), with a diameter of at least 20 F, as this allows closed-circuit, large-volume irrigation with normal saline ($\pm$aseptic additives) and the option of the instillation of fibrinolytics if required. Irrigation is continued until clear sterile fluid is recovered and the net fluid production falls below 50–100 mL day^{-1}. The instillation of fibrinolytic agents (streptokinase, urokinase) is indicated if drainage fails to clear thick pus and/or membranes and loculations are present. The value of fibrinolysis has been shown in controlled, prospective studies. 200 000–250 000 IU streptokinase, or of an equipotent dose of urokinase (50 000–100 000 IU), is instilled once or twice daily.[14] Our protocol is given in Table 17.6. Instillation of fibrinolytic agents is usually required for 5–6 days. Failure, defined as persisting clinical features or ultrasonography-demonstrated loculations after 2 weeks, occurs in about 15% of cases.[12,14] Similar results have been claimed with the use of small-bore catheters (8–14 F).[15] Contraindications to throm-

Table 17.5 *Options for empiric antimicrobial therapy in empyema and para-pneumonic effusion*

Empyema complicating	Common isolates	Empiric therapy
Community-acquired pneumonia	Pneumococci *Streptococcus* spp. *Staphylococcus aureus* *Haemophilus influenzae* *Legionella* spp. Anaerobes	2nd or 3rd generation cephalosporin or Augmentin + clindamycin or metronidazole + macrolide if *Legionella* possible
Nosocomial pneumonia	Enterobacteriaceae spp. *Pseudomonas* spp. *Staphlyococcus aureus* *Acinetobacter* *Peptostrepococcus* *Bacteroides* *Fusobacterium*	3rd or 4th generation cephalosporin (e.g. ceftazidime) + aztreonam[a] or carbapenem or acylamino-penicillin/tazobactam combination

[a]Aztreonam is recommended instead of aminoglycosides to avoid intrapleural inactivation.

sizes: diameter 20 - 28 F, length 40 cm

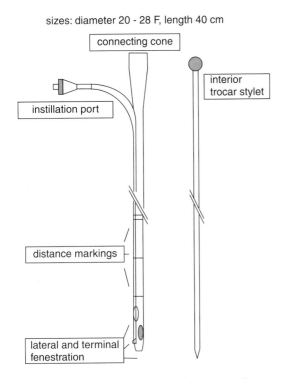

Figure 17.5 *Schematic representation of double-lumen chest tubes for irrigation and instillation therapy.*

bolytics include bronchopleural fistula, significant coagulation disorders or allergy (streptokinase). Prior use of streptokinase (e.g. in acute myocardial infarction) will not invalidate its use. The use of medical thoracoscopy to break down lung parenchymal adhesions and loculations may be helpful. Instillation of antibiotics has been suggested, with the rationale that low penetration of systemic antibiotic therapy might provide suboptimal therapy. However, with inflamed pleural membranes, concentrations well above the minimal inhibitory concentrations (MIC) have been demonstrated in empyema fluid (except aminoglycosides) in many studies.

Surgical therapy (using VATS rather than formal thoracotomy) is indicated:

- when medical treatment fails – although early (e.g. 4–7 days) intervention may be indicated in severely ill patients,
- when the empyema is encapsulated (empyema necessitans), which may be resected extrapleurally within the encapsulated empyema sack (empyemectomy),

- when empyema is traumatic or postoperative,
- for long-term open management (rib resection) of a chronically infected pleural cavity.

Even with adequate antibiotic therapy and judicious medical or surgical management, empyema remains a serious condition, with a mortality varying from 6% up to 21%, depending on case-mix. The most important late sequelae is fibrothorax with associated impairment of pulmonary function. This should occur in less than 10% of patients, in whom decortication would then be indicated.

Table 17.6 *Large-volume irrigation (LVI) and fibrinolytic therapy in the local treatment of empyema*

Drainage	Thoracoscopic/ultrasound-guided double-lumen trocar-catheter insertion, diameter 20–28 F, length 40 cm
Irrigation	1000 mL normal saline solution + 20 mL 2% polyvidone-iodine 1–2 times a day until clear irrigation fluid recovered
Fibrinolysis	200 000 IU streptokinase, tube initially clamped 4–8 hours
Duration	≤ 14 days
Side effects	Fever (> 38 °C) in 42%, pain 10%
Contraindication orcautions	Bronchopleural fistula, allergy, previous thrombolysis for myocardial infarction

PNEUMOTHORAX AND BRONCHOPLEURAL FISTULA

Aetiology

Pneumothorax is a fairly common event in respiratory intensive care. Its importance is related to the facts that many cardiorespiratory conditions that require ICU treatment can precipitate pneumothorax and that mechanical ventilation and other interventions entail both an increased incidence and complication rate. Pneumothorax is commonly divided into traumatic and spontaneous pneumothorax, the latter occurring either without apparent pre-existing lung disease (primary pneumothorax)

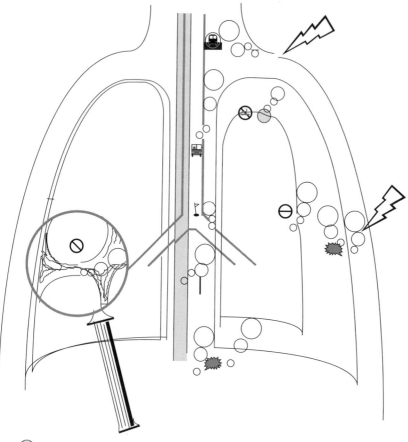

Subclavian region soft-tissue injury (soft-tissue emphysema)

Trauma to the trachea (mediastinal emphysema, soft-tissue emphysema)

Trauma to the bronchus (mediastinal emphysema, interstitial emphysema)

Alveolar rupture (interstitial emphysema)

Visceral pleura rupture (pneumothorax)

Rupture of preformed bullae or blebs (spontaneous pneumothorax)

Trauma to the external chest wall and parietal pleura (pneumothorax, soft-tissue emphysema)

Oesophagus rupture (medlastinal emphysema, soft-tissue emphysema)

Entrance of abdominal air (mediastinal emphysema, pneumothorax)

Figure 17.6 *Causes (mechanisms) of air penetration to the pleura and soft tissue and their immediate sequelae.*

or secondary to a condition involving structural damage to the lung, such as chronic obstructive lung diasease (COPD) or interstitial lung disease. Important focal pleuro-pulmonary causes include pneumonia, lung abscess, neoplasms, tuberculosis and empyema. In respiratory critical care, secondary spontaneous pneumothorax may be iatrogenic (traumatic), related to diagnostic and therapeutic interventions, or may result from barotrauma in positive pressure ventilation. Accidental pleural injuries during subclavian vein catheterization, thoracentesis, transthoracic needle aspiration and transbronchial biopsy are other important causes. The adult respiratory distress syndrome (ARDS) and opportunistic *Pneumocystis carinii* infection are particular risk factors, with a pneumothorax incidence up to 60%; bilateral occurrence is not uncommon. Aspiration pneumonia (37%) and COPD (10%) are other important causes.[1]

Respirator-associated pneumothorax combines the features of secondary and iatrogenic (traumatic) pneumothorax. The risk of pneumothorax with positive pressure ventilation has an overall incidence of 4%. Positive end-expiratory pressure (PEEP) increases the risk to approximately 17%, with a twofold to fourfold further increase in risk with PEEP > 15 cmH$_2$O.[1] Interestingly, in a large ARDS study, no relationship was found between peak airway pressure and pneumothorax risk.[16] However, only the initial period of ICU stay was reported and pneumothorax risk is greater in the later fibroproliferative stage.

The most important aspect of ventilatory pressures is the difference between plateau pressure and the level of PEEP as this determines tidal volume. The basic mechanism in respirator-associated pneumothorax is alveolar rupture due to increased shear forces resulting from inhomogeneity of lung pathology, with resulting regional over-distension and rupture of alveoli. Therefore, respirator-associated pneumothorax is more appropriately described as volutrauma rather than barotrauma.

Alveolar rupture may also lead to mediastinal emphysema, bronchopleural fistula and soft-tissue emphysema. The complications and mechanisms involved in pneumothorax are schematically depicted in Figure 17.6. Efforts to minimize the risk aim to limit pressure differences between inflation and expiration (small tidal volume) and avoid hyperinflation. The strategies for limiting airway pressure include the use of spontaneous modes of ventilation, pressure rather than volume control (de-accelerating flow) and tidal volume reduction, i.e. 'permissive' hypoventilation.[16]

Signs and diagnosis

CLINICAL SIGNS

It is important immediately to consider the possibility of pneumothorax in any patient with a known risk and compatible symptoms and signs. In the non-intubated patient, a sudden increase in dyspnoea and chest pain are the principal symptoms, with hypoxaemia and hypercapnia occurring in 16–17% of cases, cyanosis in 9% and shock in

7%.[1,17,18] In respirator-associated pneumothorax, the severity of cardiorespiratory compromise is much higher and may be disproportionate to the size of pneumothorax. The differential diagnosis includes myocardial infarction, pulmonary embolism and ruptured aneurysm. Classical signs are unilateral hyper-resonance and attenuated breath sounds (silent chest). An immobile hemi-thorax with central venous congestion and evidence of a reduced cardiac output suggest tension pneumothorax. Tension pneumothorax may also induce electrocardiogram changes due to air interposition or mediastinal displacement (e.g. dextrocardia). Ventilatory asynchrony in patients on mechanical ventilation may be recognized by a sharp rise of the peak and plateau airway pressures, a fall in tidal volume and concomitant deterioration of gas exchange.

RADIOLOGICAL SIGNS

The diagnosis is easily made in large and moderate-sized pneumothorax by standard X-ray. Problems of recognition may arise:

- with small pneumothorax and consolidated lung,
- with localized or mediastinal pneumothorax,
- in the presence of pre-existing bullous or generalized emphysema,
- with air–fluid levels (confusion with intrapulmonary cavities),
- with superimposed chest-wall artefacts.

Postural, e.g. decubitus, views and follow-up films may be helpful. Air–fluid levels, in the absence of prior chest aspiration, indicate a pulmonary leak and may be seen associated with hydrothorax, serothorax, pyothorax chylothorax and haemothorax. Standard X-ray films may also reveal additional signs of air in the mediastinum, pericardium or chest wall (surgical emphysema). The distinction between intrapulmonary and pleural air–fluid levels may require CT scanning and is important for treatment decisions.

ENDOSCOPIC DIAGNOSIS

As with pleural effusion, medical thoracoscopy can contribute significantly to diagnosis and management and is only marginally more time consuming than the standard therapeutic intervention of inserting a chest drain. The staging or classification system proposed by Swierenga and Vanderschueren[19] pro-

Table 17.7 *Endoscopic staging in spontaneous pneumo-thorax (according to Vanderschueren)*

Stage I	PTX with endoscopically normal-appearing lung (40%)
Stage II	PTX with pleuropulmonary adhesions that may be accompanied by haemothorax (12%)
Stage III	PTX with small bullae and blebs (< 2 cm in diameter) (31%)
Stage IV	PTX with numerous large bullae (> 2 cm in diameter) (17%)

vides a precise description of the endoscopic findings (Table 17.7). We recommend the incorporation of thoracoscopy into the routine management of pneumothorax, even in the mechanically ventilated patient. The advantages may be summarized as:

- better pleural and lung assessment than with CT,
- visualization of complicating bronchopleural fistula (with interventional option),
- optimum drain placement,
- ability to induce pleurodesis if required,
- assessment of need for surgical intervention.[19]

Therapeutic options

In terms of therapeutic aims, the management of pneumothorax is straightforward: re-expansion of the lung and prevention of recurrence. However, the implementation of these aims is controversial.

RE-EXPANSION

Based on a calculated pleural gas absorption rate of 1.2–1.8% day^{-1}, the indication for draining or aspirating a pneumothorax is somewhat arbitrarily set at ≥15% of the hemi-thorax volume in uncomplicated primary spontaneous pneumothorax. In secondary spontaneous pneumothorax and respirator-associated pneumothorax, however, treatment will depend more on the immediate physiological consequences or the danger of the subsequent development of a large pneumothorax in the ventilated patient. Simple aspiration may be sufficient in spontaneous pneumothorax, but the success rate (defined as complete lung expansion maintained for at least 1 month) is only 48–85% in primary and 31–80% in secondary spontaneous pneumothorax.[20] In the criti-

cal care patient, tube drainage (> 24 F) is required, particularly in the presence of a concomitant effusion (serothorax, pyothorax, chylothorax, haemothorax), with reported success rates of 96% in primary and 92% in secondary spontaneous pneumothorax.[1,18]

Low suction (10–20 cmH$_2$O) will usually suffice to achieve full lung expansion. Drainage times usually vary from 3 to 7 days. Importantly, the chest tube should not be removed prematurely. We recommend a probationary period of clamping (12 hours) before removal of the drain, but this is controversial and the patient should be closely observed. Failure of expansion to low suction pressures or early recurrence (< 7 days) indicates one of the following:

1. consolidated or atelectatic lung,
2. reduced lung compliance (stiff) or trapped lung,
3. loculated pneumothorax with adhesions,
4. pulmonary air leak (bronchopleural fistula),
5. technical problems such as kinked or plugged tube, water in the filter or excessively long connecting tubes reducing or preventing the creation of a negative pressure within the pleural cavity throughout the respiratory cycle.

Combinations of these complications may also occur and require specific management strategies. With consolidated or collapsed lung, pneumonia may be specifically treated and bronchoscopy may allow occluding mucous plugs to be removed. With stiff or trapped lung, re-expansion may eventually occur with prolonged suction at higher pressure levels and, as previously outlined, thoracoscopy may be helpful in removing fibrin or membranes when these limit re-expansion. Suction levels >20 cmH$_2$O in mal-expansion due to trapped lung must be applied in a cautious, incremental fashion and with careful observation of the patient, because negative-pressure transmission to the mediastinum may cause pain and an ipsilateral mediastinal shift with central venous obstruction.

In loculated pneumothorax, some compartments may be inadequately drained and multiple drains may be required. Bronchopleural fistula will be apparent by flow of air through the drainage tube, which may be continuous (large fistula) or discontinuous (small fistula). Air leakage may vary significantly, from <1 to 16 L min^{-1}. In the ventilated patient, quantitative assessment is easily possible by subtracting expiratory minute volume from inspiratory volume. Tube size may become critical, because an internal diameter of at least 4.72 mm ($= 20$ F drainage) is required to accommodate a flow of 10 L min^{-1} at a standard suction level of 10 mmHg, and of 5.87 mm ($= 24$ F drainage) to accommodate 15 L min^{-1} air flow.[20] Attempts to re-expand the lung using higher suction levels may merely increase the leak and it may be difficult to achieve adequate oxygenation, although the respiratory 'steal' will eliminate CO_2.

If the lung can be re-expanded, the air leak usually ceases on re-institution of pleural contact and this can usually be achieved with suction if the leak is not too large. In large pleural leaks, it may be better to avoid suction, with the drainage system acting merely as a safety valve to prevent tension pneumothorax. Lung expansion may then be attempted after closure of the defect. The management of bronchopleural fistula may require a variety of measures (summarized in Table 17.8)[21], such as reduced ventilatory pressure and attempts to close the leak bronchoscopically using fibrin sealant (which has, in our experience, a 50% success rate) or via thoracoscopy employing cautery or talc pleurodesis. Unilateral or differential bilateral ventilation can be tried, but is rarely successful and can be technically difficult. High-frequency jet ventilation and high-frequency oscillation therapy are often effective in the temporary stabilization of the difficult patient, but surgical closure may still be required when/if the patient survives the acute period of respiratory failure.

DEFINITIVE THERAPY: PREVENTION OF RECURRENCE

The recurrence rate in secondary spontaneous pneumothorax is reported to be as high as 54%.[1,20] Recurrence is most likely to occur in the immediate post re-expansion period, which is particularly relevant to the intensive care patient. Pleurodesis should be performed only after a recurrent pneumothorax in primary spontaneous cases, but should be seriously considered after the first episode in secondary spontaneous and respirator-associated pneumothorax. This is particularly true in the presence of thoracoscopy-demonstrated stage II or III pleuropulmonary changes and in the elderly patient (>50 years). The technique of pleurodesis is the same as for chronic pleural effusion, with the exception that

Table 17.8 *Ventilator-associated pneumothorax*

Barotrauma preventative strategies
  Interstitial lung disease
    BiPAP or CPAP/PCV rather than VCV ventilation
    Inverse ratio ventilation with Paw$_{max}$ < 35 or PEEP <15 cmH$_2$O
    Permissive hypercapnia
    with V <6 mL kg^{-1}
  Obstructive airway disease
    Low minute volume
    Avoiding further hyperinflation by
    limiting PEEPe $<$ PEEPi
Recognition of PTX
    Sudden increase in Paw$_{max}$ and Paw$_{plateau}$
    and deterioration in gas exchange
Treatment of PTX with bronchopleural fistula
    Large-bore drain(s)
    Postural manoeuvres: diseased side down
    Monitor size of fistula leak: $=$ inspiratory minus expiratory minute volume
    Low level suction with adjustment to minimize leak
    Reduce tidal volume, PEEP and inspiratory time
    Attempt to close fistula by occlusion of air leak with fibrin or thoracoscopic cautery or talc
    High-frequency oscillation ventilation
    Double-lumen intubation for unilateral or differential bilateral ventilation

continued pleural drainage is not relevant. The long-term success rates (up to 95%) with talc poudrage in pneumothorax closely approach those of surgical procedures such as VATS or formal thoracotomy and pleurectomy (98%).[1,20] Talc slurry may be a less-favourable agent due to unequal distribution, but tetracycline has been reported to produce long-term control in 84% of cases and thus remains a useful alternative.[1]

REFERENCES

1. Light, RW. *Pleural diseases*, 3rd edition, Williams and Wilkins, 1995.
2. Yang, PHC, Luh, KT, Chang, DB, *et al*. Value of sonography in determining the nature of pleural effusion: analysis of 320 cases. *Am J Radiol* 1992; **159**: 29–33.
3. Verschakelen, JA. Spiral CT of the chest: diaphragm, chest wall and pleura. In *Spiral CT of the chest*, ed.

M Remy-Jardin, J Remy. New York: Springer, 1996;
305–19.

4. Bittner, RC, Felix, R. Magnetic resonance (MR) imaging
of the chest: state of the art. *Eur Respir J* 1998 ; **11**:
1392–404.

5. Burgess, LJ, Maritz, FJ, Taljaard, FFJ. Comparative
analysis of the biochemical parameters used to
distinguish between pleural transudates and
exudates. *Chest* 1995; **107**: 1604–9.

6. Sahn, SA. The diagnostic value of pleural fluid analysis.
Semin Respir Crit Care Med 1995; **16**(4): 269–78.

7. Loddenkemper, R, Frank, W. Pleural effusion,
hemo-thorax, chylothorax. In *Pulmonary diseases*,
ed. C Grassi. McGraw-Hill International, 1999; 41:
391–404.

8. Valdes, L, Alvarez, D, SanJose, E, *et al.* Value of
adenosine deaminase in the diagnosis of tuberculous
pleural effusions in young patients in a region of high
prevalence of tuberculosis. *Thorax* 1995; **50**: 600–3.

9. Ferrer, J. Pleural tuberculosis. *Eur Respir J* 1997;
10: 942–7.

10. Loddenkemper, R. Thoracoscopy: state of the art. *Eur
Respir J* 1998 ; **11**: 213–21.

11. Walker-Renard, PB, Vaughan, LM, Sahn, SA. Chemical
pleurodesis for malignant pleural effusion. *Ann Intern
Med* 1994; **120**: 56–64.

12. Hamm, H, Light, RW. Parapneumonic effusion and
empyema. *Eur Respir J* 1997; **10**: 1150–8.

13. Frey, DJM, Klapa, J, Kaiser, D. Irrigation drainage
and fibrinolysis in the treatment of

parapneumonic pleural empyema. *Pneumologie*
1999; **53**: 583–642.

14. Bouros, D, Schiza, S, Patsurakis, G, *et al.* Intrapleural
streptokinase versus urokinase in the treatment of
complicated parapneumonic effusions: a prospective,
double-blind study. *Am J Respir Crit Care Med* 1997;
155: 291–5.

15. Sahn, SA. Management of complicated
parapneumonic effusions. *Am Rev Respir Dis*
1993; **148**: 813–17.

16. The Acute Respiratory Distress Syndrome Network.
Ventilation with lower tidal volumes as compared
with traditional tidal volumes for acute lung injury
and the acute respiratory distress syndrome. *N Engl
J Med* 2000; **342**: 1301–8.

17. Shields, TW, Oilschlager, GA. Spontaneous
pneumothorax in patients 40 years of age and
older. *Ann Thorac Surg* 1966; **2**: 377–83.

18. Seremetis, MG. The management of spontaneous
pneumothorax. *Chest* 1970; **8**: 57–65.

19. Vanderschueren, RG. The role of thoracoscopy in the
evaluation and management of pneumothorax. *Lung*
1990; Suppl., 1122–5.

20. Baumann, MH. Treatment of spontaneous
pneumothorax, a more aggressive approach?
Chest 1997; **112**: 789–804.

21. Baumann, MH, Sahn, SA. Medical management
and therapy of bronchopleural fistulas in the
mechanically ventilated patient. *Chest* 1990;
97: 721–28.

18

Acute interstitial lung disease

RICHARD MARSHALL

INTRODUCTION

The term interstitial lung disease (ILD) encompasses a group of disorders in which there are varying degrees of inflammation and fibrosis in the interstitial space and distal airway. Many of these disorders present with a progressive decline in respiratory function, permitting management in the out-patient setting. Less commonly, they present acutely with more severe respiratory failure and may reach the attention of critical care physicians. Their incidence in the intensive care unit (ICU) is largely unknown, but it is likely that a number of cases are misclassified as either diffuse infection or acute respiratory distress syndrome (ARDS), with which they share many features.

ILD often generates understandable nihilism amongst clinicians, the result of complex classification systems and a perceived paucity of therapeutic options, which can act as a deterrent to further understanding and investigation. In this chapter, a pragmatic approach is adopted to both the classification and management of acute ILD. In particular, although often essential for accurate diagnosis, suitable biopsy material is seldom available in the ICU setting, and an emphasis on pathological description

is avoided as far as possible. Similarly, a detailed discussion of potential pathological mechanisms may be found elsewhere.[1]

Clinical suspicion is the key to diagnosis and must remain high if these conditions are not to be missed and delays in administering appropriate therapy are to be avoided.

TERMINOLOGY

The study and management of ILD suffer from an over-complex and changeable classification system. ILD presenting acutely may broadly be considered as interstitial pneumonias, organizing pneumonias or diseases primarily of the small airways. By this definition, ARDS itself is a form of ILD, but is considered elsewhere (see Chapters 11 and 12).

Interstitial and organizing pneumonias are parenchhymal lung diseases characterized by a mononuclear cell and proteinaceous infiltrate distal to the terminal bronchiole. All have the capacity to progress to established fibrosis to a varying degree.[1] A number of subtypes have been classified on the basis of histological appearance. At present, it is useful to think of the following clinical disease entities.[2]

- *Usual interstitial pneumonia* (UIP): a subtype of cryptogenic fibrosing alveolitis (CFA), also known as idiopathic pulmonary fibrosis (IPF). This is a progressive, fibrotic lung disease that may rapidly accelerate in a minority of patients. Generally, there is a poor response to current therapy.
- *Desquamative interstitial pneumonia* (DIP) and *non-specific interstitial pneumonia* (NSIP): further CFA subtypes that appear to have a better prognosis than UIP.
- *Diffuse alveolar damage* (DAD): this is the characteristic histological pattern seen in ARDS (see Chapter 11).
- *Acute interstitial pneumonia* (AIP): pathologically very similar to ARDS, but idiopathic. It was previously known as the Hamman–Rich syndrome.
- *Organizing pneumonia* (OP): a pathological description in which small airway and alveolar granulation tissue predominates. It has a number of known causes, particularly drug toxicity and collagen vascular disease, and is sometimes referred to as bronchiolitis obliterans organizing pneumonia (BOOP) in this context. A cryptogenic form (COP) is described. OP usually demonstrates an excellent response to corticosteroids.

MAKING THE DIAGNOSIS

The presentation of acute ILD is typified by the development of respiratory failure in the presence of widespread radiological opacification on chest X-ray (CXR). The diagnosis must often be made in the absence of histological analysis or specific diagnostic tests, and is more often based upon a composite of clinical, radiological and laboratory features. In such cases, the diagnosis is one of exclusion and, in particular, differentiating acute ILD from pulmonary infection and ARDS. It is because of this overlap that the presence of non-ARDS ILD may be overlooked. A classification system for ILD based upon aetiology is perhaps more useful in this context (Table 18.1).

Clinical features

Obtaining an adequate history remains vital. A more prolonged symptomatic period prior to hospital admission is an important clue and includes fever,

malaise and anorexia, which may precede pulmonary symptoms by weeks or even months. The presence of non-pulmonary symptoms, clinical evidence of systemic disease (such as with vasculitis) and unusual radiological features should also alert suspicion (Table 18.1). Pulmonary signs, including the ubiquitous coarse crepitations, are non-specific. In practice, it may be the failure of antimicrobial therapy that prompts the search for ILD. An approach to diagnosis is outlined in Figure 18.1.

Radiology

Plain films should be reviewed regularly with a radiologist. The pattern of opacification, its distribution and changes over time are important. A computerized tomography (CT) scan should also be performed where possible to help to resolve the pattern of disease (i.e. reticular, alveolar or bronchocentric) and to uncover unexpected pathology such as malignancy, lymphadenopathy, pre-existing ILD, pleural effusions or pneumothoraces. Occasionally, prognostic information may also be obtained.

Radionucleotide imaging is not usually possible in mechanically ventilated patients, but may be considered in the less severe cases. [99m]TcDTPA clearance, where available, is superior to ^{67}Ga scanning in the detection of an interstitial inflammatory process at early stages, being a more sensitive index of epithelial integrity. The results are usually non-specific, but may have prognostic value, at least in chronic forms of ILD.[2]

Bronchoalveolar lavage

Although sampling secretions from the lower respiratory tract is routine in ventilated patients, more formal assessment of alveolar lining fluid by bronchoalveolar lavage (BAL) is variable in its use. This may partly depend upon local experience of the technique, but perhaps more so on its perceived usefulness and safety. Competency on the part of the operator is vital to ensure safety and improve diagnostic yield. Although it is not always possible to extrapolate results published by large centres to general ICU practice, the safety of BAL has been demonstrated repeatedly in the literature,[3] and its use should be considered early in the diagnostic

Table 18.1 *Classification of interstitial lung disease by cause*

Cause	Disease	Key distinguishing features
Trauma/sepsis/haemorrhage/ surgery/burns etc.	ARDS	
Infection	Miliary TB, RSV, CMV	Presence of immunosuppressive factors
	HIV	Serology
	Invasive aspergillosis	
Pulmonary oedema	Cardiac failure	Presence of left ventricular
	Rapid lung re-expansion	impairment (echocardiography,
	Fluid overload	previous history etc.)
Allergy	Eosinophilic pneumonia	History, Eosinophilia on BAL
		Peripheral, migratory opacification on CXR
Drug induced	Amiodarone lung	
	Cytotoxic agents	History
Inhalation injury	Smoke	History
	Chlorine	Bronchoscopic appearance
Pulmonary haemorrhage	Wegener's granulomatosis	History
	Goodpasture's syndrome, Behçet's syndrome	Presence of systemic disease Serology
	Acute SLE	Radiological appearance
Vasculitis	Acute SLE	Presence of systemic disease
	Rheumatoid pneumonitis	Serology
		Prodromal symptoms
Idiopathic	Eosinophilic pneumonia	Prodromal symptoms
	Acute interstitial pneumonia	Absence of causative agents
	COP	

ARDS, acute respiratory distress syndrome; TB, tuberculosis; RSV, respiratory syncytial virus; CMV, cytomegalovirus; HIV, human immunodeficiency virus; BAL, bronchoalveolar lavage; CXR, chest X-ray; SLE, systemic lupus erythematosus; COP, cryptogenic organizing pneumonia.

pathway. BAL will aid the exclusion of a typical infection, but may also yield specific diagnostic features, e.g. eosinophilia.

Biopsy

Trans-bronchial biopsy is to be avoided on the ICU. Its diagnostic yield in ILD is usually poor and it carries a significant risk of morbidity. Open lung biopsy is clearly not available to most intensive care physicians, yet, as with BAL, published series attest to its usefulness and safety.[4] Many issues surround the decision to perform an open lung biopsy, not least its tolerance by the patient, the potential to precipitate the need for intubation, and the impact of the information obtained on management decisions. As a general rule, if clinical and radiological features are non-specific and blind immunosuppressive therapy is contemplated, a biopsy should be strongly considered.

Additional tests

An assessment of immunological markers may be of great help, including: microbial antigens, antinuclear antibodies (ANAs) and anti-cytoplasmic antibodies (ANCAs), helping to exclude infection and identify autoimmunity. Evidence of systemic disease should also be sought, including an examination of the urine for proteinuria, and casts, an assessment of the peripheral blood film and further radiological imaging of affected tissues. A markedly elevated or normal erthrocyte sedimentation rate or C-reactive protein may steer the clinician towards

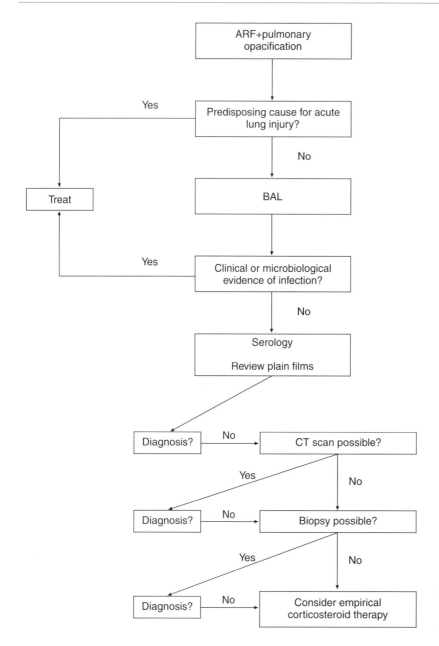

Figure 18.1 *Diagnostic algorithm for acute interstitial lung disease. ARF, acute respiratory failure; BAL, bronchoalveolar lavage; CT, computed tomography.*

systemic disease or infection, but both are non-specific. They may be of use in monitoring the course of the disease and the response to intervention.

THERAPY

Once infection is excluded, as far as is possible, treatment falls into two main categories: supportive and immunosuppressive (there are currently no therap-

ies that effectively target fibroproliferative pathways). Acute ILD is uncommon and the evidence supporting specific therapy is poor. There have been no randomised, controlled trials.

Setting the ventilator

Given the clinical and pathological features that many causes of acute ILD share with ARDS, it would seem reasonable to adopt a comparable approach to ventilator management. Ventilator-induced lung injury is likely to be an issue for all patients with severe respiratory failure, and the avoidance of high tidal volumes (6–10 mL kg^{-1}) coupled with a level of positive end-expiratory pressure (PEEP) titrated to FiO$_2$ would seem prudent. Permissive hypoxia (8–10 kPa) and hypercapnoea (6–10 kPa) may also be preferable, although the evidence for either is weak at present. Interestingly, hyperoxia rapidly induces lung injury *in vivo*[5] and may interact synergistically with NO.[6] Although there is little documentation of its effects in humans, it at least suggests that limiting FiO$_2$ may be theoretically beneficial.

The role of other ventilatory strategies, such as rotational therapy and nitric oxide (NO), is unclear. Neither has a sufficient evidence base to be recommended unequivocally, but their use in patients with severe hypoxaemia seems as pertinent to other forms of acute respiratory failure as it is to ARDS. Their use will also depend on the availability of suitable resources and expertise in individual centres.

Immunosuppression

The use of immunosuppressive agents remains the mainstay of treatment for all ILD. In the absence of infection, these should only be given blindly when a biopsy is not possible or has been non-diagnostic, and only when all other serological tests have been requested.

Again, the evidence from randomised, controlled trials for any therapy is weak at best and limited to patients with less severe disease than will be encountered on the ICU. High-dose systemic corticosteroids form the mainstay of initial therapy. Methyl-prednisolone has less mineralocorticoid activity, dexamethasone requires a smaller volume for administration, but otherwise there is little evidence to support the use of one agent over the other. Other immunosuppressants, e.g. cyclophosphamide and azathioprine, may be added as steroid-sparing agents in prolonged therapy or may be specifically indicated, i.e. in Wegener's granulomatosis.[7]

ACUTE INTERSTITIAL PNEUMONIA

Clinical features

Hamman and Rich, at the Johns Hopkins Hospital, described three cases of 'acute diffuse fibrosis of the lung' over a period of 3 years. They had to wait 10 years for a fourth case before publishing their report in 1944. These initial cases were acute in onset and produced a rapidly fatal course. Although the Hamman–Rich syndrome has been synonymous with IPF in the past, it is no longer a useful term and is now referred to as AIP, which it resembles clinically and radiologically.[8]

Confusion occurs as to its relationship with ARDS. AIP in reported cases occurs at a mean age of 49 years (range 7–83). It presents with a rapid deterioration, usually over a few days; however, in contrast to ARDS, a flu-like prodrome is characteristically present and no predisposing cause is found. AIP is thus, by definition, idiopathic. In addition, although almost all patients require mechanical ventilation, one does not observe the profound systemic inflammatory response and multi-organ failure more typical of ARDS.

Pathology

Histologically, AIP is characterized by a pattern known as DAD, which is also seen in ARDS (see Chapter 11). An initial profound exudation of fluid and protein into the lung accompanied by neutrophilic infiltration is followed by intense fibroproliferation and, subsequently, established fibrosis. Hyaline membranes consisting of organized fibrin clot are typical. These changes are spatially uniform, which may distinguish AIP from the more intra-alveolar and patchy distribution seen in OP.[9]

Investigations

Radiologically, widespread infiltration of the lung is seen, with ground-glass opacification and consolidation in the absence of the cystic changes and gross parenchymal distortion seen in more chronic forms of ILD (Fig. 18.2).

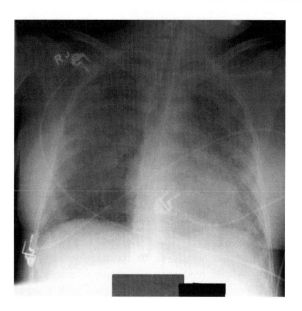

Figure 18.2 *Acute interstitial pneumonia. This 34-year-old man presented with a 3-day history of flu-like symptoms. Severe respiratory failure ensued. A thorough screen for pulmonary infection (including bronchoalveolar lavage) was negative. He later died despite immunosuppressive therapy.*

CT scan appearances mirror those found on the CXR. It is most useful in the early stages of illness to differentiate AIP from an acute acceleration of underlying IPF, which may mimic the condition. Honeycombing or traction bronchiectasis in the early phase strongly suggests the latter, although their presence has been described in late AIP, but only after many weeks of illness. The differential diagnosis also includes diffuse infection, lymphoproliferative infiltration, OP, pulmonary vasculitis and toxic pulmonary reactions to drugs or inhaled agents. Although OP cannot be easily be distinguished radiographically from AIP, it is generally characterized as a patchy, migratory infiltrate with more diffuse involvement of all lobes.

Additional tests such as serology, erythrocyte sedimentation rate (ESR), C-reactive protein (CRP) and BAL, although likely to be abnormal, are not specific to AIP, but are helpful to exclude infection and other causes of ILD.

Treatment and prognosis

The reported mortality is 78%, although, as with ARDS, this may have improved recently.[10] Given this poor prognosis, the early use of corticosteroids is probably justified, provided infection and ARDS can be excluded. Few data exist, but intravenous prednisolone (250 mg day^{-1}), cyclophosphamide (1.5 g day^{-1}) and vincristine (2 mg) have been reported to halt the otherwise rapid progression of the disease.[11]

Lung-protection strategies, including low tidal volume ventilation and high PEEP, are also likely to be beneficial in AIP given the pathological similarities with ARDS. One case of lung transplantation has been reported in which there was an improvement in the native lung. This is probably the result of a more intense immunosuppressive regimen and has also been reported in patients with IPF.

In summary, AIP could be considered as an idiopathic form that mimics ARDS, but which may be more susceptible to immunosuppression early in its course and which carries a worse prognosis. The presence of a prodromal syndrome and a clinical picture of ARDS for which no predisposing cause can be identified are the most useful diagnostic features.

CRYPTOGENIC ORGANIZING PNEUMONIA

OP is a histological feature of pulmonary inflammation, comprising buds of granulation tissue filling the alveolar space and terminal bronchiole. There are varying degrees of accompanying interstitial inflammation and fibroproliferation. OP may have a definable cause (e.g. infectious pneumonia, bronchiectasis, IPF, drug reactions) or occur in the context of another disease (e.g. collagen vascular disease, ulcerative colitis, leukaemia).[12] Here, we are concerned with the cryptogenic form. The term BOOP is probably best avoided because it is easily confused with bronchiolitis obliterans, which predominantly affects small airways and presents with airways obstruction.

Clinical features

A subacute presentation is usual, which will immediately distinguish COP from ARDS and AIP. The mean age at presentation is 55–60 years, but it has been described in all adult age groups. A flu-like illness coupled with non-productive cough, chest pain and arthralgia is the typical picture. In severe cases, the differential diagnosis includes ARDS, AIP, acute eosinophilic syndromes and vasculitic lung disease. Importantly, there is no evidence of systemic disease, and immunological testing will be non-specific in COP. Thus, these investigations are of value only in excluding underlying autoimmune and collagen vascular disease.

Radiology

Migrating peripheral air-space opacification is characteristic of COP, and an examination of sequential CXRs is crucial (Fig. 18.3). Other patterns include diffuse bilateral infiltration, a single opacity (which may cavitate and which is usually associated with a more prolonged illness) and, less commonly, crescentic opacities, subpleural bands or even a pneumatocoele. A CT scan can be invaluable in establishing the diagnosis.

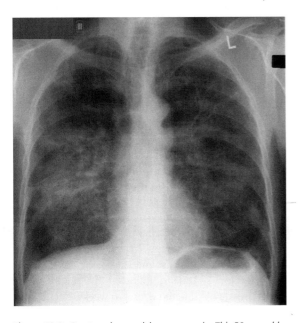

Figure 18.3 *Cryptogenic organizing pneumonia. This 56-year-old man complained of progressive dyspnoea over a 2-week period. His condition deteriorated despite broad-spectrum antibiotics. There was no previous history of drug exposure. Organizing pneumonia was diagnosed by open lung biopsy and responded to corticosteroids. No aetiological agent was identified.*

Lung function and histology

The prime abnormality on lung-function testing is a restrictive pattern. Severe hypoxia results from right-to-left shunting and the alveolar–arterial O_2 difference will be increased on 100% O_2. BAL changes are usually non-specific.

If clinical and radiological features are unhelpful, a biopsy is indicated. This is largely because of the excellent response of this condition to corticosteroids, which can be started earlier in the presence of a histological diagnosis. A biopsy will also help ensure against the potential hazards of immunosuppression in infectious disease. Granulation tissue fills the alveolar space, often 'budding' into adjacent alveoli via the pores of Kohn. Of note, bronchiolitis obliterans is clearly bronchocentric by comparison. A diagnosis of COP also demands that the granulation tissue is the predominant lesion and not merely in association with other features of vasculitis or granuloma. In severe cases, large areas of lung tissue will be involved, but care should be taken to ensure imaging is performed immediately prior to biopsy, due to the migratory and transient nature of the lesions.

Therapy and clinical course

Occasional spontaneous improvement occurs, but this is unlikely in severe cases. Generally, patients respond rapidly to corticosteroid therapy (e.g. 0.75 mg kg^{-1} day^{-1} prednisolone). Some show improvement in hypoxaemia within 48 hours and almost all will have improved within 7 days. Although COP that is refractory to corticosteroids has been reported, it is more likely that these cases represent alternative diagnoses, including ARDS, AIP or a rapid acceleration of IPF. In severe, biopsy-proven COP, one to three intravenous boluses of cyclophosphamide may also be considered.

Treatment is usually required for between 6 and 12 months. Corticosteroids should be tapered after 1–3 months, depending on the speed of resolution. Relapses occur in some individuals and the dose may have to be temporarily elevated or prolonged in such instances. The prognosis of COP with patchy alveolar opacities is excellent providing the diagnosis is made. On the ICU, diagnostic delay and secondary pathology – notably infection – are potential hazards.

EOSINOPHILIC PNEUMONIA

The term 'pulmonary eosinophilia' is commonly used to describe any condition in which pulmonary opacities are associated with a peripheral eosinophilia. This is misleading because it includes conditions in which there is a blood eosinophilia and an increased susceptibility to non-eosinophilic pneumonia. The term eosinophilic pneumonia is preferable because it implies the presence of pulmonary rather than peripheral eosinophilia. The eosinophilic pneumonias are classified on the basis of cause and the length of the clinical presentation into simple, acute and chronic forms.

The term simple eosinophilic pneumonia should now be used to describe the disorders originally encompassed by Loeffler's syndrome, which was characterized by peripheral eosinophilia and pulmonary opacities and was either idiopathic or caused by a variety of agents including drugs and parasites. Such cases are usually mild and transient.

Acute eosinophilic pneumonia (AEP) is a relatively new entity, first described in 1989 and increasingly reported in the literature.[13] Characteristically, it affects younger individuals (mean age 30 years). A number of reports from Japan describe a strong association with tobacco-smoke inhalation, but only a proportion of patients are smokers. The severity is variable and, from the list of other agents (Table 18.2) implicated in its aetiology, there is clearly potential overlap with simple eosinophilic pneumonia. However, the short clinical course and absence of recurrence in AEP are distinguishing features. Radiologically, more peripheral, migratory air-space opacification may help differentiate AEP from other ILD, but the distribution may be variable (Fig. 18.4).

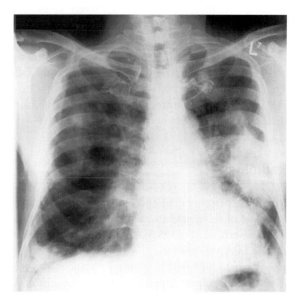

Figure 18.4 *Acute eosinophilic pneumonia (AEP). This chest radiograph demonstrates peripheral, patchy, air-space shadowing typical of AEP. This 64-year-old woman presented with a 2-day history of fever and dyspnoea and deteriorated rapidly after this chest X-ray was obtained. Subsequently, bronchoalveolar lavage revealed 38% eosinophilia. Corticosteroid therapy led to a full recovery.*

Clinical course and treatment of acute eosinophilic pneumonia

The presentation is typically less than 1 month in duration, with fever and malaise being the prominent symptoms. Peripheral blood eosinophilia is variable, but BAL eosinophilia is generally diagnostic, with the demonstration of increased cellularity and 20–50% eosinophils. The histological features are those of DAD with profound eosinophilic infiltration. Histologically diagnosed AEP without BAL eosinophilia has been reported.

The prognosis is excellent, with a good clinical response to steroid therapy. Treatment should initially be with methylprednisolone at 1 mg kg^{-1} every 6 hours for 2–3 days, followed by prednisolone 40–60 mg day^{-1} tapered over 4–6 weeks. Recurrence has not been reported to date.

Chronic eosinophilic pneumonia presents with general malaise, weight loss and fever. Investigations reveal a marked peripheral blood eosinophilia with a polymorph leucocytosis, anaemia and a raised ESR. The cause is unknown, but there is a good response

Table 18.2 *Factors associated with acute eosinophilic pneumonia*

Tobacco smoking	Carbamazepine
Heroin smoking	Clomipramine
Ranitidine	Venlafaxine
Pentamidine	Trazadone
Aspirin	Minocyline

to corticosteroid therapy. Admission to an ICU is rarely necessary.

DRUG-INDUCED INTERSTITIAL LUNG DISEASE

The list of agents associated with pulmonary ILD continues to expand. The more common associations are considered here by way of example, particularly those that may present with more severe respiratory failure.

General considerations

Clinical signs, radiological features and lung-function tests are non-specific and thus clinical suspicion is the main diagnostic prompt. A detailed history and thorough search of the medical notes should be made to identify agents associated with pulmonary syndromes. Symptoms may develop weeks, months or even years after drug administration and after the drug responsible has been stopped. Changes in diffusing capacity may precede the onset of symptoms and radiographic changes by days or weeks, at which time the agents are discontinued to halt progression. BAL is useful primarily to exclude infection, but may also reveal eosinophilia. Once suspected, a thorough search for infection should be made and all potentially responsible drugs should be stopped and, if clinically indicated, an alternative agent substituted.

Most patients will recover from drug-induced pulmonary disease, although, in a minority of cases, respiratory symptoms will persist or even progress after drug withdrawal. Treatment for these individuals is largely supportive.

Pathology

Drug reactions present with a variety of pulmonary pathologies, including interstitial pneumonia, OP, eosinophilic pneumonia and diffuse reticular fibrosis (Table 18.3). These different patterns may occur in response to the same drug.

The mechanisms of drug-induced lung injury are poorly understood. Sequestration or metabolism of the drug in the pulmonary circulation/parenchyma makes toxicity more likely. Although severe reactions

Table 18.3 *Patterns of acute pulmonary drug reactions*

Pattern	Typical agents implicated
Interstitial pneumonitis	Methotrexate, nitrofurantoin, β-blockers
Organizing pneumonia	Amiodarone, bleomycin, cytotoxics
Interstitial fibrosis	Bleomycin, amiodarone, cytotoxics
Eosinophilic pneumonia	Antibiotics, NSAIDS, cytotoxics
Pulmonary oedema	Aspirin, opiates, drug overdose
Diffuse alveolar haemorrhage	Quinidine, thrombolytics, anticoagulants

NSAIDS, non-steroidal anti-inflammatory drugs.

are not common, subclinical evidence of toxicity can be found in a much larger proportion of individuals. This suggests modifying factors that influence the progression from subtle injury to clinically manifest disease. Hypotheses concerning the mechanisms of injury include direct cellular toxicity, immunological reaction, redox imbalance, phospholipidosis (amiodarone), apoptosis and DNA scission.

Chemotherapeutic agents

The increasing use of cytotoxic therapy, particularly bleomycin, cyclophosphamide and methotrexate, has led to an increased incidence of pulmonary drug toxicity. Cumulative dose and concomitant therapy are factors that have been associated with an increased susceptibility to pulmonary drug reactions and, although genetic factors are proposed, none has been described to date. Interestingly, cyclophosphamide has been used to treat not only non-drug induced ILD but also methotrexate and amiodarone pneumonitis, highlighting the complex interaction between external and internal environments.

Fever, a dry cough and progressive dyspnoea over days or weeks may precede more severe respiratory compromise. In the immunocompromised patient, the major differential diagnosis is infection. Patients presenting with respiratory failure in the absence of neutropenia should alert particular suspicion. Diffuse malignant infiltration by the underlying disease is also a possibility, but an open lung biopsy is necessary to confirm the diagnosis. The diagnostic yield is approximately 50% for malignancy-associated pulmonary infiltrates, but this is highly variable and will almost certainly depend on the adequacy of samples obtained, the size and choice of site of the biopsy, the skill of operator, the stage of illness and the strength of clinical suspicion. The decision to undertake open lung biopsy in such cases should be considered on an individual basis, but its early use, prior to broad-spectrum antimicrobial therapy, is to be recommended.

In addition to the withdrawal of the drug, treatment is supportive. Evidence for the use of corticosteroids is variable.

Bleomycin

This is the chemotherapeutic agent that most commonly causes pulmonary ILD. There is a significant increase of bleomycin-related pulmonary disease in patients over 70 years of age and in those who have received a cumulative dose $\geq$550 U. Prior or concomitant thoracic radiotherapy increases the incidence of severe pulmonary toxicity and there is a synergistic effect between prior bleomycin exposure and subsequent exposure to high O_2 concentrations.[14]

Intense screening with pulmonary function tests, CT scanning and ^{67}Ga scanning suggests as many as 40% of bleomycin-treated patients develop pulmonary disease, but this is clinically relevant in approximately 5–20%. Frequent monitoring of the CO-diffusing capacity may predict toxicity. CT may also be useful in establishing an early diagnosis. Up to 3% of those treated with bleomycin may die from severe drug-induced fibrosis.[15]

Diffuse pneumonitis, OP and severe progressive fibrosis with honeycombing are the pulmonary pathologies most frequently seen with bleomycin. Treatment is supportive and the changes may be reversible if detected at an early stage. However, if significant fibrosis has already developed, the process may progress despite corticosteroid therapy.[16]

Cyclophosphamide

The incidence of cyclophosphamide-induced pneumonitis is certainly underestimated. There is no clear-cut relationship between toxicity and dose.

Clinical features include dyspnoea, fever, cough, new parenchymal infiltrates and pleural thickening. Two patterns have been defined. Early-onset pneumonitis occurs within the first 6 months of therapy and generally responds to withdrawal of the drug. In contrast, late-onset pneumonitis commences after many months or years of cyclophosphamide therapy and manifests with progressive pulmonary fibrosis and bilateral pleural thickening. The late-onset variety has a minimal response to withdrawal of the drug or the use of corticosteroid therapy.

Methotrexate

Pneumonitis is one of the most serious complications of methotrexate therapy. This reaction is unrelated to dose. Dyspnoea, non-productive cough and fever usually develop a few days to several weeks after starting treatment and, in rare cases, even several months or years later. Diffuse pulmonary infiltrates with or without hilar lymphadenopathy and pleural effusions may be seen on CXR. Peripheral and/or pulmonary eosinophilia is seen in over half of the cases. The process is almost always reversible with or without the addition of corticosteroids and only a few deaths have been reported.[17]

Nitrofurantoin

Nitrofurantoin is one of the commonest causes of drug-induced pulmonary ILD, although the clinical use of this antibiotic is waning. The incidence is estimated at between 1 in 500 and 1 in 5000 individuals treated. The onset of symptoms is usually within hours to several days after the initiation of therapy and is not dose related. Fever and dyspnoea are almost always present and pleuritic chest pain is reported in about one-third of patients. Other common findings include a peripheral leucocytosis, eosinophilia and a high ESR.

The CXR shows an alveolar and/or interstitial process and there may be a pleural effusion, which is usually unilateral. There are no specific laboratory tests to confirm the presence of acute nitrofurantoin pneumonitis. It is not known whether corticosteroids accelerate the resolution. One per cent of nitrofurantoin pulmonary reactions are fatal.[18]

Amiodarone

This anti-arrhythmic agent has become an important cause of drug-induced ILD in recent years. Pneumonitis occurs in up to 6% of patients. The time from starting treatment to onset is inversely proportional to the dose and it is uncommon in patients taking less than 200 mg day^{-1}. The majority of the patients have been receiving the drug for at least a month, usually at a dose of at least 400 mg day^{-1}. The average time to onset is 1–2 years. Recently, cases have been described of ARDS developing within a few days of cardiac surgery in patients previously receiving amiodarone (Fig. 18.5)[19] and this may be an unsuspected cause of ARDS.[20]

Most patients complain of dyspnoea, non-productive cough and, occasionally, a low-grade fever. Pleuritic chest pain occurs in 10% of patients. The pathogenesis is uncertain, but there is evidence of increased oxidant stress, and amiodarone-induced apoptosis in alveolar epithelial cells has been demonstrated *in vitro*. The pulmonary toxicity appears to be related to its sequestration in the lung.

As withdrawal of the drug may precipitate life-threatening arrhythmia, the diagnosis should be confirmed by thorough investigation, but may remain one of exclusion. Laboratory studies show a normal to mildly elevated leucocyte count, generally without eosinophilia, and an elevated ESR. Pulmonary function studies reveal hypoxaemia, with a decreased total lung capacity and CO-diffusing capacity. ^{67}Ga lung scanning may be useful in differentiating amiodarone pneumonitis from congestive heart failure, but echocardiography and an assessment of pulmonary capillary wedge pressure may also be required. Cardiac failure is also distinguishable by its clinical response to conventional therapy.

Although helpful in excluding infection, BAL is non-diagnostic in amiodarone pneumonitis as cellular patterns range from normal to lymphocytic, neutrophilic and mixed pictures. The *absence* of foamy cells (phospholipid-filled macrophages) eliminates the diagnosis, whereas their presence only confirms exposure to the drug and does not necessarily indicate toxicity. Recently, KL-6, a mucin-like glycoprotein secreted by type II alveolar cells, was found to be elevated in amiodarone pneumonitis[21] and interstitial pneumonitis. This is likely to be a non-specific but potentially useful marker of type II cell injury.

Amiodarone pneumonitis is primarily an interstitial or alveolar process seen on CXR (Fig. 18.5). CT

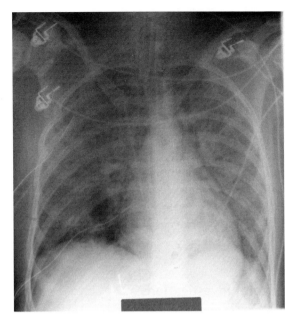

Figure 18.5 *Amiodarone pneumonitis. This 62-year-old woman developed an acute respiratory distress syndrome-like respiratory failure following coronary bypass surgery, but had also been on amiodarone for over 2 years. Bronchoalveolar lavage revealed a 23% eosinophilia. No evidence of infection was found and her condition dramatically improved on withdrawal of the amiodarone.*

scanning may provide further definition because amiodarone is iodinated and consequently radio-opaque, making the lesions of amiodarone pneumonitis denser than the surrounding soft tissue in the chest wall.

A biopsy is not usually necessary to establish the diagnosis. Histological features include foam cells as evidence of abnormal phospholipid turnover, OP and diffuse interstitial fibrosis, which develops in 10% of affected patients.

Eighty per cent of patients respond to stopping the drug and treatment with steroids, which are usually required for at least 2–6 months. Approximately 25% of patients will demonstrate long-term pulmonary sequelae in the form of persistent radiological or lung-function abnormalities. A few individuals show recurrence of pulmonary opacities, usually as the corticosteroids are withdrawn. There are many case reports of patients who have continued on amiodarone because it was the only drug that controlled their ventricular dysrhythmia, and who were concurrently given corticosteroids to suppress amiodarone pneumonitis. The overall mortality is about 20% and includes death from respiratory and cardiac causes.

ACUTE VASCULITIC LUNG DISEASE

Pulmonary involvement has been described in association with all the systemic vasculitides, including systemic lupus erythematosus (SLE), rheumatoid arthritis, dermatomyositis/polymyositis, Sjögren's syndrome, polyarteritis, giant cell arteritis, microscopic polyarteritis, Wegener's granulomatosis and Henoch–Schonlein purpura. Pathology varies both within and between diseases. Most cases present subacutely, but pulmonary involvement, characterized by OP, pneumonitis, DAD or diffuse alveolar haemorrhage (DAH), can present with acute respiratory failure.

General investigations

There may be a preceding history of joint/other organ involvement, but a vasculitis may present primarily with pulmonary pathology. Clinical evidence for systemic vasculitis should be sought and serological tests, including ANA and ANCA requested. The presence of ANA suggests collagen vascular disease. Immune complex deposition, hypergammaglobulinaemia and complement consumption are also features of these disorders.

The ANCA-positive vasculitides are Wegener's granulomatosis, microscopic polyarteritis and Churg–Strauss syndrome. ANCA is positive in 90% of patients with acute Wegener's, is usually positive in microscopic polyarteritis and Churg–Strauss syndrome, but will be negative in collagen vascular diseases.

Collagen vascular disease

SLE may present acutely as lupus pneumonia, diffuse pulmonary haemorrhage or OP, but all are uncommon. BAL will exclude infection and determine the presence or absence of DAH in such individuals. Both lupus pneumonia and OP will generally respond to steroids, although some patients will require the addition of cyclophosphamide. DAH, by contrast, is associated with a high mortality. Its response to immunosupression is variable.

Other collagen vascular diseases may present acutely, rarely as OP or accelerating interstitial pneu-

monia. Both respond to increased immunosuppression and generally have a better prognosis than when no cause is found.

ANCA-associated vasculitis

Wegener's granulomatosis may present solely in the lung. Its manifestation depends on whether the predominant pathological lesion is granulomatous or vasculitic. Radiological appearances are often distinct from other causes of acute ILD. Most patients present with either large opacities (70%) or multiple small opacities that change over time. The clinical picture will be one of systemic upset and progressive respiratory failure, usually over weeks or months. Mechanical ventilation may be required in severe cases, particularly those with DAH (see below).

In suspected cases, a histological diagnosis should be made from the most accessible tissue affected (nose, skin, kidney or lung being the most common sites for biopsy). BAL adds little to the specific diagnosis of ANCA-associated vasculitis, but may be helpful in excluding other diagnoses. Untreated, the disease is rapidly fatal. Treatment is with corticosteroids and cyclophosphamide. If severe, parenteral therapy may be required, usually with three doses of cyclophosphamide.

Churg–Strauss syndrome occurs at a mean age of 35 years, initially presenting as asthma. Untreated, it progresses to eosinophilic pneumonia with high peripheral blood eosinophilia. Rarely, it presents late in the disease course as severe pulmonary disease due to overwhelming vasculitis. The response to steroids is excellent.

DIFFUSE ALVEOLAR HAEMORRHAGE

DAH is a clinical diagnosis and may occur in association with a number of disorders, including Wegener's granulomatosis, Goodpasture's syndrome, microscopic polyarteritis, SLE, rheumatoid arthritis, polymyositis, lymphangioleiomyomatosis, pulmonary vascular occlusive disease and lung allograft rejection. Of importance is the absence of haemoptysis as a presenting symptom in approximately one-third of patients. Progressive pulmonary infiltrates, a falling haemoglobin level and a haemorrhagic

BAL with the presence of haemosiderin are usually diagnostic. In subacute cases, there may be an increase in diffusion capacity on pulmonary function testing and this may also herald recurrence in previously diagnosed cases. The radiological appearance is one of diffuse air-space shadowing (Fig. 18.6).

Screening for ANCA, ANA, rheumatoid factor, anti-phospholipid antibodies, complement, cryoglobin and coagulation abnormalities may help identify an underlying associated syndrome such as Goodpasture's syndrome or collagen vascular disease. In most cases, the diagnosis of the collagen vascular disease pre-dates the occurrence of DAH. Renal involvement may be present secondary to vasculitis and collagen vascular disease.

Histology may show small-vessel vasculitis or bland pulmonary haemorrhage. Characteristically, DAH is characterized by an oedematous interstitium with fibrinoid necrosis, infiltration of neutrophils and leakage of red blood cells into the alveolar space.

The outcome of DAH depends on the underlying disease, with an early mortality approaching 50% in

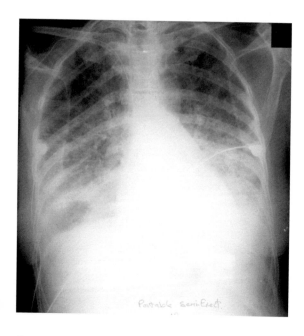

Figure 18.6 *Diffuse alveolar haemorrhage. A 72-year-old man presented with a 2-month history of progressive dyspnoea, anaemia and leucocytosis. Bronchoalveolar lavage was positive for Heme and also revealed a lymphocytosis (26%). Antinuclear cytoplasmic antibody (ANCA) testing was positive and a renal biopsy confirmed Wegener's granulomatosis. The patient continued to deteriorate despite methylprednisolone and cyclophosphamide.*

SLE and a 5-year survival of only 20%. In contrast, isolated vasculitis enjoys a better prognosis, with 25% early mortality and a 5-year survival of over 50%.

DAH is treated by controlling the underlying vasculitis with cyclophosphamide and prednisolone. In severe cases, other therapies, including plasmapheresis and pooled intravenous immunoglobulins, have been used, but such therapy remains empirical.

SUMMARY

The broader differential diagnosis of acute ILD should be considered in all patients presenting with acute respiratory failure and radiological opacities. As individual entities, these disorders are rare, but collectively they form an important diagnostic differential together with ARDS and severe pulmonary infection. In particular, the absence of a predisposing factor for ARDS coupled with a prodromal phase should alert suspicion. A vigorous and prompt search for infection should be made to avoid delay in commencing immunosuppressive therapy, to which many of these disorders respond well. It is probable that patients with acute ILD will benefit from similar ventilatory strategies and adjunctive therapies to those currently used in ARDS. Because these are rare diseases, improvements in diagnosis and therapy will be slow to materialize, but developments in the treatment of ARDS and the chronic forms of ILD may provide valuable insights into the stereotypical responses of the lung to diffuse injury.

REFERENCES

1. Phan, S, Thrall, R, eds. *Pulmonary fibrosis*. New York: Marcel Dekker, 1995.
2. Wells, AU, Hansell, DM, Harrison, NK, Lawrence, R, Black, CM, du Bois, RM. Clearance of inhaled [99mTc]-DTPA predicts the clinical course of fibrosing alveolitis. *Eur Respir J* 1993; **6**: 797–802.
3. Steinberg, KP, Mitchell, DR, Maunder, RJ, Milberg, JA, Whitcomb, ME, Hudson, LD. Safety of bronchoalveolar lavage in patients with adult respiratory distress syndrome. *Am Rev Respir Dis* 1993; **148**: 556–61.
4. Papazian, L, Thomas, P, Bregeon, F, *et al.* Open-lung biopsy in patients with acute respiratory distress syndrome. *Anesthesiology* 1998; **88**: 935–44.

5. de los Santos, R, Seidenfeld, JJ, Anzueto, A, *et al*. One hundred percent oxygen lung injury in adult baboons. *Am Rev Respir Dis* 1987; **136**: 657–61.

6. Capellier, G, Maupoil, V, Boillot, A, *et al*. L-NAME aggravates pulmonary oxygen toxicity in rats. *Eur Respir J* 1996; **9**: 2531–6.

7. Fauci, AS, Wolff, SM, Johnson, JS. Effect of cyclophosphamide upon the immune response in Wegener's granulomatosis. *N Engl J Med* 1971; **285**(27): 1493–6.

8. Bouros, D, Nicholson, AC, Polychronopoulos, V, du Bois, RM. Acute interstitial pneumonia. *Eur Respir J* 2000; **15**: 412–18.

9. Primack, SL, Hartman, TE, Ikezoe, J, Akira, M, Sakatani, M, Muller, NL. Acute interstitial pneumonia: radiographic and CT findings in nine patients. *Radiology* 1993; **188**: 817–20.

10. Suntharalingam, G, Regan, K, Keogh, BF, Morgan, CJ, Evans, TW. Influence of direct and indirect aetiology on acute outcome and 6-month functional recovery in acute respiratory distress syndrome. *Crit Care Med* 2001; **29**: 562–6.

11. Vourlekis, JS, Brown, KK, Cool, CD, *et al*. Acute interstitial pneumonitis. Case series and review of the literature. *Medicine (Baltimore)* 2000; **79**: 369–78.

12. Cordier, JF. Organising pneumonia. *Thorax* 2000; **55**: 318–28.

13. Allen, JN, Pacht, ER, Gadek, JE, Davis, WB. Acute eosinophilic pneumonia as a reversible cause of noninfectious respiratory failure. *N Engl J Med* 1989; **321**: 569–74.

14. Tryka, AF, Godleski, JJ, Brain, JD. Differences in effects of immediate and delayed hyperoxia exposure on bleomycin-induced pulmonary injury. *Cancer Treat Rep* 1984; **68**: 759–64.

15. White, DA, Stover, DE. Severe bleomycin-induced pneumonitis. Clinical features and response to corticosteroids. *Chest* 1984; **86**: 723–8.

16. Maher, J, Daly, PA. Severe bleomycin lung toxicity: reversal with high dose corticosteroids. *Thorax* 1993; **48**: 92–4.

17. Emery, P, Breedveld, FC, Lemmel, EM, *et al*. A comparison of the efficacy and safety of leflunomide and methotrexate for the treatment of rheumatoid arthritis. *Rheumatology (Oxford)* 2000; **39**: 655–65.

18. Jick, SS, Jick, H, Walker, AM, Hunter, JR. Hospitalizations for pulmonary reactions following nitrofurantoin use. *Chest* 1989; **96**: 512–15.

19. Van Mieghem, W, Coolen, L, Malysse, I, Lacquet, LM, Deneffe, GJ, Demedts, MG. Amiodarone and the development of ARDS after lung surgery. *Chest* 1994; **105**: 1642–5.

20. Ashrafian, H, Davey, P. Is amiodarone an underrecognized cause of acute respiratory failure in the ICU? *Chest* 2001; **120**: 275–82.

21. Endoh, Y, Hanai, R, Uto, K, *et al*. KL-6 as a potential new marker for amiodarone-induced pulmonary toxicity. *Am J Cardiol* 2000; **86**: 229–31.

19

Pulmonary embolism and pulmonary hypertension

GRAHAM F PINEO, RUSSELL D HULL AND GARY E RASKOB

INTRODUCTION

Venous thromboembolism is a common disorder with an estimated annual incidence of symptomatic venous thromboembolism of 117 per 100 000 population.[1] The incidence increases with each decade over the age of 60. Accordingly, with an ageing population, it is an increasingly important problem for the health services in many countries.

Venous thrombosis commonly develops in the deep veins of the leg, but may occur in the arm or in the superficial veins of the limbs. Superficial venous thrombosis is a relatively benign disorder unless extension into the deep venous system develops. Thrombosis involving the deep veins of the leg is divided into two prognostic categories:

1. thrombi that remain confined to the deep calf veins (calf-vein thrombosis),
2. proximal-vein thrombosis involving the popliteal femoral or iliac veins.

Pulmonary embolism (PE) originates from thrombi in the deep veins of the leg in 90% or more of patients. Other less common sources include the deep pelvic veins, renal veins, inferior vena cava, right side of the heart or the axillary veins. Although most clinically important emboli arise from proximal deep-vein thrombosis (DVT) of the leg, upper-extremity thrombosis may be the source.[2] DVT and/or PE are referred to collectively as venous thromboembolism.

AETIOLOGY AND PATHOGENESIS

Venous thrombi are composed mainly of fibrin and red blood cells, with a variable platelet and leucocyte component. The formation, growth and breakdown of venous thromboemboli represent a balance between thrombogenic stimuli and protective mechanisms. The thrombogenic stimuli are venous stasis, activation of blood coagulation and vein damage. The protective mechanisms are:

- the inactivation of activated coagulation factors by circulating inhibitors (e.g. antithrombin, protein C),
- clearance of activated coagulation factors and soluble fibrin polymer complexes by the reticulo-endothelial system and by the liver,
- lysis of fibrin by fibrinolytic enzymes derived from plasma, endothelial cells and leucocytes.

CLINICAL FACTORS PREDISPOSING TO THE DEVELOPMENT OF VENOUS THROMBOEMBOLISM

Epidemiologic studies, particularly in hospitalized patients, have identified a number of clinical factors that predispose to DVT. Common risk factors are shown in Table 19.1. When designing clinical trials for the prevention of DVT, these risk factors are usually taken into account, but, in some studies, high-risk patients are excluded, making the results less generalizable. The identification of natural inhibitors that predispose to DVT is important in cancer, pregnancy and the use of the oral contraceptive pill. Patients with cancer have been known, since the days of Trousseau, to be at risk for the development of DVT, but it has been difficult to understand why patients with minimal disease develop thrombosis whereas others with advanced malignancy do not. Similarly, although DVT is relatively uncommon in users of oral contraceptive pills or in pregnancy, it is now clear that the presence of an inhibitor deficiency markedly increases the likelihood of DVT.

The known inhibitor deficiencies predisposing to thrombosis include antithrombin, protein C deficiency, protein S deficiency, activated protein C resistance, the prothrombin mutant and decreased fibrinolytic activity. These disorders have been reviewed and an attempt has been made to identify the incidence, the ethnic distribution and the degree of risk in pregnancy, surgery and cancer, and recommendations have been made for prophylaxis and treatment.[3,4] Homocysteinaemia (sometimes referred to as hyperhomocysteinaemia) predisposes to both venous and arterial thrombosis through mechanisms that are poorly understood. The same applies to patients with the antiphospholipid syndrome and heparin-induced thrombocytopenia.

Activated protein C resistance is the most common abnormality predisposing to DVT. The defect is due to substitution of glutamine for arginine at residue 506 in the factor V molecule, making factor V resistant to proteolysis by activated protein C. The gene mutation is known as factor V Leiden and follows autosomal dominant inheritance. Factor V Leiden is present in approximately 5% of the normal population, in 16% of patients with a first episode of DVT and in up to 35% of patients with idiopathic DVT.[3] Prothrombin G20210 A is a recently identified gene mutation predisposing to DVT. It is present in approximately 2% of apparently healthy individuals and in 7% of those with DVT. In approximately 60% of patients with idiopathic DVT, an inherited abnormality cannot be detected, suggesting that other gene mutations are present and may have an aetiological role.

CLINICAL FEATURES

PE occurs in 50% of patients with objectively documented proximal-vein thrombosis. Many of these emboli are asymptomatic. The clinical importance of PE depends on the size of the embolus and on the patient's cardiorespiratory reserve. Usually, only part of the thrombus embolizes and 70% of patients with PE demonstrated by angiography have detectable DVT at presentation. DVT and PE are not separate disorders, but a continuous syndrome in which the initial clinical presentation may be with symptoms of either DVT or PE. Strategies for detection include tests for PE – lung scanning, pulmonary angiography or spiral computerized tomography (CT) – and tests for DVT – ultrasound, impedance plethysmography or venography.

The clinical features of venous thrombosis include pain, tenderness and swelling, a palpable cord (i.e. a thrombosed vessel that is palpable as a cord), discoloration, venous distension and prominence of the superficial veins and cyanosis. The clinical diagnosis of DVT is non-specific because symptoms or signs may be caused by non-thrombotic disorders. The rare exception is the patient with phlegmasia cerulea dolens (swollen leg with cyanosis of the skin due to marked obstruction of venous outflow), in whom the diagnosis of massive ileofemoral thrombosis is usually obvious. This syndrome occurs in <1% of patients with symptomatic DVT. In most, the symptoms and signs are non-specific and yet, in 50–85%,

Table 19.1 *Clinical risk factors predisposing to the development of venous thromboembolism*

	Inherited or acquired abnormalities
Surgical and non-surgical trauma	Activated protein C resistance
Previous venous thromboembolism	Prothrombin polymorphism
Immobilization	Protein C deficiency
Malignant disease	Protein S deficiency
Heart disease	Antithrombin deficiency
Leg paralysis	Anticardiolipin syndrome
Age > 40	Heparin-induced thrombocytopenia
Obesity	
Oestrogens	
Parturition	
Varicose veins	

thrombosis will not be confirmed by objective tests. Patients with extensive DVT may have minor symptoms and signs. Conversely, patients with florid leg pain and swelling may have no objective evidence of DVT. Patients can be assigned pre-test probabilities of DVT based on their clinical features and history. However, these pre-test probabilities are neither sufficiently high to give anticoagulant treatment nor sufficiently low to withhold treatment without performing objective testing.

The clinical scenarios of acute PE include the following syndromes, which may overlap:

- transient dyspnoea and tachypnoea,
- the syndrome of pulmonary infarction including pleuritic chest pain, haemoptysis and pleural effusion and infiltrates on chest radiograph
- right-sided heart failure with severe dyspnoea and tachypnoea,
- cardiovascular collapse with hypotension, syncope and coma (massive PE),
- less common and non-specific presentations, including unexplained arrhythmia, resistant cardiac failure, wheezing, cough, pyrexia, anxiety/apprehension and confusion.

All of these clinical scenarios are non-specific and may be caused by a variety of cardiorespiratory disorders. Objective testing is therefore mandatory to confirm or exclude the presence of PE. Classifying patients into categories of pre-test probability (low, intermediate or high) is useful in a minority of patients when combined with lung-scan findings. Pre-test clinical probabilities for PE have not been as reproducible as they have been for the diagnosis of DVT.

LABORATORY FEATURES

Venous thromboembolism is associated with non-specific laboratory changes of the acute-phase response. This response includes elevated levels of fibrinogen and factor VIII, increases in the leucocyte and platelet counts, systemic activation of blood coagulation, fibrin formation and breakdown, and increases in the plasma concentrations of prothrombin fragment 1.2, fibrinopeptide A, complexes of thrombin–antithrombin and D-dimer. All of these are non-specific and may occur as the result of surgery, trauma, infection, inflammation or infarction. None can reliably be used to predict the development of DVT.

The fibrin breakdown fragment D-dimer can be measured by an enzyme-linked immunosorbent assay (ELISA) or by a latex agglutination assay. Some of these assays have a rapid turnaround time and some are quantitative. The D-dimer may be useful as a test for exclusion of patients with suspected DVT or PE (see below). A positive result is non-specific.

DIAGNOSIS

The differential diagnosis in DVT includes muscle strain, lymphangitis, popliteal cyst rupture and cellulitis. Without objective testing, it is impossible to confirm or exclude DVT. Diagnosis can often be determined once DVT has been excluded, although in 25% the cause remains uncertain, even after careful follow-up.[5]

Objective tests for deep-vein thrombosis

The tests of value in clinically suspected DVT are ultrasound imaging, impedance plethysmography and venography.[6] Each has been validated by clinical trials, including prospective studies with long-term follow-up. These have established the safety of withholding anticoagulant treatment in patients with negative test results.[6] Ultrasound imaging or impedance plethysmography (IP) are both effective in detecting proximal-vein thrombosis. They have limited sensitivity for calf-vein thrombosis and require serial testing to detect extension into the popliteal vein or more proximally. When performed serially, these tests can safely replace venography in symptomatic patients. Venography continues to have an important role in selected patients, such as those for whom serial testing is impractical and those with abnormal non-invasive test results who have conditions known to produce false-positive results. The wide availability of ultrasound has meant that it has supplanted IP as the principal non-invasive test for DVT in most centres. Venography remains useful in patients with suspected acute recurrent DVT. A diagnostic approach for a patient with a first episode of DVT is shown in Figure 19.1. Ultrasound imaging has two practical advantages. It is more sensitive than IP for small, non-occlusive thrombi and this enables serial testing to be limited to a single repeat test done 5–7 days after presentation. Also, it is not influenced by congestive cardiac failure or by disorders that impair deep-venous filling (e.g. peripheral arterial disease), which may produce false-positive IP results. In the absence of these conditions, IP has a similar high positive predictive value (>90%) to ultrasound imaging, but clinical examination of the patient is required to exclude potential causes of false-positive results.

IP is a valuable test for patients with suspected recurrent DVT because it returns to normal earlier than ultrasonography in proximal-vein thrombosis.[7] Compression ultrasound may remain abnormal for 2 years or more due to persistent non-compressibility of the vein caused by fibrous organization of the original thrombus. A normal IP result obtained at the time of completing anticoagulant treatment provides a useful baseline for future comparison. An IP result that has changed from normal to abnormal is

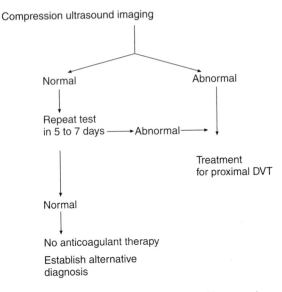

Figure 19.1 *Diagnosis and therapy of patients with suspected first-episode deep-vein thrombosis (DVT). (For details see text and reference 3.)*

highly predictive of acute recurrent proximal-vein thrombosis. The finding of a *new* non-compressible venous segment by ultrasound imaging is probably predictive of acute recurrent thrombosis, but this criterion is of limited value because many patients have persistently non-compressible venous segments due to the initial episode. To date, no ultrasound imaging criteria have been validated by prospective follow-up studies to establish the safety of withholding anticoagulant treatment in patients with recurrent DVT.

Studies have demonstrated a high negative predictive value of D-dimer for acute DVT.[8] The measurement of plasma D-dimer may be useful in patients with initially negative ultrasound imaging to exclude the presence of DVT and to avoid the need for repeated testing. However, this is less important in patients with suspected first-episode DVT, because the need for repeat testing has been reduced to a single test at 5–7 days.[9] Most require a follow-up clinic visit anyway, so the return visit is not a major inconvenience. The value of D-dimer is potentially greater in patients with suspected acute *recurrent* DVT. However, the safety of withholding anticoagulant treatment in such patients with negative D-dimer results has not been established by adequately designed clinical trials.

Differential diagnosis of pulmonary embolism

The differential diagnosis is wide, depending upon the clinical scenario. It includes pneumonia, pneumothorax, pulmonary oedema, pericarditis, rib fracture, myocardial infarction, and septicemia. The key tests include echocardiography, spiral CT, pulmonary angiography, ventilation perfusion (VQ) lung scanning, magnetic resonance imaging (MRI) and objective tests for proximal DVT.[6] A diagnostic approach is summarized in Figure 19.2.

Objective testing for DVT is useful in patients with suspected PE, particularly those with non-diagnostic lung-scan results (indeterminate, intermediate or low probability categories).[6] The detection of proximal DVT provides an indication for anticoagulant treatment, regardless of the presence or absence of PE. A negative result does not exclude PE. If the patient has adequate cardiorespiratory reserve, serial ultrasound imaging may be used as an alternative to pulmonary angiography. The rationale is that the clinical objective in such patients is to prevent *recurrent* PE, which is unlikely in the absence of proximal-vein thrombosis. For patients with inadequate cardiorespiratory reserve, the clinical objectives are to prevent death and morbidity from an existing embolus and to allow further testing for the presence or absence of PE.

OBJECTIVE TESTS

The value of echocardiography has recently been firmly established and has four main advantages:

- it is non-invasive and easily available,
- it can exclude other causes of cardiogenic shock, e.g. extensive left ventricular infarction, pericardial tamponade or dissecting aortic aneurysm,
- it allows an estimate of pulmonary artery pressure and so provides information on the severity of pulmonary artery obstruction,
- it can be used serially to assess response to treatment.

The echocardiographic findings are not specific and reflect the response of the right heart to acute pulmonary artery hypertension. They consist of distension of the pulmonary artery trunk, right ventricular (RV) dilatation and hypokinesis, reduced left ventricular (LV) size and an increased RV/LV diameter, diastolic and systolic flattening of the intraventricular septum and paradoxical systolic wall motion. This pattern is mimicked, in particular, by RV infarction associated with LV dysfunction.

Scoring systems have been developed that correlate well with the angiographic severity index, and the value of serial echocardiography has been demonstrated in patients treated with thrombolytic agents. Rarely, RV thrombus may be visualized, a clinical situation associated with a high mortality rate, 30% of such patients succumbing as a result of massive pulmonary thromboembolism.

There are several limitations to the applications of echocardiography. At least 40% of the pulmonary vascular bed needs to be obstructed to produce detectable features. Co-existent cardiorespiratory disease also limits its value because of the non-specific nature of the abnormalities and because

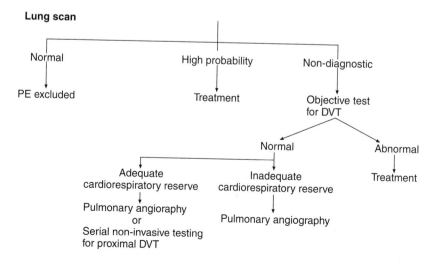

Figure 19.2 *Diagnosis and therapy of patients with suspected pulmonary embolism (PE). DVT, deep-vein thrombosis. (For details see text and reference 3.)*

imaging via the transthoracic route may be difficult. Transoesophageal echocardiography may be valuable in this situation, particularly in making a full haemodynamic assessment in the shocked, intubated patient.

Both spiral CT imaging and MRI are now of proven value in PE. Spiral CT imaging is highly sensitive for large emboli (segmental or greater arteries), but is less sensitive for emboli in subsegmental pulmonary arteries.[10] These smaller emboli may still be clinically important in patients with inadequate cardiorespiratory reserve. MRI is highly sensitive for PE. However, one study documented significant inter-observer variation in the sensitivity, ranging from 70% to 100%.[11] The safety of withholding anticoagulant treatment in patients with negative results by spiral CT imaging or MRI has not been established by prospective clinical trials.

The assay for plasma D-dimer is potentially useful to exclude PE, based on a high negative predictive value reported from centres with research expertise.[8] However, further studies are required to establish the place of D-dimer testing and, in particular, to evaluate the safety of withholding anticoagulant treatment in patients with a negative result.

TREATMENT OF VENOUS THROMBOEMBOLISM

The objectives of treatment are:

- to prevent death,
- to prevent recurrent DVT and PE,
- to prevent the post-phlebitic syndrome.

Anticoagulant drugs constitute the mainstay of treatment, and graduated compression stockings (for 24 months) significantly decrease the incidence of the post-thrombotic syndrome.

Heparin therapy

The anticoagulant activity of unfractionated heparin depends upon a unique pentasaccharide that binds to antithrombin and potentiates the inhibition of thrombin and activated factor X (Xa) by antithrombin. About one-third of all heparin molecules contain the unique pentasaccharide sequence, regardless of whether they are low or high molecular

weight (HMWH) fractions.[12] It is the pentasaccharide sequence that confers the molecular high affinity for antithrombin. In addition, heparin catalyses the inactivation of thrombin by another plasma cofactor (co-factor II), which acts independently of antithrombin.

Heparin has a number of other effects. These include the release of tissue factor pathway inhibitor, binding to proteins located on platelets, endothelial cells and leucocytes, suppression of platelet function and an increase in vascular permeability. The anticoagulant response to a standard dose of heparin varies widely amongst patients. This makes it necessary to monitor the anticoagulant response, using either the activated partial thromboplastin time (aPTT) or heparin levels, and to titrate the dose to the individual patient.

Conventional therapy comprises a combination of continuous intravenous heparin and oral warfarin.[6] The length of the initial intravenous heparin therapy can be reduced to 5 days, thus shortening the hospital stay. The simultaneous use of initial heparin and warfarin has become standard practice in medically stable patients. Exceptions include patients who may require immediate interventions such as in thrombolysis or insertion of a vena cava filter or patients at very high risk of bleeding. Heparin is continued until the INR has been within the therapeutic range (2–3) for 2 consecutive days.

The efficacy of heparin therapy depends upon achieving a critical therapeutic level of heparin within the first 24 hours of treatment. Data from three consecutive, double-blind clinical trials indicate that failure to achieve the therapeutic aPTT threshold by 24 hours is associated with a 23.3% subsequent recurrent venous thromboembolism rate, compared with 4–6% for the patient groups who reached therapeutic anticoagulation at 24 hours.[13] The recurrences occurred throughout the 3-month follow-up period and could not be attributed to inadequate oral anticoagulant therapy. The critical therapeutic level of heparin, as measured by the aPTT, is 1.5 times the mean of the control value or the upper limit of the normal aPTT range. This corresponds to a heparin blood level of 0.2–0.4 U mL^{-1} by the protamine sulphate titration assay and 0.35–0.70 U mL^{-1} by the anti-factor Xa assay.

There is a wide variability in the aPTT and in heparin blood levels with different reagents and even with different batches of the same reagent. It is therefore vital for each laboratory to establish the minimal therapeutic level of heparin, as measured by the aPTT, that will provide a heparin blood level of at least 0.35 U mL^{-1} by the anti-factor Xa assay for each batch of thromboplastin reagent being used, particularly if the batches of reagent are provided by different manufacturers.

Although there is a strong correlation between subtherapeutic aPTT values and recurrent thromboembolism, the relationship between supra-therapeutic aPTT and bleeding (aPTT ratio 2.5 or more) is less definite. Indeed, bleeding during heparin therapy is more closely related to underlying clinical risk factors. A lower body weight and age > 65 are independent risk factors for bleeding on heparin.[14,15]

Numerous audits indicate that administration of intravenous heparin is difficult and that the clinical practice of using an *ad hoc* approach to heparin dose titration frequently results in inadequate therapy. For example, an audit of physician practices at three university-affiliated hospitals documented that 60% of patients failed to achieve an adequate aPTT response (ratio 1.5) during the initial 24 hours of therapy and that 30–40% of patients remained 'sub-therapeutic' over the next 3–4 days.[16] Several practices were identified that led to inadequate therapy. The common theme is an exaggerated fear of bleeding complications on the part of clinicians. Consequently, it has been common practice for many clinicians to start treatment with a low heparin dose and to increase this dose cautiously over several days to achieve the therapeutic range. The use of a protocol has been evaluated in two prospective studies involving patients with venous thromboembolism.[17,18] In one, for the treatment of proximal DVT, patients were given either intravenous heparin alone followed by warfarin or intravenous heparin and simultaneous warfarin.[17] The heparin nomogram is summarized in Tables 19.2 and 19.3. Only 1% and 2% of the patients were under-treated for more than 24 hours in the heparin group and in the heparin and warfarin group, respectively. Recurrent DVT (objectively documented) occurred infrequently in both groups (7%). In the other trial, a weight-based heparin dosage nomogram was compared with a standard-care nomogram (Table 19.4).[18] Patients on the weight-adjusted heparin nomogram received a starting dose of 80 U kg^{-1} as a bolus and 18 U kg^{-1} h^{-1} as an infusion. The heparin dose was adjusted to maintain an aPTT of 1.5–2.3 times control. In the weight-adjusted group, 89% of patients achieved the therapeutic range within 24 hours, compared with 75% in the standard-care group. The risk of recurrent thromboembolism was more frequent in the standard-care group. The weight-based nomogram has gained widespread acceptance.

COMPLICATIONS OF HEPARIN THERAPY

The main adverse effects of heparin therapy include bleeding, thrombocytopenia and osteoporosis.

Table 19.2 Heparin protocol

1. Administer initial intravenous heparin bolus: 5000 U
2. Administer continuous intravenous heparin infusion: commence at 42 mL h^{-1} of 20 000 U (1680 U h^{-1}) in 500 mL of two-thirds dextrose and one-third saline (a 24-h heparin dose of 40 320 U), except in the following patients, in whom heparin infusion is commenced at a rate of 31 mL h^{-1} (1240 U h^{-1}, a 24-h dose of 29 760 U):
   (a) patients who have undergone surgery within the previous 2 weeks
   (b) patients with a previous history of peptic ulcer disease or gastrointestinal or genitourinary bleeding
   (c) patients with recent stroke (i.e. thrombotic stroke within previous 2 weeks)
   (d) patients with a platelet count <150 × 10^9 L^{-1}
   (e) patients with miscellaneous reasons for a high risk of bleeding (e.g. hepatic failure, renal failure or vitamin K deficiency)
3. Adjust heparin dose by use of the aPTT. The aPTT test is performed in all patients as follows:
   (a) 4–6 hours after commencing heparin; the heparin dose is then adjusted
   (b) 4–6 hours after the first dosage adjustment
   (c) then as indicated by the nomogram for the first 24 hours of therapy
   (d) thereafter, once daily, unless the patient is sub-therapeutic,[a] in which case the aPTT test is repeated 4–6 hours after the heparin dose is increased

[a]Sub-therapeutic = aPTT < 1.5 times the mean normal control value for the thromboplastin reagent being used.
aPPT, activated partial thromboplastin time.
Adapted from Hull, RD, *et al. Arch Intern Med* 1992; **152**: 1589–95, with permission.[17]

Table 19.3 *Intravenous heparin dose titration nomogram according to the activated partial thromboplastin time (aPTT)*

aPTT (s)	Rate change (mL h^{-1})	Dose change (IU/24 h)[a]	Additional action
≤45	+6	+5760	Repeated aPTT[b] in 4–6 h
	+3	+2880	
46–54	0	0	Repeated aPTT in 4–6 h
55–85	−3	−2880	None[c]
			Stop heparin sodium treatment
			or 1 hour; repeated aPTT
			4–6 hours after re-starting
86–110	−6	−5760	heparin treatment
			Stop heparin treatment for
			1 hour; repeated aPTT 4–6 hours
>110			after re-starting heparin treatment

[a]Heparin sodium concentration 20 000 IU in 500 ml = 40 IU ml^{-1}.
[b]With the use of Actin – FS thromboplastin reagent (Dade, Mississauga, Ontario, Canada).
[c]During the first 24 h, repeated aPTT in 4–6 h. Thereafter, the aPTT will be determined once daily, unless sub-therapeutic.
Adapted from Hull, RD, *et al. Arch Intern Med* 1992; **152**: 1589–95, with permission.[17]

Table 19.4 *Weight-based nomogram for initial intravenous heparin therapy*

	Dose (IU kg^{-1})
Initial dose	80 bolus, then 18 h^{-1}
aPTT <35 s (<1.2×)	80 bolus, then 4 h^{-1}
aPTT 35–45 s (1.2–1.5×)	40 bolus, then 2 h^{-1}
aPTT 46–70 s (1.5–2.3×)	No change
aPTT 71–90 s (2.3–3.0×)	Decrease infusion rate by 2 h^{-1}
aTT >90 s (>3.0×)	Hold infusion 1 h, then decrease infusion rate by 3 h^{-1}

Figures in parentheses show comparison with control.
aPTT, activated partial thromboplastin time.
Adapted from Raschke, RA, *et al. Ann Intern Med* 1993; **119**: 874–81, with permission.[19]

Patients at risk of bleeding include those who have had recent surgery or trauma or who have other clinical factors that predispose to bleeding, such as active peptic ulcer, liver disease, haemostatic defects or age >65 years. The management of bleeding will depend on its severity, the risk of recurrent venous thromboembolism and the aPTT. Heparin should be discontinued temporarily or permanently and insertion of an inferior vena cava filter considered. If urgent reversal of heparin effect is required, protamine sulphate can be administered.

Heparin-induced thrombocytopenia is a well-recognized complication, usually occurring 5–10 days after heparin treatment has started. Approximately 1–2% of patients receiving unfractionated heparin will experience a fall in platelet count to less than the normal range. In the majority, this mild to moderate thrombocytopenia appears to be a direct effect of heparin on platelets and is of no consequence. However, approximately 0.1–0.2% of patients develop an immune thrombocytopenia mediated by IgG antibody directed against a complex of PF4 and heparin (HIT). This may be accompanied by arterial or venous thrombosis, which may lead to death or limb amputation.[19] The diagnosis of HIT, with or without thrombosis, must be made on clinical grounds, because the assays with the highest sensitivity and specificity are not readily available and have a slow turnaround time.

When the diagnosis of heparin-induced thrombocytopenia is made, heparin in all forms must be stopped immediately. This is a particularly difficult problem in the critically ill, in whom thrombocytopenia is usually the result of a variety of more common causes, e.g. sepsis, bleeding or other intravascular or extravascular consumption. Typically, HIT is sudden in onset, with a precipitous fall in platelet count. Therefore, a slowly falling count may not necessitate the complete cessation of all heparin (e.g. arterial flushes). In those patients requiring on-going anticoagulation, several alternatives exist; the agents most extensively used are the heparinoid Danaparoid and Hirudin.[19]

Osteoporosis has been reported in patients receiving unfractionated heparin in dosages of 20 000 U day^{-1} (or more) for more than 6 months. Demineralization can progress to the fracture of vertebral bodies or long bones and the defect may not be entirely reversible.

LOW MOLECULAR WEIGHT HEPARIN

Heparin currently in clinical use is polydispersed, unmodified heparin, with a mean molecular weight ranging from 10 to 16 kD. In recent years, low molecular weight derivatives of commercial heparin have been prepared that have a mean molecular weight of 4–5 kD.

The low molecular weight heparins (LMWHs) that are commercially available are made by different processes (such as nitrous acid, alkaline or enzymatic depolymerization) and they differ chemically and pharmacokinetically. The clinical significance of these differences is unclear and there have been very few studies comparing different LMWHs with respect to clinical outcomes. The doses of the different LMWHs have been established empirically and are not necessarily interchangeable.

The LMWHs differ from unfractionated heparin in numerous ways. Of particular importance are the following:

- increased bio-availability (>90% after subcutaneous injection),
- prolonged half-life and predictable clearance, enabling once or twice daily injection,
- predictable antithrombotic response based on body weight, permitting treatment without laboratory monitoring.

Other possible advantages are their ability to inactivate platelet-bound factor Xa, resistance to inhibition by platelet factor IV and their decreased effect on platelet function and vascular permeability (possibly accounting for fewer haemorrhagic effects at comparable antithrombotic doses).

There has been a hope that LMWHs will have fewer serious complications than unfractionated heparin. Evidence is accumulating that these complications are indeed less serious and less frequent. LMWHs cross-react with unfractionated heparin and cannot therefore be used as alternative therapy in patients who develop HIT. The heparinoid Danaparoid possesses a 10–20% cross-reactivity and can be used instead.

In a number of clinical trials, LMWH by subcutaneous or intravenous injection was compared with continuous intravenous unfractionated heparin, with repeat venography being the primary endpoint. These studies demonstrated that LMWH was at least as effective as unfractionated heparin. Subcutaneous unmonitored LMWH has also been compared with continuous heparin in a number of clinical trials.[20,21] These studies indicate a significant advantage for LMWH in the reduction of major bleeding and mortality. Three recent studies indicated that LMWH used predominantly out of hospital was as effective and safe as intravenous unfractionated heparin given in hospital,[21] and LMWH is as effective as intravenous heparin in the treatment of patients presenting with PE. Economic analysis has also shown that LMWH is cost-effective.

Oral anticoagulant therapy

Oral anticoagulant treatment is continued for 3–6 months in patients with a first-episode DVT or PE.[22] Stopping oral anticoagulant treatment at 4–6 weeks results in a high incidence (12–20%) of recurrence during the following 12–24 months.[23] Warfarin should be continued for 1 year to indefinitely in patients with a second episode of objectively documented DVT or PE. Stopping treatment at 3 months in these patients results in a 20% incidence of recurrent DVT and a 5% incidence of PE.[24]

Patients at high risk of recurrent thromboembolism are those with idiopathic thrombosis, homozygous factor V Leiden gene mutation or cancer.[22]

MASSIVE PULMONARY EMBOLISM

Patients with acute massive PE usually have a dramatic presentation with sudden onset of severe shortness of breath, hypoxaemia and right ventricular failure. Symptoms include central chest pain, often identical to angina, severe dyspnoea and, frequently, syncope, confusion or coma. Examination reveals a patient in severe distress with tachypnoea, cyanosis and hypotension. The marked increase in pulmonary vascular resistance leads to acute right ventricular failure, with the presence of large A-waves in the jugular veins and a right ventricular diastolic gallop. With pulmonary hypertension, there is marked right ventricular dilatation with a shift of the intraventricular septum, decreasing cardiac output and further decreasing coronary perfusion, which may result in cardiorespiratory arrest. If patients with a massive PE survive, they are at great risk from further thromboembolism.

The emergency management of massive PE includes the use of intravenous heparin, O_2, mechanical ventilation, volume resuscitation and the use of inotropic agents or even vasodilators. In addition to these supportive measures, specific treatment options for massive PE include:

- thrombolysis,
- pulmonary thrombectomy, with or without cardiopulmonary bypass support,
- transvenous catheter embolectomy or clot dissolution,
- insertion of an inferior vena cava filter.

Thrombolytic therapy

Several studies have demonstrated that the mortality from PE can be decreased by heparin. Treatment with intravenous heparin and oral anticoagulants reduces the mortality rate to less than 5% and this may be further reduced with the use of LMWH. In the prospective investigation of PE diagnosis (PIOPED) trial,[25] only 10 of 399 (2.5%) patients who had angiographically confirmed PE died. However, patients who present with acute massive PE and hypotension have a mortality rate of approximately 20%. For such patients, the appropriate use of thrombolytic agents has a role.

Several trials have compared thrombolytic drugs with heparin.[26] Outcome measures for accelerated thrombolysis included quantitative measures on repeat pulmonary angiograms, quantitative scores on repeat pulmonary perfusion scans and measures of pulmonary vascular resistance. Although all studies demonstrated superiority of thrombolysis (and in particular with tPA) in radiographic and haemodynamic abnormalities within the first 24 hours, this advantage was short lived.[26] Repeat perfusion scans at 5–7 days revealed no significant difference between the patients treated with thrombolytic agents or with heparin. However, at 1 year, those receiving thrombolytic therapy had higher CO diffusion capacity and lung blood capillary volume compared to patients receiving heparin. Follow-up of 23 patients at 7 years showed that patients who had

been treated with thrombolytic therapy had lower pulmonary artery pressure and pulmonary vascular resistance. The clinical relevance of these findings, however, must await further prospective studies.[26]

Three thrombolytic agents have been approved by the Federal Drug Administration (FDA) for the treatment of acute PE. The dosage schedules are as follows:

- streptokinase 250 000 units over 30 min, followed by 100 000 units h^{-1} for 24 h,
- urokinase 4400 units kg^{-1} over 10 min, followed by 4400 units kg^{-1} h^{-1} for 12–24 hours (now withdrawn from the market),
- recombinant tissue plasminogen activator (rt-PA) 100 mg administered over 2 h.

Anticoagulation with heparin or LMWH is usually commenced when the aPTT is less than two times the control.

In weighing the risks and benefits of thrombolytic therapy, the main concern relates to bleeding. Data from five randomized trials indicate that the frequency of intracranial haemorrhage following thrombolytic therapy is 1.9% (95% confidence interval, 0.7–4.1%).[27] Diastolic hypertension was identified as a risk factor. The incidence of major bleeding has decreased, particularly with the use of bolus or short-term infusions and of newer thrombolytic agents, but intracerebral haemorrhage continues to occur more frequently than with heparin.

The role of thrombolytic agents in massive PE remains controversial. Until there is a clearly demonstrated benefit in terms of both morbidity and mortality, the question of risk/benefit will remain. In the meantime, the use of thrombolytic agents has become simpler with the use of echocardiography[28,29] or spiral CT to confirm the diagnosis, the use of short-term or bolus infusion into peripheral veins, the elimination of monitoring by laboratory tests and treatment in high dependency units (HDUs) rather than in ICUs. The fact that a high percentage of acute massive PE occurs following surgery indicates that greater efforts must be made to ensure that prophylactic measures are applied.

PULMONARY EMBOLECTOMY

Pulmonary embolectomy is occasionally indicated in the management of massive PE. It is usually only considered if there is >50% obstruction of the pulmonary vasculature, the patient is in shock and the PaO_2 is <9.0 Kpa. In some centres, patients who have contraindications to thrombolytic therapy are candidates for thrombectomy. On the other hand, it could be argued that a patient who survives the first 2 hours will probably survive with adequate medical management if no further PE occurs. It is unlikely that a randomized trial comparing thrombolytic therapy with pulmonary embolectomy is possible.

Early experience with the Trendelenburg procedure revealed unacceptably high mortality (>50%). With the use of cardiopulmonary bypass support, mortality rates between 16% and 57% have been reported. In a review of 651 patients undergoing emergency pulmonary embolectomy, the survival rate was 59.3% with cardiopulmonary bypass support and 47.7% without it.[30] Patients' with chronic pulmonary hypertension, other medical disorders, or with symptoms of more than 7 days' duration have higher mortality rates, as do patients who have sustained a cardiac arrest before embolectomy.[31] Care to avoid vasodilatation at the initiation of anaesthesia is important. Pulmonary haemorrhagic infarction with reperfusion has been reported. Pulmonary embolectomy is usually accompanied by insertion of a vena cava filter.

The role of pulmonary embolectomy remains unclear and will depend on the availability of a surgical team. Patients who are not candidates for thrombolysis (e.g. those who have had recent surgery) or who have not responded to maximal medical therapy may be candidates. However, a recent report of successful thrombolysis with intrapulmonary urokinase in patients treated within 10 days of surgery[32] casts further doubt on the need for this radical procedure.

PERCUTANEOUS CLOT EXTRACTION OR DISRUPTION

Pulmonary embolectomy via a catheter suction device or mechanical disruption has been used in the treatment of patients with acute massive PE who have contraindications to anticoagulants or thrombolysis. Mortality rates were 27% and 28%.[33] The commonest cause of death is cardiac arrest from ventricular arrhythmia, right heart failure and pulmonary haemorrhage. Some patients in whom clot extraction or disruption was not possible have gone on to successful pulmonary embolectomy on bypass. Attempts have been made to fragment PE using conventional cardiac catheters or a catheter guide wire in conjunction with pulmonary thrombolytic therapy. Catheter clot extraction is currently confined to a few centres and its role is unclear.

INFERIOR VENA CAVAL INTERRUPTION

Early approaches to inferior vena caval interruption included ligation or plication using external clips. Both procedures were accompanied by an operative mortality rate of 12–14%, a recurrent pulmonary emboli rate of 4–6% and an occlusion rate of 67–69%.[34] These complications gave rise to the development of catheter-inserted intraluminal filters. An ideal filter is one that is easily and safely placed percutaneously, is biocompatible and mechanically stable, able to trap emboli without causing occlusion of the vena cava, does not require anticoagulation and is not ferromagnetic (i.e. does not cause artefacts on MRI). Although there is as yet no ideal filter, several types are available. These include the Greenfield stainless-steel filter, titanium Greenfield filter, bird's nest filter, Vena Tech filter and Simon–Nitinol filter. In experienced hands, these devices can be quickly and safely inserted under fluoroscopic control. One filter (for example, Antheor™Tu 50–125 Medi-Tech, Boston Scientific Corp.) can be inserted temporarily in conjunction with thrombolytic therapy and then removed. The follow-up data available to date show that the Greenfield filter has had the best performance record and any future comparative studies should use this filter as the standard.[34]

The main indications for caval filters are contraindications to anticoagulants, recurrent PE despite adequate anticoagulation and prophylactic placement in high-risk patients.[34] In the last category are patients with cor pulmonale or a previous history of PE who are placed in high-risk situations such as acetabular fracture or who have cancer. More controversial indications for the prophylactic insertion of a filter include emergency surgery occurring within the first 4 weeks of commencing anticoagulant therapy following thrombolytic therapy.[34]

In the past, the detection of a free-floating thrombus by ultrasound examination has been considered an indication for either thrombectomy or insertion of an inferior vena cava filter. An important study compared the clinical outcomes of patients who had either the presence or absence of a free-floating thrombus in a proximal leg vein.[35] There was no difference in the incidence of PE or death between the two groups. The authors conclude that the routine insertion of inferior vena cava filters in patients with free-floating thrombi cannot be supported. This is in keeping with an earlier observation[36] that free-floating thrombi become attached to the vein wall rather than embolizing. In a further study, patients with proximal DVT were randomized to receive an inferior vena cava filter or anticoagulant treatment alone.[37] All patients were treated with heparin, followed by oral anticoagulant therapy for 3 months. At 10 days, there was a significant difference in the incidence of PE, but no difference in mortality. Extended follow-up at 1–2 years showed a (non-significant) increase in the incidence of PE in the control group, but a higher incidence of recurrent DVT in the vena cava filter group and no difference in mortality.

CHRONIC THROMBOEMBOLIC PULMONARY HYPERTENSION

In a small number of patients, the emboli fail to resolve and undergo fibrovascular organization to produce chronic obstruction to pulmonary arterial blood flow and progressive right ventricular failure, hypoxaemia and death. Many of these patients have been found to have thrombophilia such as the factor V Leiden mutation or the antiphospholipid antibody syndrome and, in some, decreased fibrinolytic activity can be demonstrated at the endothelial cell level. At the present time, there is no unifying concept for the pathophysiology of chronic thromboembolic pulmonary hypertension. The clinical presentation is variable. Patients will be short of breath on exertion. Other symptoms relate to decreased cardiac output, fatigue, syncope on exercise or in other situations leading to a fall in systemic vascular resistance, such as taking a hot shower. Chest pain, due to pleuritic involvement or to cardiac ischaemia, may be experienced. There may be a history of previous DVT and/or PE, but frequently this is missing. Ultimately, patients develop severe hypoxia and right

heart failure with acute decompensation often following trivial insult, e.g. urinary tract infection.

The physical findings are those of severe pulmonary hypertension. The diagnosis can be made by a combination of echocardiography, right heart catheterization and pulmonary angiography and can be further assessed with optic angioscopy, ultra-fast CT scanning or MRI. Supportive therapy consists of anticoagulation, insertion of a vena cava filter, O_2 and the judicious use of diuretics. Medical therapy aims to produce pulmonary vascular dilatation using intravenous prostacyclin, oral calcium channel blockers or inhaled nitric oxide. These may be of benefit in preventing some of the secondary changes such as endothelial cell dysfunction, accelerated growth of pulmonary vascular smooth muscle cells and vascular remodelling. The only definitive management available is pulmonary thromboendarterectomy (or transplantation). This former procedure is compli-cated and carries a high risk for post-operative complications.[38]

CONCLUSION

Over the past 20 years, a large number of trials have been carried out on the diagnosis, prevention and treatment of venous thromboembolism. Clinical practice has dramatically changed in response. A number of studies are currently underway to explore new approaches to diagnosis and treatment. These include the use of pre-test clinical probabilities, the role of spiral CT and MRI and trials to determine the optimal management using LMWH and newer anticoagulants such as pentasaccharide and specific antithrombin agents.[5] Longer duration of anticoagulant therapy with LMWH or warfarin is aimed at decreasing recurrent DVT and PE and decreasing the incidence of the post-thrombotic syndrome. Clinical trials aimed at the prevention of DVT in high-risk medical and surgical patients continue. Many of the remaining questions regarding management should be answered in the near future.

REFERENCES

1. Anderson, FA, Wheeler, HB, Goldberg, RJ, *et al.* A population-based perspective of the hospital incidence and case-fatality rates of deep vein thrombosis within a

defined urban population. The Worcester DVT Study. *J Intern Med* 1992; **232**: 155–60.

2. Prandoni, P, Polistena, P, Bernardi, E, *et al*. Upper extremity deep-vein thrombosis risk factors, diagnosis, and complications. *Arch Intern Med* 1997; **157**: 57–62.

3. Lane, DA, Mannucci, PM, Bauer, KA, *et al*. Inherited thrombophilia: Part 1. *Thromb Haemost* 1996; **76**(5): 651–62.

4. Lane, DA, Mannucci, PM, Bauer, KA, *et al*. Inherited thrombophilia: Part 2. *Thromb Haemost* 1996; **76**(6): 824–34.

5. Hull, RD, Pineo, GF. Clinical features of deep venous thrombosis. In *Venous thromboembolism in an evidence-based atlas*, ed. RD Hull, G Raskob, GF Pineo. Armonk, New York: Futura Publishing Co, 1996; 87–100.

6. American Thoracic Society. The diagnostic approach to acute venous thromboembolism – clinical practice guideline. *Am J Respir Care Med* 1999; **160**: 1043–66.

7. Huisman, M, Buller, H, ten Cate, JW. Utility of impedance plethysmography in the diagnosis of recurrent deep-vein thrombosis. *Arch Intern Med* 1988; **148**: 681–3.

8. Perrier, A, Desmarais, S, Miron, MJ, *et al*. Non-invasive diagnosis of venous thromboembolism in outpatients. *Lancet* 1999; **353**(9148): 190–5.

9. Birdwell, BG, Raskob, GE, Whitsett, TL, *et al*. Predictive value of compression ultrasonography for deep vein thrombosis in symptomatic outpatients: clinical implications of the site of vein noncompressibility. *Arch Intern Med* 2000; **160**(3): 309–13.

10. Rathburn, SW, Raskob, GE, Whitsett, TL. Sensitivity and specificity of helical computed tomography in the diagnosis of pulmonary embolism: a systematic review. *Ann Intern Med* 2000; **132**(3): 227–32.

11. Meaney, JFM, Weg, JG, Chenevert, TL, *et al*. Diagnosis of pulmonary embolism with magnetic resonance angiography. *N Engl J Med* 1997; **336**: 1422–7.

12. Hirsh, J, Warkentin, TE, Shaughnessy, SG, *et al*. Heparin and low-molecular-weight heparin: mechanisms of action, pharmacokinetics, dosing considerations, monitoring, efficacy, and safety. *Chest* 2001; **119**(Suppl. 1): 64S–94S.

13. Hull, RD, Raskob, GE, Brant, RF, *et al*. The importance of initial heparin treatment on long-term clinical outcomes of antithrombotic therapy. *Arch Intern Med* 1997; **157**(10): 2317–21.

14. Campbell, NR, Hull, RD, Brant, R, *et al*. Different effects of heparin in males and females. *Clin Invest Med* 1998; **21**(2): 71–8.

15. Campbell, NR, Hull, RD, Chang, SC, *et al*. Aging and heparin-related bleeding. *Arch Intern Med* 1996; **156**(8): 857–60.

16. Wheeler, A, Powell, L, Jaquiss, RD, Newman, JH. Physician practices in the treatment of pulmonary embolism and deep-venous thrombosis. *Arch Intern Med* 1988; **148**: 1321–5.

17. Hull, RD, Raskob, GE, Rosenbloom, DR, *et al*. Optimal therapeutic level of heparin therapy in patients with venous thrombosis. *Arch Intern Med* 1992; **152**: 1589–95.

18. Raschke, RA, Reilly, BM, Guidry, JR, *et al*. The weight-based heparin dosing nomogram compared with a 'standard care' nomogram. *Ann Intern Med* 1993; **119**: 874–81.

19. Warkentin, TE. Heparin-induced thrombocytopenia and its treatment. *J Thromb Thrombolysis* 2000; Suppl. 1: S29–35.

20. Hull, RD, Raskob, GE, Pineo, GF, *et al*. Subcutaneous low-molecular-weight heparin compared with continuous intravenous heparin in the treatment of proximal-vein thrombosis. *N Engl J Med* 1992; **326**: 975–82.

21. Gould, MK, Dembitzer, AD, Doyle, RL, Hastie, TJ, Garber, AM. Low-molecular-weight heparins compared with unfractionated heparin for treatment of acute deep vein thrombosis – a meta-analysis of random-ized, controlled trials. *Ann Intern Med* 1999; **130**: 800–9.

22. Hyers, TM, Agnelli, G, Hull, RD, *et al*. Antithrombotic therapy for venous thromboembolic disease. *Chest* 2001; **119**(Suppl. 1): 176S–93S.

23. Schulman, S, Rhedin, AS, Lindmarker, P, *et al*. A comparison of six months of oral anticoagulation therapy after a first episode of venous thromboem-bolism. *N Engl J Med* 1995; **332**: 1661–5.

24. Schulman, S, Granqvist, S, Holmstrom, M, *et al*. The duration of oral anticoagulant therapy after a second episode of venous thromboembolism. *N Engl J Med* 1997; **336**: 393–8.

25. A Collaborative Study by the PIOPED Investigators. Value of the ventilation/perfusion scan in acute pulmonary embolism diagnosis (PIOPED). *JAMA* 1990; **263**: 2753–9.

26. Arcasoy, SM, Kreit, JW. Thrombolytic therapy of pulmonary embolism. *Chest* 1999; **155**(6): 1695–707.

27. Kanter, DS, Mikkola, KM, Patel, SR, *et al*. Thrombolytic therapy for pulmonary embolism. Frequency of intracranial hemorrhage and associated risk factors. *Chest* 1997; **111**: 1241–5.

28. Goldhaber, SZ, Haire, WD, Feldstein, ML, *et al*. Alteplase versus heparin in acute pulmonary embolism: randomized trial assessing right ventricular function and pulmonary perfusion. *Lancet* 1993; **341**: 507–11.

29. Come, PC, Kim, D, Parker, JA, *et al*. and participating investigators. Early reversal of right ventricular dysfunction in patients with acute pulmonary embolism after treatment with intravenous tissue plasminogen activator. *J Am Coll Cardiol* 1987; **10**: 971–8.

30. del Campo, C. Pulmonary embolectomy: a review. *Can J Surg* 1985; **28**: 11.

31. Dehring, DJ, Arens, JF. Pulmonary thromboembolism: disease recognition and patient management. *Anesthesiology* 1990; **73**: 146.

32. Molina, JE, Hunter, DW, Yedlicka, JW, *et al*. Thrombolytic therapy for postoperative pulmonary embolism. *Am J Surg* 1992; **163**: 375.

33. Timsit, JF, Reynaud, P, Meyer, G, *et al*. Pulmonary embolectomy by catheter device in massive pulmonary embolism. *Chest* 1991; **100**: 655.

34. Greenfield, LJ. Evolution of venous interruption for pulmonary thromboembolism. *Arch Surg* 1992; **127**: 622.

35. Pacouret, G, Alison, D, Pottier, JM, *et al*. Free floating thrombus and embolic risk in patients with angiographically confirmed proximal deep venous thrombosis. *Arch Intern Med* 1997; **157**: 305.

36. Baldridge, ED, Martin, MA, Welling, RE. Clinical significance of free floating venous thrombi. *J Vasc Surg* 1990; **11**: 62–9.

37. Decousus, H, Leizorovitcz, A, Parent, F, *et al*. A clinical trial of vena caval filters in the prevention of pulmonary embolism in patients with proximal deep-vein thrombosis. *N Engl J Med* 1998; **338**(7): 409–15.

38. Jamieson, SW, Nomura, K. Indications for and the results of pulmonary thromboendarterectomy for thromboembolic pulmonary hypertension. *Semin Vasc Surg* 2000; **13**(3): 236–44.

20

Organizational issues in respiratory critical care

ADRIAN J WILLIAMS

INTRODUCTION

Intensive care is the first part of a continuum of progressive care (followed by intermediate care, self-care, long-term care and home care) that provides services for patients with potentially recoverable conditions who can benefit from a higher level of observation and treatment than is available on a general hospital ward. This approach is usually considered to have originated with the polio epidemic of the 1950s,[1] during which patients who developed respiratory failure were managed with negative-pressure ventilation using 'iron lungs'.[2] Initially, these ventilators were located throughout the hospital and, amongst those with concomitant pharyngeal paralysis, mortality was over 90% in those early days, largely due to problems with aspiration, but also due to the lack of expertise with assisted ventilation and the lack of monitoring. Ibsen measured arterial blood gases and showed that the patients were dying from ventilatory failure. The improved understanding of the ventilatory status of patients, and the need for airway protection, led to the use of cuffed tracheostomy tubes and positive-pressure ventilation. The increased invasiveness of this treatment prompted centralized care and, with this, mortality fell below

40%. Respiratory intensive care was established. To quote Gilbertson:[3]

> Ibsen's contribution in 1952, leading to a 50% reduction in mortality from combined respiratory and pharyngeal paralysis, was a great step forward. Its particular importance was that it revolutionised the treatment of respiratory failure caused by the scourge of the day, paralytic polio. The earlier practitioners, with their 'Iron Lungs' and cuirasses, saved a large number, if not a large proportion, of patients with respiratory paralysis due to polio, and many patients with previously fatal respiratory depression from other causes. Intensive therapy has since moved forward from simply providing respiratory support to the management of multi-system failure, but there can be no doubt that the modern specialty owes its origins to the demonstration that patients with failure of a vital organ could be kept alive by mechanical support with skilled round-the-clock nursing and medical care and could recover.

In subsequent years, intensive care remained largely defined by the need to provide invasive assisted ventilation against a backdrop of variable and often multiple organ system failures, occurring as complications of severe sepsis, trauma and major surgery. Different units were managed either independently, often the case with the specialist surgical units, or by a team with both general physicians and anaesthetists. In the USA in the 1980s, however, respiratory physicians became ever more involved with the clinical practice of critical care, and training programmes rapidly evolved to encompass the specialties of both respiratory medicine and critical care. This development was paralleled by the expansion of the critical care assembly of the American Thoracic Society to become the largest of eight assemblies, and in January 1994, under the editorial guidance of Robert Klock, the *American Review of Respiratory Diseases* became the *American Journal of Respiratory and Critical Care Medicine*. The journal welcomed manuscripts dealing with all aspects of critical care medicine, not just those related to the lungs. The respiratory physician with a background in ventilation is increasingly well placed to understand the critically ill patient and, in particular, to provide respiratory critical care.

This chapter makes the case that the respiratory physician should be involved in the delivery of all levels of critical care. With the increasing use of acute non-invasive ventilation (NIV), and with outreach teams identifying respiratory and circulatory failure much earlier on the wards, there is a growing need for the respiratory physician to be trained and involved in critical care. Respiratory medicine skills, particularly in NIV and bronchoscopy, can be supplemented with training in airway management and the circulation through training programmes such as those existing in the USA. The respiratory physician will then be well placed to provide a bridge between acute medicine and critical care.

DEFINITIONS

In the UK, the Department of Health has outlined categories of organ system monitoring and support in the following way, all of which should be available in intensive care.

- Advanced respiratory support: the provision of mechanical ventilation via endotracheal tube or tracheostomy, excluding mask ventilation unless complicated by other significant problems, or the potential need for intubation such as with impending respiratory failure and/or retained bronchial secretions.

- Patients who require $FiO_2 > 0.4$, those who may deteriorate and require increasing FiO_2 and/or 2-hourly chest physiotherapy, those recently extubated and those requiring respiratory support with continuous positive airways pressure (CPAP) or NIV by facemask. Some patients intubated for airway protection and otherwise stable would also require this form of monitoring and support.

- Circulatory support: the use of vasoactive drugs, the monitoring of circulatory instability due to hypovolaemia not responding to modest volume replacement, and following cardiac arrest.

- Neurologic monitoring and support: in the setting of central nervous system (CNS) depression and with the capability of invasive intracranial monitoring.

- Renal support: acute renal replacement treatment via various routes such as peritoneal dialysis and haemofiltration.

The intensive care unit (ICU) is characterized by a designated area where the minimum nurse:patient ratio is 1:1 (not including the nurse in charge of the shift) and with 24-h resident medical cover. There is the ability to provide advanced respiratory support and to support other organ system failures such as circulatory and renal failure as well as the management of co-morbidities.

In contrast, a high dependency unit (HDU) is defined as an area capable of providing support of one organ system excluding invasive ventilatory support, a level of care intermediate between that of a general ward and the ICU. The HDU is characterized by a designated area with a minimum nurse:patient ratio of 1:2, appropriate monitoring facilities and the continuous availability of medical staff. This concept of specialized high dependency care had already been applied with the development of coronary care units (CCUs) and renal dialysis units in the 1950s in the USA and in the 1960s in the UK. The ubiquitous presence of CCUs has meant that cardiac disease in general (and myocardial infarction in particular) is dealt with separately in almost all hospitals. Renal dialysis units are less common and, in their absence, this procedure usually falls under the aegis of the ICU rather than the HDU. Another specialized unit that has existed in the USA for more than 25 years is the respiratory intensive care unit (RICU) or the pulmonary acute care unit. Here, complex respiratory support, including invasive ventilation, can be provided for cases of isolated respiratory failure and also limited circulatory support. The advantages of such an environment include the ability to cultivate respiratory expertise in ancillary staff and to develop and utilize weaning strategies. The existence of these units is in part due to the fact that lone respiratory failure accounts for 5–15% of a typical medical service's emergency work. They have also spawned regional weaning centres where patients who have proved difficult to liberate from assisted ventilation continue to be treated outside the more expensive ICU and with an improved chance of weaning.[4]

ADMISSION, DISCHARGE AND RE-ADMISSION POLICIES

Standards, policies and practice guidelines define expectations for clinical practice, create consistency and promote continuity. *Standards* are defined as the level of performance that can or should be expected. *Policies* are a non-negotiable requirement representing conditions that must exist to facilitate care of the standard expected. They are directions for the unit's operation. *Practice guidelines* (also referred to as clinical protocols) represent appropriate pathways for the management of a specific clinical problem. The American Society of Critical Care Medicine provides expert consensus recommendations on which 'best practice' may be based. The needs for such directives are many, not least to reduce unnecessary expenditure by providing a defence for limiting diagnostic testing and management strategies. By promoting the use of best evidence, they should be viewed as an important part of a total quality management programme and not simply a cookbook.

Admission, discharge and re-admission policies are crucial to the efficient running of the ICU, HDU and RICU. The aim of admission guidelines is to exclude patients who are well enough to be adequately cared for in a general ward, or those who are hopelessly ill. Suggested admission and discharge criteria were first published in the USA in 1988. In 1996, the Department of Health NHS Executive published *Guidelines on admission to and discharge from intensive care and high dependency units*.[5]

Admission criteria

Referral to the ICU for specialist care may be made from many clinical areas, including the accident and emergency department, general medicine and surgical wards, high dependency areas and occasionally from other ICUs. It is usually considered appropriate for patients requiring advanced respiratory support alone, or with combinations of two or more other organ system failures. Sufficient information must be made available to allow an assessment of potential reversibility, always erring on the side of optimism, and of comorbidities. Chronic impairment of one or more organs sufficient to restrict daily activities will weigh against admission. However, patients may accept limitations that others may not. The need or potential need for ventilatory support or for other complex organ system monitoring and/or support will be evident. High-risk surgical patients are another group deserving of intensive care, particularly because there are ample data indicating that ensuring appropriate intravascular volume resuscitation and maintaining blood pressure and O_2 delivery reduce morbidity and mortality in the early postoperative period.[6] Perioperative optimization has also been shown to improve outcome in a number of recent studies.

Admission to the HDU is appropriate for support of a single organ system, excluding *invasive* ventilation, although non-invasive positive-pressure ventilatory support (NIPPV) can be instituted provided suitable monitoring is available. However, the limited availability of such beds, in the UK in particular, means that many patients who may benefit from the services of the HDU may have to be admitted to a general ward. This widespread practice in the UK is reflected by the fact that ethically approved studies have been conducted on the use of NIV on the general ward in the treatment of patients with acute respiratory failure.[7] The advent of NIPPV has revolutionized the management of respiratory failure, but has produced a problem in identifying suitable locations for treating patients in this way and has provided added impetus to the concept of the RICU. One-third of acute admissions to hospital are with respiratory problems and one-third of these are in patients with acute or acute-on-chronic respiratory failure. Those patients not requiring imminent intubation and ventilation may benefit from early NIPPV, and an environment with expertise in this therapy may limit progression of the condition, thereby preventing the need for ICU admission. If respiratory failure remains the only major problem, then such RICUs can provide invasive ventilation with the advantages of a focused group of carers, nurses and therapists who are familiar with NIV, and this minimizes the period of intubation, partly due to the use of therapist-supervised protocols. The experience when both ICUs and RICUs are available is frequently that NIPPV is used to a greater extent in RICUs, perhaps for the reasons stated and due to the thoracic training of the medical personnel.

Discharge criteria

Patients must be discharged sensibly from scarce ICU beds to make room for more severely ill patients. The reported mortality after discharge from intensive care is 9–27%.[8,9] It may be assumed, although it is as yet unproven, that the dominant factor determining the risk of hospital death is the physiological risk score, and a reduction to acceptable levels should form the basis of a discharge. The importance of this has recently been reported by Daly et al.,[10] who developed a predictive model (with reference to patients' age, chronic health points, acute physiology points at discharge from the unit, length of stay in the unit and whether or not cardiac surgery had been performed) with a cut-off of 0.6 predicting subsequent mortality at 14% versus 1.5%. Those identified as at risk have a mortality of 25% and, if the model is valid, mortality after discharge from intensive care would be reduced by more than one-third if those patients stayed an extra 2 days in intensive care.

Re-admission criteria

ICU outcome studies have identified re-admission rates ranging from 4% to 10%, with 7.9% in the UK. It is important to identify patients at high risk of re-admission to allow them longer ICU stays or transfer to an appropriate HDU (or RICU). The original diagnoses most frequently associated with a re-admission are hypoxic respiratory failure, inadequate pulmonary toilet and gastrointestinal bleeding. The first two again raise the question of whether some of these patients should be managed from the outset in a specialized RICU.

ORGANIZATION AND ACTIVITY

The design and organisation should reflect the special needs of each specific group of critically ill patients. Current guidelines from national societies are available, but it is recognized that these may change. Open ward bays of four to eight beds are most common, with additional single rooms in an appropriate ratio to provide facilities for barrier nursing. The special HDU or single-discipline ICU may be best placed close to the general ICU to enable sharing of facilities (such as laboratory and technical staff). The patient area needs to be spacious enough to allow bedside services, hand-wash sinks should be prolific, and X-ray viewing boxes and emergency trolleys evident. Nursing stations will be integral, and other staff areas, as well as support and storage facilities, are necessary.

Activity will in large part determine staffing, and the relationship between the two is linked through levels of care. At a conference at Bethesda in 1983, levels of care were defined on the basis of average nursing workload measured by means of a Therapeutic Intervention Scoring System (TISS).[11] This provides the following levels of care:

- 40–45 TISS = 1 patient:1 nurse = ICU,
- 20–39 TISS = 1.5 patients:2 nurses = HDU,
- 10–19 TISS = medium/high level care.

The TISS concept remains valuable and was redefined by Reis Miranda et al.[12] as 1 point = 10.8 min of nurse work, therefore one nurse shift = 46 TISS points, a revalidation of the ICU/HDU nursing guidelines. Although each patient:nurse ratio represents a level of care, it is possible to aggregate the various levels of care to three: level I: ratio >3; level II: ratio average 2.5; level III: ratio <1.6.

Units might therefore be labelled not as ICU/HDU etc., but as in Table 20.1.

The actual activities involved in respiratory intensive care consist of regular and repetitive assessment designed to detect events that might result in patient harm. They invariably include:

- arterial blood gases for respiratory and metabolic acid–base status,
- pulse oximetry for arterial O_2 saturation,
- transcutaneous monitoring of CO_2,
- aspects of ventilation, respiratory muscle function and respiratory mechanics.

Table 20.1 *Levels of care defined according to nurse dependence, resource usage and Acute Physiology Score*

	P/N	Mean TISS	Mean SAPS
Grade III	<1.6	>28	>38
Grade II	1.7–2.9	27–16	37–25
Grade I	>3	<15	<24

P/N, patient/nurse ratio; TISS, Therapeutic Intervention Scoring System; SAPS, Simplified Acute Physiology Score.

Pulmonary artery catheterization may result in useful information at the expense of complications. When this should be performed is a balance of reasonable expectation that an event or change might occur and need to monitor therapy. Unnecessary monitoring can create patient 'harm', with attendant costs, device-related injury and, importantly, inappropriate clinical response.

Funding of intensive care is variable across the UK and Europe and inevitably this has led to rationing, with a consequent increase in the severity of illness of patients admitted to the ICU. Admission of patients to the general wards until their condition deteriorates to the point that intensive care is mandatory creates a situation in which too little is done too late and where the chance of reversing organ dysfunction is remote. This leads to inefficient use of resources for treating those who are no longer able to benefit. Part of the reason for insufficient funding may be the multiple-specialty status that exists in Europe, which leads to intensive care being a part of other specialty budgets. However, changes are afoot, both in continental Europe and in the UK, to allow intensive care to develop as a multidisciplinary subspecialty as in the USA. The variability in organizational structures within European intensive care was evident from the EURICUS study,[13] which also underscored the lack of independent specialty status for intensive care.

Partly as a result of these funding issues, important modifications in the practice of respiratory intensive care have recently emerged. The first of these is non-invasive ventilation in the acute care setting. The recent increase in the use of NIPPV in the acute care setting has been driven by the hope of reducing the complications of invasive ventilation and the costs. In patients with exacerbations of chronic obstructive airways disease, the largest single diagnostic category, an average success rate in avoiding intubation with survival of 83% has been demonstrated in five randomised, controlled trials,[14–18] compared with 61% in controls. Predictors of outcome have been assessed,[19] and secretions, an edentulous state and cardiovascular instability have been found to be negative influences. However, if assisted ventilation is indicated, it should first be attempted non-invasively using a facemask or nasal mask. The use of NIPPV has been extended to other causes of acute respiratory failure, and an international consensus conference[20] felt that 'NIPPV has the potential for reducing the morbidity and possibly the mortality, associated with hypercarbic or hypoxaemic respiratory failure'; also that, 'available studies indicate that NIPPV can be initiated outside the intensive care unit' and 'shortening weaning time and avoiding reintubation represent promising indications for NIPPV' (see also Chapters 13 and 22).

In a recent meta-analysis, Keenan *et al.*[21] concluded that the evidence supports the use of NIPPV in chronic obstructive pulmonary disease (COPD). A remaining question is where such therapy might be instituted. Some studies have used the ICU,[22] which limits the potential value in the 'real world', and another has examined the use of the general respiratory ward.[7] In the last-mentioned study, 232 patients with COPD and a respiratory acidosis (pH 7.25–7.35) in 14 UK hospitals were randomized to either NIPPV or 'usual' treatment and a reduced need for ventilation was demonstrated in the intervention group (15% versus 27%).

An alternative approach is to use specialized high dependency areas (the RICU) such as exist in Italy,[23] where more than one-half of the patients admitted to 26 units countrywide are treated with N1PPV as a first line of treatment. RICUs have not been widely developed in the UK, but in our experience they do have a valuable part to play.

This changing clinical scene provides both the need and the opportunity for the respiratory physician to be trained in critical care and to provide a bridge between acute medicine and intensive care. Indeed, the potential benefits of respiratory support outside the ICU include earlier intervention to prevent further respiratory deterioration and access to support for those who would not otherwise be admitted to the ICU. The selection of such patients requires a skilled team, including a respiratory physician, and adequate monitoring.

New indications for NIPPV may include help with weaning from mechanical ventilation and the avoidance of re-intubation. The respiratory physician practised in the art of NIPPV, if also competent in the management of the ventilated patient, is ideally placed to provide this. Although the majority of studies have been conducted in ICUs, NIPPV provides an opportunity for delivering ventilatory support in RICUs or HDUs, where other acute physicians would also be involved.

Another development has been the creation of centres for weaning from mechanical ventilation. Ventilatory dependency in the ICU occurs in 20% of patients. Resolution of the disease process preventing weaning from respiratory support may still be possible, but the economic pressure to transfer the patients from the ICU as soon as possible is ever present. Choosing the appropriate facility to which ICU patients should be discharged will depend on the patient's clinical condition, the resources of the transfer destination and whether weaning attempts will continue. Experience with continued attempts at liberation in long-term acute care facilities is accumulating.[24, 25]

Weaning centres in the USA such as exist in Los Angeles at Barlow Hospital have demonstrated economic viability, with the same benefits being suggested in Italy, where these patients constitute 12% of admissions to the RICUs.[23]

MULTIDISCIPLINARY CRITICAL CARE

Effective and efficient care needs the complementary knowledge and skills of physicians, nurses and administrators. For the ICU, there should be a single medical director as well as intensivists helped by senior trainees and residents. The nursing complement also needs an identified lead nurse, with accredited intensive care nurses, nurses in training and nursing assistants. Pharmacists, physiotherapists and other therapists also have an important part to play. The background of the medical and support teams varies across hospitals and across countries. In the UK, most critical care facilities are staffed by anaesthetists. In many, though not all, instances the responsible consultants continue to have regular sessions in the operating theatre, which prevent them from providing full-time ICU cover. At present, few units have full-time respiratory physician intensivists. However, as the training of respiratory physicians

comes to include intensive care, these physicians, when appointed to consultant posts, may have links with or input into the intensive care. Some will also extend their ICU training to include a period of anaesthesia, currently recommended in the UK to be a minimum of 6 months, which will allow accreditation in intensive care medicine and the opportunity to direct an ICU.

In contrast, in the USA, 80–85% of medical ICUs are staffed by respiratory physicians with additional credentials (Boards in Critical Care Medicine). In larger (regional and/or teaching) hospitals, intensive care medicine is subdivided by specialty (medical, coronary, obstetric, paediatric, surgical, with further subdivisions of surgery into cardiac versus general, and even organ transplantation specific), so that the respiratory critical care physician will usually only be responsible for strictly medical problems, being invited to consult on medical issues in the other units. The training of respiratory critical care physicians takes account of the limited experience of the medical ICU by including rotations through other surgical and specialist critical care areas. In smaller hospitals, intensive care patients may be cared for in the same unit, although by different specialists. Such units will usually have a respiratory medical care physician as medical director, with powers to override the management decisions of the specialists as clinical need dictates.

Nursing expertise in critical care environments includes familiarity with mechanical ventilation and invasive monitoring. The one-to-one or one-to-two nurse:patient ratio permits the nurse the time to provide a wide range of treatments, including respiratory therapy. This has tended to limit the development of the physiotherapy practitioner in the ICU. In some institutions, specialization as a respiratory physiotherapist is encouraged, such therapists being more acquainted with mechanical ventilation and bronchoscopy, although still without authority to alter ventilation management (see Chapter 6). The further specialization of such individuals into respiratory therapists has not happened in the UK as it has in the USA. In the USA, respiratory therapists supervise the ventilatory management of patients under the direction of a physician and are permitted to alter ventilatory strategies according to strict protocols. Such 'therapist-implemented protocols' have been used to extubate or wean patients in the ICU setting, with evidence of a significant reduction in the period of dependence or mechanical ventilation.[12,24]

At the other extreme, recent reviews of adult critical care services in the UK have re-emphasized the concept of the 'patient at risk', for whom delay in the recognition of their condition and transfer to an appropriate area result in a poorer outcome. Better training of junior medical and nursing staff, early-warning scoring systems and 'outreach' critical care has been advocated.[19] Goldhill has shown that physiologic abnormalities are common in the 24 hours preceding admission to the ICU.[23] Inadequate input from experienced clinicians has been noted,[24] as has the inadequate training in acute medicine that physicians in general have.[25] The respiratory physician with intensive care training is ideally placed to address these issues and to be part of, or even to direct, intensive care teams that provide outreach services.

REFERENCES

1. Lassen, HCA. A preliminary report of the 1952 epidemic of polio in Copenhagen with special reference to the treatment of acute respiratory insufficiency. *Lancet* 1953; **I**: 37–41.

2. Williams, AJ. Iron lung. In *The Oxford companion to the body*, ed. C Blakemore. Oxford: Oxford University Press, 2001; 406–7.

3. Gilbertson, AA. Before intensive therapy? *J R Soc Med* 1995; **88**: 459–63.

4. Sirio, CA, Angus, DC, Rosenthal, GE. Cleveland Health Quality Choice [CHQC] – an ongoing collaborative, community-based outcomes assessment program. *New Horiz* 1994; **2**: 321–5.

5. Department of Health. *Guidelines on admission to and discharge from intensive care and high dependency units*. London: NHS Executive, 1996.

6. Bishop, MH, Shoemaker, WC, Appel, PL, *et al*. Prospective randomised trial of survivor values of cardiac index, oxygen delivery and oxygen consumption as resuscitation endpoints in severe trauma. *J Trauma* 1995; **38**: 780–7.

7. Plant, PK, Owen, JL, Elliott, MW. Early use of non-invasive ventilation for acute exacerbations of COPD on general respiratory wards. A multicentre randomised controlled trial. *Lancet* 2000; **355**: 1931–5.

8. Munn, J, Willatts, SM, Tooley, MA. Health and activity after intensive care. *Anaesthesia* 1995; **50**: 1017–21.

9. Goodhill, DR, Sumner, A. Outcome of intensive care patients in a group of British intensive care units. *Crit Care Med* 1998; **26**: 1337–45.

10. Daly, K, Beale, R, Chang, RWS. Reduction in mortality after inappropriate early discharge from intensive care unit: logistic regression triage model. *BMJ* 2001; **322**: 1274–6.

11. Cullen, DJ, Ferrara, IC, Briggs, BA, *et al*. Survival, hospitalisation charges and follow-up results in critically ill patients. *N Engl J Med* 1976; **294**: 982–7.

12. Reis Miranda, D, Ryan, DW, Schaufeli, WB, *et al*. *Organisation and management of intensive care. A prospective study in 12 European countries*. Berlin: Springer, 1997.

13. Soohoo, G, Santiago, S, Williams, AJ. Nasal mechanical ventilation for hypercapnoeic respiratory failure in COPD. *Crit Care* 1994; **22**: 1253–61.

14. Keenan, SP, Kernerman, PD, Cook, DJ, *et al*. The effect of non-invasive positive pressure ventilation on mortality in patients with acute respiratory failure: a metaanalysis. *Crit Care Med* 1997; **25**: 1685–92.

15. Jasmer, RM, Luce, JM, Matthay, JA. Non-invasive positive pressure ventilation with standard medical therapy in hypercapnoeic acute respiratory failure. *Chest* 1997; **111**: 1672–8.

16. Confalonieri, M, Gorini, M, Ambrerino, C, *et al*. Respiratory intensive care units in Italy: a national census and prospective cohort study. *Thorax* 2001; **56**: 373–8.

17. Scheinhorn, DJ, Chao, DC, Stearn-Hassenpflug, M, *et al*. Outcomes in post ICU mechanical ventilation. A therapist-implemented weaning protocol. *Chest* 2001; **119**: 236–42.

18. Hamid, S, Noonan, YM, Williams, AJ, Davidson, AC. An audit of weaning from mechanical ventilation in a UK weaning centre. *Thorax* 1999; **54**: 86.

19. Jaeschke, RZ, Meade, MO, Guyatt, GH, *et al*. How to use diagnostic tests in the ICU; diagnosing weanability using f/Vt. *Crit Care Med* 1997; **25**: 1514–21.

20. Department of Health. *Comprehensive critical care – a review of adult critical care services*. Report. London: Department of Health, May 2000.

21. Department of Health and NHS Executive. Health Service Circular [HSC] 2000/17. *Modernising critical care services*. London: Department of Health, 23 May 2000.

22. Audit Commission. *Critical to success*. Report. London: HMSO, October 1999.

23. Goldhill, DR, White, SA, Sumner, A. Physiologic values and procedures in the 24 hours before ICU admission from the ward. *Anaesthesia* 1999; **54**: 529–34.

24. Neale, G. Risk management in the care of medical emergencies. *J R Coll Phys Lond* 1998; **32**: 125–9.

25. Federation of Medical Royal Colleges Acute Medicine. *The physician's role. Proposals for the future.* Report. London: Federation of Royal Colleges, Publications Unit RCP, February 2000.

21

Ethical issues in the intensive care unit

SEAN P KEENAN AND WILLIAM J SIBBALD

INTRODUCTION

The purpose of this chapter is to summarize ethical issues experienced on a regular basis by healthcare professionals working in the intensive care unit (ICU). Ethics has been defined as the discipline that deals with what is good and what is poor practice and includes moral duty or obligation. While this definition is open to interpretation, there is an added factor, generally recognized within medicine, of the obligation to conform to accepted professional standards of conduct. The interpretation of good and poor practices will vary among healthcare systems and will partially depend upon the values of the society in which they exist. As a starting point, the ethical principles that operate and influence clinical decision making are:

- patient *autonomy*, or the respect for a patients' right to self-direction, regardless of the opinion of healthcare providers,
- *beneficence*, or the obligation of healthcare workers to make decisions in the patient's best interest,
- *non-maleficence*, or the moral obligation to do no harm to the patient,
- *justice*, a concept originally attributed to Aristotle, that reminds us that everyone should be treated equally and not be discriminated against.

Other chapters in this book provide information that respiratory critical care physicians need to make important patient care decisions. To make good decisions, one requires both the knowledge of the underlying pathophysiology of the critically ill and the evidence (from the medical literature) regarding the potential benefit or harm of diagnostic and therapeutic options. Many decisions made in caring for the critically ill do not require the clinician to spend much time considering ethical principles, for example in the decision whether or not to perform a bronchoscopy for suspected ventilator-associated pneumonia or simply to initiate antibiotics. This chapter focuses on those decisions that do call for consideration of ethical principles and, therefore, require a different expertise. The following questions are covered.

- Should this patient be admitted to the ICU?
- Once in the ICU, should life-support measures be continued or extended?
- What role do advance directives play in decisions about ICU admission and care?
- Under what circumstances is consent required in the ICU and how should it be obtained?

SHOULD THIS PATIENT BE ADMITTED TO THE INTENSIVE CARE UNIT?

The ethics of intensive care unit admission

Various societies, including the Society of Critical Care Medicine, have addressed triaging critically ill patients to the level of care that best meets their needs.[1] Decisions regarding admission to the ICU incorporate all four ethical principles. One could reasonably include the principles of beneficence and non-maleficence in all decisions that medical practitioners make because our aim is always to help, not harm, our patients. We also respect patient autonomy, doing our best to follow a patient's wishes or those expressed by his or her surrogate decision maker. At times, however, the principle of justice may appear to be at odds with the others. ICU is a limited resource and, as such, there are times when we find ourselves acting not only as patient advocates but also as administrators who must 'manage' this scarce resource. From the perspective of a physician manager, therefore, it may be appropriate to deny admission to the ICU, despite the requests of family or fellow clinicians, if it appears that a patient will not benefit from this admission. But how do we know?

What is the role of the intensive care unit?

Although this may seem an odd question, it is a reasonable place to start when trying to define who should be admitted to an intensive care unit. Generally, intensive care units exist:

- to provide *life support*,
- to provide *intensive monitoring* for patients who do not currently require life support but who require interventions that may avoid the need for life support, for example a patient with an active gastrointestinal bleed or a brittle diabetic with severe ketoacidosis.

Each ICU admission comes with its own unique set of ethical issues. While it is often apparent which patient requires life support to continue to survive in the short term, whether life support should be provided for a specific patient may require serious ethical deliberation. Prior to instituting life-support measures, the following factors should, ideally, be satisfied.

- Is the institution of life support consistent with the patient's wishes (patient autonomy)?
- Will the patient benefit from the institution of life support in the short or long term (beneficence, non-maleficence)?

To answer the first question, a clinician (usually not an intensivist) should have the opportunity to discuss life support with the patient, either during a previous clinical encounter or at the time of presentation. In the latter case, patient competence must be considered. Critically ill patients, even while conscious, may not be able to give truly informed consent; there may be impaired cognitive function as a result of the critical illness or of medications, such as analgesics and sedatives. In these circumstances, a surrogate, such as a family member or general physician, may act on the patient's behalf. It is important to note that the person who can act as surrogate varies amongst different healthcare systems. Each practitioner must review with local authorities the legislation that defines the appropriate surrogate for their patients. When decisions have to be made quickly in the absence of explicit directions, the default is to provide resuscitation and life support until appropriate discussions can take place, i.e. presume 'life'.

The second question of patient benefit from life support is more difficult and often cannot be fully assessed prior to instituting life-support measures. Resuscitation may be required immediately (to sustain life) and before the clinician has a full understanding of the process underlying the patient's acute presentation. In other cases, however, there will be time for discussion of the benefits and detriments of initiating life support. A patient's prognosis may be so poor that the initiation of life support may be inappropriate; the patient may therefore be considered too ill for an ICU admission. Deciding not to admit a patient to the ICU on the grounds that he or she is too ill to benefit from admission is an increasingly common scenario for the critical care physician. The factors to take into account in considering admission to an ICU include the following:[1]

- the likelihood of a successful outcome,
- the patient's life expectancy due to the disease(s),

- the anticipated health status of the patient,
- the wishes of the patient (or surrogate),
- the burdens for those affected, including financial and psychological,
- missed opportunities to treat other patients,
- health and other needs of the community,
- individual and institutional moral and religious values.

Another group of patients considered for admission to the ICU are those who require intensive monitoring (versus life-support) measures. These patients are increasingly considered for triaging to a level of care other than the ICU – an example is a high dependency unit (HDU). In the past decade, we have seen the introduction of intermediate care units designed specifically to care for patients requiring more intensive monitoring than is available on the general ward. When such a resource is not available, decision making becomes more complex. The availability of ICU beds, alternate areas of care and the flexibility of the nurse:patient ratio on the general ward will often dictate local practice. What may be an inappropriate admission to the ICU in one institution may be justifiable in another.

Today's ICU physician, therefore, needs to be constantly alert to the ethical principles of patient autonomy, beneficence and non-maleficence when admitting patients. However, as the role of the ICU physician has expanded from being a care provider to 'administrating' or 'managing' critical care beds, we find ourselves forced to consider the fourth principle of justice to a greater degree. This is not necessarily a bad thing: realizing that we cannot admit everyone to the ICU, we have been forced to learn more about the prognosis of different patient groups. In the end, knowledge of prognosis, driven by the principle of justice, should lead to decisions that are also in our patients' best interests.

ONCE IN THE ICU, SHOULD LIFE-SUPPORT MEASURES BE CONTINUED OR EXTENDED?

Withholding and withdrawal of life support

A major ethical decision confronting critical care professionals is whether, at some point in the patient's ICU stay, life-support measures should be limited or withdrawn. Just as with an ICU admission, this decision also incorporates the four ethical principles. Care for the critically ill patient is invasive, stressful and at times uncomfortable and painful. In some circumstances, continuing full life support could be considered contrary to the principle of non-maleficence – but it could be justified if the eventual outcome is considered to be good (beneficence). With an increasing understanding of the natural history and prognosis of critical illness, critical care professionals may find themselves caring for patients they know to have little chance of survival.

Some patients die early in their ICU stay despite aggressive therapy and before there is any need to reach a consensus that the outlook is hopeless, but these are a minority. More often in the ICU we become aware that a patient's outcome is extremely poor after the institution of life support, and this same patient may require addition of further life support measures to 'survive' in the short term. At this time a decision must be made about whether the process of *adding* or *continuing* life-support measures is appropriate. Just as before, we act in the patient's best interest (beneficence), while avoiding harm (non-maleficence), and are guided by the patient's wishes (patient autonomy). Possible decisions in this setting include:

- continuing full aggressive management,
- continuing all measures, but limiting resuscitation in the event of a cardiac arrest,
- maintaining, but not escalating, the current level of life support (withholding life support),
- withdrawal of some, or all, current life support.

In most cases, discussion with other clinicians and family members leads to a consensus that is consistent with autonomy, beneficence and non-maleficence. At times, however, differences of opinion arise and clinicians find themselves in a situation in which patient autonomy, expressed by surrogate decision makers, is at odds with perceived principles of beneficence, non-maleficence and justice. Justice could then be violated when resources needed by other patients are dedicated to someone who has no chance of recovery. Sometimes, the pressure to continue care comes from other clinicians rather than from family members. This may particularly be the case following iatrogenic complications or critical illness following routine surgery.

What is happening now?

In a landmark paper, Smedira and colleagues documented end of life care for two San Francisco ICUs in the late 1980s.[2] At that time, 51% of deaths followed the decision either to withhold or withdraw life support (although this high figure was partly due to the fact that brain-dead patients were included in the study). In a follow-up study 5 years later, the same group documented a significant increase to 90% in the proportion of patients who died following withholding or withdrawal of life support.[3] Reports from many centres over the past decade note that approximately 70–80% of patients die following limiting or withdrawal of life support. Because such studies do not provide a complete view of practice in general, Cook and colleagues used hypothetical clinical case scenarios to demonstrate the variation among healthcare professionals in decision making about life-support limitation.[4] Factors considered most important included: the likelihood of the patient surviving the current episode, the likelihood of long-term survival, pre-morbid cognitive function and patient age.

In a related study by the same group, healthcare workers choosing either extreme levels of care (full aggressive management) or comfort measures with in the same patient scenario were equally confident in their decision.[5] This scenario-based study reported what clinicians say they would do (rather than what they actually do), but it was consistent with another study that included data from 131 different ICUs from 38 US states.[6] After excluding brain-dead patients, this study reported that 26% of patients died despite full aggressive therapy, 24% died without cardiopulmonary resuscitation, 14% died following limitation of life support and 36% died following the withdrawal of life support. The most interesting findings were the differences amongst institutions. For example, death following the withdrawal of life support varied from 0% to 79%. It is interesting that the rate of withdrawal of life support was lowest in the two US states with strict legal standards for surrogate involvement in the decision-making process (New York and Missouri). The medico-legal environment may therefore lead to practices that might be considered not to be in the patients' best interest.

Another US survey also found variation in practice among respondents. In this survey, 12% stated that they had withdrawn life support without the knowledge of the family and 3% had withdrawn life support against the objections of the family.[7] These findings highlight the potential ethical dilemma that arises when physicians feel that their obligation to the principles of beneficence and non-maleficence run contrary to the wishes of the family. Whereas it is generally believed that physicians are not obligated to provide futile care, many are probably uncomfortable acting in opposition to family requests. However, this survey demonstrates that physicians will act against family wishes if they believe both that further care is futile and that they are supported by their healthcare system.

The withholding and withdrawal of life support have been deemed to be ethically the same by the United States President's Commission, a position endorsed by most professional societies (including the Society of Critical Care Medicine, the British Medical Society and the American College of Chest Physicians). Despite these endorsements, a significant number of healthcare workers do not view these two actions as being equivalent. In a survey by the Ethics Committee of the Society of Critical Care Medicine, 43% of respondents believed that withholding life support was more acceptable than withdrawing life support, and 26% admitted to being more disturbed by withdrawing life support than by simply withholding it. We found that withholding life support was more common in community hospitals than in teaching centres, consistent with findings that greater experience with end of life decision making is associated with a higher level of withdrawal of life support.[8]

If one considers the withholding and withdrawal of life support to be ethically the same, then continuing some life-support measures (but not others) could be perceived as acting contrary to the patient's best interests, violating the principles of beneficence and non-maleficence.

Once a decision has been reached to withdraw life support, which modalities should be withdrawn and in what order? We have noted that official statements of professional societies and ethicists suggest *all* forms of withdrawal of life support are ethically the same. Despite this, analysis of current practice clearly shows that there is more widespread comfort in withdrawing haemofiltration or inotropic support versus ventilation, nutrition and fluid therapy. Some practitioners may feel that the withdrawal of fluid therapy is cruel, but there is no evidence that patients suffer as a result if the process is accompanied by careful attention to the use of sedation and narcotics. In the UK, the British Medical Association affirms that withholding fluids and nutrition does not constitute the removal of basic medical care (which should always be provided) as nasogastric feeding is seen as artificial, i.e. a therapy. Nevertheless, it recommends resort to the courts, for the time being, before such removal in cases of persistent vegetative state and stresses the need for multi-professional agreement to such discontinuation of therapy.[9]

The approach used to withdrawing life support has also been found to vary. In general, patients receive adequate medication in the form of opiates, with or without sedation, and life-support modalities are withdrawn at varying rates, sequentially or all together. While the ethically most correct approach continues to be debated, we support an approach that is as rapid as patient (and sometimes family) comfort will allow.

The approach to limiting or withdrawing life support also varies among healthcare systems. This section has focused primarily upon practice as reported in North American centers. Compared to the USA, critical care physicians in both the UK and Australia historically seem to have adopted a more paternalistic approach to decision making. This may now change as a result of implementation of the European Human Rights Act. Guidance from the British Medical Association on withdrawing and withholding[9] provides a clear analysis of the ethical issues involved, especially for incompetent individuals (through illness or lack of understanding) and, compared with previous practice, is more patient centred.

In a study examining the attitudes of critical care physicians, ethical questions were approached differently in 16 different European countries.[10] Differences were partially related to geography, with southern countries tending to be more conservative than the northern ones. This may reflect differences in religious bias, with southern countries comprising a greater proportion of Catholics compared to Protestants. 'Do not resuscitate' orders after a cardiac arrest are more common in the north, with the Netherlands leading the way at 91%, compared to a low of 8% in Italy. Similar differences in geography were found concerning the frequency of withholding

and withdrawal of life support and the use of drug administration to precipitate death. It should be noted that although physicians may claim a specific religious affiliation, they may or may not adhere to its beliefs. Both withdrawal of life support and the administration of drugs to hasten death were less common among physicians viewing themselves as religious.

WHAT ROLE DO ADVANCE DIRECTIVES PLAY IN DECISIONS ABOUT ICU ADMISSION AND CARE?

An important development is the increased prevalence of advanced care planning and the documents that have been developed around this issue.[11] The latter are referred to as 'advanced directives' and are comprised of an individual's wishes, in writing, regarding the use of life-support measures that should/should not be provided in the event that he or she is no longer able to participate in such decisions. In the interests of the ethical principle of patient autonomy, the development of advanced directives provides a means for patients to discuss potential health scenarios and to express their wishes regarding the use of life-support measures. In general, advanced directives designate a surrogate decision maker for a patient who is either unconscious or deemed incompetent.

In theory, advanced directives are a good idea and ensure patient autonomy, but problems still remain. An advanced directive is only useful if it is extensive enough to cover all potential scenarios. For an advanced directive to be effective requires both considerable time on the part of the physician (often more than is available) and physician knowledge of the clinical scenarios (which may be beyond his or her area of expertise).

Whereas some advanced directives are comprehensive, others provide less specific statements, such as 'I do not wish to be kept alive on life support if there is no hope of recovery'. (Perhaps it is a sign of how far we have progressed that most ICU physicians would find such a statement to be unhelpful!) The days of protracted life support for patients without hope of recovery have largely disappeared in North America and Europe. ICU physicians are generally comfortable with advising the withdrawal of care under such circumstances, and society is generally supportive. However, a statement of patient's wishes when there is no hope of recovery is only a starting point. In reality, critical care professionals work in a setting that deals in probabilities rather than certainties. The question is: in the scenario with such-and-such a probability of surviving hospital stay, with such-and-such a range of potential health status, and knowing the prior quality of life, would the patient want life support continued, resuscitation, etc? To make the situation more difficult, the scenario changes with time and alters the prognosis.

Although there are potential pitfalls in advanced directives, they are clearly important and will become increasingly useful as those involved (physicians, lawyers, family and patients) work together. There is clearly a desire among both physicians and the general public for their development. A SUPPORT study[12] underlined the fact that physicians are often not aware of their patients' wishes regarding resuscitation and life-support measures. One helpful development in advanced directives is the introduction of *decision aids*. These consist of well-thought-out scenarios that allow future patients to make decisions in the setting of uncertainty that reflects the reality of medicine. Although still not perfect, they add information about how patients feel about the use of life-support measures.

UNDER WHAT CIRCUMSTANCES IS CONSENT REQUIRED IN THE ICU AND HOW SHOULD IT BE OBTAINED?

Consent in medicine is generally sought for two different reasons:

- to administer a therapy or to conduct a diagnostic test for clinical reasons,
- to enroll a patient in a research protocol.

In both cases, permission is ideally sought from a competent patient. However, critically ill patients who are not conscious or are clearly disoriented and confused are appropriately considered incompetent and cannot give informed consent. Other critically ill patients who may appear alert and oriented, and thus competent, may not recall any events from their ICU stay. It is not possible to foresee which patients will or

will not recall conversations. Although these patients are usually considered competent to give consent, it may be best to involve family members in the process (assent) to ensure that decisions are felt to be consistent with the patient's pre-morbid character.

Patients who are considered incompetent require a surrogate decision maker. In some US states and Canadian provinces, legislation exists that clearly defines how to identify an appropriate surrogate. As mentioned previously, advanced directives can help to identify the patient's chosen surrogate. In the setting in which no family exists, these states or provinces will appoint a surrogate to act on the patient's behalf. Where there are no formal procedures for the designation of a surrogate decision maker, the issue of consent is approached in a variety of ways, but usually involves physicians acting on the patient's behalf.

The issue of consent to participate in a research study requires even greater care, as there is no evidence that critically ill patients will benefit from their involvement in the study, and they may even be harmed. The principles of patient autonomy (respect for patient choice, obtaining informed consent and maintaining confidentiality), beneficence (favourable balance of potential benefit and harm) and justice (all must be equally likely to be involved) must be applied.[11] In addition, the study must be scientifically valid, address a question of sufficient value, be conducted honestly and be reported accurately and promptly.[11]

SUMMARY

This chapter highlights the main ethical issues that are involved in caring for the acutely unwell. Clearly, on-going study of practice and how we make these sometimes difficult decisions is required. Researchers in this area have provided us with a framework, but further work is needed to understand how we can best serve our patients. Our decisions will become easier as the public becomes more aware of what current medical technology can and cannot achieve. Although practice will always vary among healthcare systems, and even amongst physicians, it is hoped that greater attention to ethical issues will make these decisions less difficult for all in the future.

REFERENCES

1. Society of Critical Care Medicine Ethics Committee. Consensus statement on the triage of critically ill patients. *JAMA* 1994; **271**: 1200–3.

2. Smedira, NG, Evans, BH, Grais, LS, *et al*. Withholding and withdrawal of life support from the critically ill. *N Engl J Med* 1990; **322**: 309–15.

3. Prendergast, TJ, Luce, JM. Increasing incidence of withholding and withdrawal of life support from the critically ill. *Am J Respir Crit Care Med* 1997; **155**: 15–20.

4. Cook, DJ, Guyatt, GH, Jaeschke, R, *et al*. Determinants in Canadian health care workers of the decision to withdraw life support from the critically ill. *JAMA* 1995; **273**: 703–8.

5. Walter, SD, Cook, DJ, Guyatt, GH, *et al*. Confidence in life-support decisions in the intensive care unit: a survey of healthcare workers. *Crit Care Med* 1998; **26**: 44–9.

6. Prendergast, TJ, Claessens, MT, Luce, JM. A national survey of end-of-life care for critically ill patients. *Am J Respir Crit Care Med* 1998; **158**: 1163–7.

7. Asch, DA, Hansen-Flaschen, J, Lanken, PN. Decisions to limit or continue life-sustaining treatment by critical care physicians in the United States: conflicts between physicians' practices and patients' wishes. *Am J Respir Crit Care Med* 1995; **151**: 288–92.

8. Keenan, SP, Busche, KD, Chen, LM, *et al*. Withdrawal of withholding of life support in the intensive care unit: a comparison of teaching and community hospitals. *Crit Care Med* 1998; **26**: 245–51.

9. *Withholding and withdrawing life-prolonging medical treatment. guidance for decision making*, 2nd edition. London: BMJ Books, 2001.

10. Vincent, JL. Forgoing life support in western European intensive care units: the results of an ethical questionnaire. *Crit Care Med* 1999; **27**: 1626–33.

11. Singer, PA. *Bioethics at the bedside: a clinician's guide*. Ottawa: Canadian Medical Association, 1999.

12. The SUPPORT Principal Investigators. A controlled trial to improve care for seriously ill hospitalized patients: the study to understand prognoses and preferences for outcomes and risks of treatments (SUPPORT). *JAMA* 1995; **274**: 1591–8.

13. The Acute Respiratory Distress Syndrome Network. Ventilation with lower tidal volumes for acute lung injury and the acute respiratory distress syndrome. *N Engl J Med* 2000; **342**: 1301–8.

22

Respiratory failure: new horizons, new challenges

A CRAIG DAVIDSON AND DAVID F TREACHER

INTRODUCTION

This final chapter reviews the current management of acute respiratory failure and discusses some of the areas of controversy identified in the preceding chapters. The management of acute respiratory failure is, at present, undergoing re-evaluation in the light of recent research and technological developments. Similar to the way in which 'clot-busting' therapy has impacted on cardiology, non-invasive ventilation (NIV) is acting as the catalyst for this change. 'Patient at-risk teams' (PART)[1] and 'medical emergency teams'[2] have developed in response to the evidence that the care of the ward patient whose condition is deteriorating may be inadequate and the delay in referral to the intensive care unit (ICU) may be fatal. An important aspect of the experience of PART teams is that respiratory distress is recognized as a frequent feature of the deteriorating ward patient.[3, 4] Its presence should trigger medical review and prompt a decision regarding the need for respiratory support and whether the use of non-invasive respiratory support in the high dependency area is appropriate or whether referral to intensive care is necessary. Recommendations for 'seamless' care and dissolution of the historical barriers between ICUs and general wards are compelling.[5] The details of delivery will inevitably vary amongst hospitals and amongst different countries, but, at the interface between the admitting clinician and the ICU, a system needs to be in place that identifies 'at-risk' patients, monitors their well-being, appropriately 'steps up' care when necessary and carefully observes patients following their discharge from the ICU.

RECOGNIZING RESPIRATORY FAILURE

Classical medical teaching divides respiratory failure into two forms (Table 22.1). Both are characterized by a low PaO_2 (by definition, < 8 Kpa or 60 mmHg). In type 1 there is alveolar hyperventilation and in type 2 alveolar hypoventilation. The patient with type 1 respiratory failure will usually present with obvious respiratory distress, whereas recognition of type 2 failure may be more difficult. Assessment of severity, which will be necessary to determine care, depends on both the response to an increase in the inspired oxygen concentration (FiO_2), because this reflects the size of the disturbance of gas exchange (the $A - a$ gradient), and the underlying cause of respiratory distress along with any other associated

Table 22.1 *Causes of respiratory failure*

Type 1 respiratory failure (primary abnormality: ventilation/perfusion mismatch)
  Acute lung injury/acute respiratory distress syndrome
  Cardiogenic pulmonary oedema
  Pneumonia
  Pulmonary embolism
  Pneumothorax
  Asthma (moderate)
  Interstitial lung disease
Type 2 respiratory failure (primary abnormality: respiratory pump failure)
  Central nervous system encephalopathy, e.g. cerebrovascular accident, opiates, head injury
  Peripheral neurological causes, e.g. myasthenia gravis, Guillain–Barré, cervical spine injury, poliomyelitis
  Muscle disease, e.g. muscular dystrophy, critical illness myopathy
  Chest-wall disease, e.g. scoliosis, thoracoplasty, trauma
  Severe left ventricular failure or asthma
  Chronic obstructive airways disease

chronic illnesses. For instance, if the young man with pneumonia requires an FiO_2 of 60% to maintain SaO_2 >90% and he has associated organ dysfunction, e.g. hypotension, his care demands ICU admission. On the other hand, in the patient with a malignant pleural effusion, a similar degree of respiratory distress would indicate the urgent need for pleurocentesis rather than transfer to a higher dependency area.

The patient with type 2 respiratory failure is frequently more difficult to identify and it can be particularly difficult to judge the risk of deterioration with the final outcome of respiratory arrest. In patients with chronic neuromuscular or chest wall disease, the onset of respiratory failure may be insidious. Life-threatening episodes can be precipitated by minor illness, yet the presentation is often with confusion and hypersomnolence rather than breathlessness. Examination of arterial blood gases is therefore critical in evaluation. In the patient with chronic respiratory failure, renal compensation will be evident by an increase in buffer capacity. Back titration to a normal pH then provides a guide to the 'normal' PCO_2. As a rough guide, an acute increase in $PaCO2$ of 1 kPa decreases pH by 0.06 units, whereas in chronic hypercapnia, with renal adjustment, it decreases pH by 0.02 units.[6] In our experience, confusion often arises when there is a co-existent circulatory or septic cause for acidosis – hence the importance of calculating the anion gap, measuring serum lactate and testing for urinary ketones to exclude diabetic ketoacidosis.

If respiratory failure develops as a result of central nervous system (encephalopathy, trauma, infection etc.) or peripheral nerve disease (Guillain–Barré, myasthenia gravis), hypoxaemia develops at a later stage in the presence of a normal A–a gradient. It is caused by marked hypoventilation as the vital capacity (VC) falls below 1 L and is reflected by progressive hypercapnia. Clinical suspicion and monitoring of serial VC and arterial blood gases are therefore important aspects of the care of such patients. It is in the 'yet to be diagnosed' patient that the risk of sudden deterioration is greatest. Here, the unsupervised, or unthinking, use of supplemental O_2 may make appropriate assessment *less* likely as the nurse, or junior doctor, is falsely reassured by a 'normal' oximeter reading.

RECOGNIZING THE NEED FOR ASSISTED VENTILATION IN CHRONIC OBSTRUCTIVE PULMONARY DISEASE

Confusion arising from the use of inappropriate O_2 therapy is more commonly a feature of advanced respiratory failure resulting from chronic obstructive pulmonary disease (COPD). The mechanisms of O_2 toxicity in these circumstances remain controversial. Three factors are implicated: a reduction in central drive, a deterioration in gas exchange resulting from increased shunt, secondary to relief of hypoxic vasoconstriction, and a change to a less fatiguing but excessively rapid breathing pattern all contribute.[7–9] The pathophysiological mechanisms of CO_2 retention in COPD include hyperinflation impairing pump efficiency, an abnormal respiratory pattern, with additional dynamic hyperinflation as expiratory time shortens, and resistive work resulting from air flow obstruction. Although minute ventilation is increased, alveolar ventilation falls as load exceeds the capacity of the ventilatory pump. Worsening respiratory failure disturbs sleep so that *in extremis* it is difficult to distinguish central fatigue from electrophysiological respiratory muscle failure. Untreated, the tachypnoeic agitated patient lapses into confusion, with a fall in respiratory effort and terminal bradycardia and asystolic cardiac arrest. At what stage in this process should the clinician initiate ventilatory support?

The risk of death or of reaching the point of unequivocal need for endotracheal intubation is better predicted by pH and PCO_2 than by the degree of hypoxaemia For instance, in trials assessing the impact of NIV, pH has been found to be predictive. In the Brochard *et al.* study, [10] 74% of patients with a mean pH 7.26 who were managed conventionally required intubation and the subsequent in-hospital mortality was 29%. In the Plant *et al.* study, [11] 27% of those with pH 7.25–7.35 reached the intubation criteria and had a hospital mortality of 20%. In another survey of outcome, Soo Hoo *et al.* reported a 54% intubation rate, which increased to 72% when pH <7.2.[12] Subsequent multivariate analysis from the Plant study revealed that pH and PCO_2 both contribute to risk, although the sensitivity and specificity of these factors alone do not allow sufficiently accurate prediction for application on an individual basis.[13] For instance, the odds ratio for a patient with pH 7.30 and PCO_2 8 kPa was 3.84, compared to 16.8 for pH 7.25 and PCO_2 10 kPa. Data from this study also showed that pH often improves between the accident and emergency department and ward admission with conventional non-ventilator management. In the absence of a clear need for intubation, such as a Glasgow Coma Score <8, respiratory rate >40 or <10 min^{-1}, conservative therapy should therefore be initially employed. It is the failure to improve, or further deterioration, that signals the need for assisted ventilation.

In Chapter 5, Dr Schönhofer reviewed the evidence for using NIV in respiratory failure for both COPD and non-COPD causes. What is becoming apparent is that the patient whose condition stabilizes or improves with NIV has a better prognosis.[14] Part of the benefit clearly arises from avoidance of the complications of intubation and the risks involved with intensive care admission. Failure with NIV is an adverse prognostic sign, presumably because it indicates more serious underlying pathophysiology. However, there is the danger, however, that inappropriate use of NIV, and delayed recourse to intubation when it is failing, might also be responsible. One of the recommendations made by the British Thoracic Society in its guidelines for acute NIV, [15] and in a consensus document on NIV, [16] is that clear limits should be set to define what constitutes a 'trial of therapy'. Explicit in these recommendations is the requirement to determine the appropriateness of aggressive management, including intubation and admission to the ICU.

DETERMINING APPROPRIATENESS OF ASSISTED VENTILATION

Guidelines have been published to assist clinicians in the UK in the difficult area of limiting or withholding therapy.[17] It is an area, as described in Chapter 21, that is culturally and religiously determined and that is fast changing. Despite the considerable investment in time and training required, a more open discussion with patients to determine their wishes is to be encouraged.[18] In many cases, however, this may not be possible because the patients' condition renders them 'non-competent'. In the absence of advance directives, decision-making then rests with the clinician. What guidance is available? In a large European and US study, involving 1426 patients, survival following mechanical ventilation for respiratory failure (all causes) was 55%.[19] Depending upon the severity of lung injury, survival ranged from 18% to 67%; multi-organ failure carried a 90% mortality rate. Outcome is critically dependent on the population of patients included in studies and this is particularly the case in COPD. Of those admitted to hospital, and therefore including milder cases, approximately 10% will die and the 1 year survival is reported at 58%.[20] Of those not requiring ventilatory support, 57–88% are reported to survive to 1 year, [21] falling to 34–56% following intubation and a period of mechanical ventilation.[22, 23]

A better outcome (58–87%) has been reported following mechanical ventilation with NIV.[13, 24, 25] Age, severity of airflow obstruction and presence of chronic respiratory failure largely determine survival in COPD. It remains to be seen whether prognosis is really affected by avoidance of intubation by NIV and whether prognosis can be further improved with domiciliary NIV in these at-risk patients.[26, 27]

WEANING IN TYPE 2 RESPIRATORY FAILURE

In Chapter 13, Dr Nava and colleagues considered the weaning process through which patients are liberated from mechanical ventilation. Although protocols allow earlier identification of the patient ready to breath spontaneously, and possibly speed the process,[28, 29] there is no evidence to indicate that any one method is indisputably superior to another in speeding the process – although synchronized intermittent mandatory ventilation (SIMV) seems to be the least favoured. Again, NIV is changing practice. For COPD patients, there is often a 'window of opportunity' early in their ICU stay, when the acute physiology has been corrected, sleep restored and dynamic hyperinflation and airway obstruction reduced and before sedative drugs have accumulated, when they may be extubated onto NIV. Although the evidence is at present limited, NIV may allow speedier extubation at a time when more conventional indices of 'weanability' are not satisfied.[30, 31] Physiological studies certainly show that NIV offloads the respiratory muscles as effectively as invasive pressure support and is preferred by patients.[32] Even if extubation criteria are met, patients with underlying COPD have a an incidence of post-extubation failure of over 20%, and again NIV may be useful in preventing re-intubation.[33] Sometimes, glottic or supraglottic narrowing contributes to post-extubation respiratory distress and these aspects will not be detected by conventional extubation criteria . In addition to treating upper airway narrowing, with steroids or nebulized adrenaline, helium/O_2 mixtures may be useful.[34] Certainly, avoiding re-intubation is important. Such patients have a higher mortality and this is, to some extent, explained by exposure to the risks of further nosocomial infection. Re-intubation almost invariably leads to the insertion of a tracheostomy and, with this, poten-

tially a more prolonged ICU stay. In these circumstances, the availability of a coordinated weaning service is helpful and, if available, a respiratory intensive care unit (RICU) or a high dependency unit (HDU) would be the most suitable location for continued weaning and rehabilitation.

Although severe COPD is a common reason for delayed weaning, underlying neuromuscular or chest-wall disease, and co-morbidity with cardiovascular or central nervous system problems complicating the initial reason for ICU admission, are also frequent reasons for patients remaining ventilator dependent.[35] In 153 weaning referrals to our specialist respiratory ICU between 1998 and 2000, there was a 73% overall survival to discharge, with 1-year and 2-year survivals of 63% and 50%, respectively. Interestingly, 54% of patients referred from outside hospitals required ventilatory support at discharge, compared with 22% for 'in-house' referrals, reflecting both the longer duration of ICU stay before referral and the higher incidence of neuromuscular disease among outside referrals.[36] It would be useful if there were reliable prognostic features for predicting eventual success at weaning in this type of patient. The obvious factors, such as age, presence of co-morbidity and pre-morbid level of functioning, are not sufficiently predictive and we therefore place more importance on patient motivation and family support. In the UK, if weaning eventually proves unsuccessful, the option of continued invasive mechanical ventilation in an institution is limited, and domiciliary care is critically dependent upon the provision of suitable carers and acquiring sufficient funding. Long-term care facilities are available in the USA,[37] and it would appear that support in the rest of Europe for these patients is better and more centrally co-ordinated than in the UK. Provision varies considerably amongst countries, with few COPD patients receiving mechanical ventilation at home in the Netherlands but contributing a rapidly rising proportion to the total home-care population in France and Germany.

REFRACTORY HYPOXAEMIA

For the purpose of this discussion, refractory hypoxaemia is defined as an arterial oxygen tension that is ≤10 kPa (75 mmHg), with an inspired oxygen tension (FiO_2) of at least 0.6, which has failed to respond to routine respiratory therapy. These levels correspond to a hypoxaemia index (PaO_2/FiO_2) of ≤ 125 mmHg (16.7 kPa). The conventional definition of hypoxaemia as PaO_2 <8 kPa when breathing air (FiO_2 of 0.21) represents a hypoxaemia index <285 mmHg (38 kPa).

It is important to note that the currently used American European Consensus Guidelines for defining hypoxaemia in acute lung injury and ARDS[38] take no account of the positive end-expiratory pressure (PEEP) level or other set ventilatory parameters when the hypoxaemia index is derived. It seems both misleading and likely to cause heterogeneity in study populations if the level of PEEP is not standardized before the calculation of this index. In this discussion it is assumed that optimum ventilator management includes a PEEP level of at least 10 cmH$_2$O and that other general aspects of management, including drainage of large pleural air or fluid collections, have been addressed.

The following issues related to the management of refractory hypoxaemia are discussed:

- 'appropriate' target levels for arterial oxygenation and inspired O_2 concentration,
- 'appropriate' fluid balance targets and circulatory management – the attempt to identify the 'correct' balance between an adequate intravascular volume and increased lung oedema,
- additional therapies that should be considered when the optimum ventilatory, fluid balance and circulatory strategies have failed to improve oxygenation.

What are the appropriate target levels for arterial PaO_2 and FiO$_2$: pulmonary oxygen toxicity or permissive hypoxaemia?

Appropriately for a book on respiratory critical care, considerable space has been devoted to the causes and management of patients with primary lung pathologies that result in severe hypoxaemia. However, the issue of oxygen delivery has not been addressed.

Because the prime function of the lungs is to oxygenate the blood and, together with the circulation, to ensure that the oxygen supply to the tissues meets their individual and fluctuating require-

ments, it is important to consider this component of the O_2 cascade.

The delivery of O_2 from the external environment via the lungs to the mitochondria within individual cells is summarized in Figure 22.1, with values quoted for a 75-kg individual undertaking normal activity. The delivery of O_2 from the environment to the systemic circulation is the part of the O_2 cascade that is best understood, but there remains much to be learnt about the factors that control regional delivery, diffusion and the cellular uptake and utilization of O_2.[39]

Global O_2 delivery (DO$_2$) is the product of cardiac output and the arterial O_2 content (CaO$_2$), which is itself determined by the O_2 saturation and haemoglobin concentration of the arterial blood. Over the past two decades, there has been considerable debate over what constitutes an 'adequate' global DO$_2$. Maintaining an 'appropriate' DO$_2$ by ensuring 'adequate' intravascular volume replacement followed by the 'judicious' use of vasoactive agents is undoubtedly important in preventing organ failure, particularly in the peri-operative period[40] and in the early stages of critical illness.[41] These issues have been reviewed elsewhere,[39] but the level of FiO$_2$ and corresponding value of PaO_2 that are accepted are particularly relevant to the management of the patient with refractory hypoxaemia, because this represents a balance between the risks of pulmonary O_2 toxicity and permissive hypoxaemia.

Of the four phases in the transport of O_2 from the external environment to the tissue cells, two are convective and two diffusive:

(i) The convective or 'bulk flow' phases involve the movement of O_2 from the environment to alveoli by ventilation and its transport from the pulmonary to the systemic tissue capillaries: these are the active, energy-requiring stages that rely on work performed by the respiratory and cardiac 'pumps'.

(ii) The diffusive phases involve the passage of O_2 from alveolus to pulmonary capillary and from systemic capillary to tissue cell: these stages are passive and depend on the gradient of O_2 partial pressures, the tissue capillary density (which determines diffusion distance), the position of the O_2 dissociation curve (P_{50}) and the ability of the cell to take up and use O_2 (Fig. 22.2).

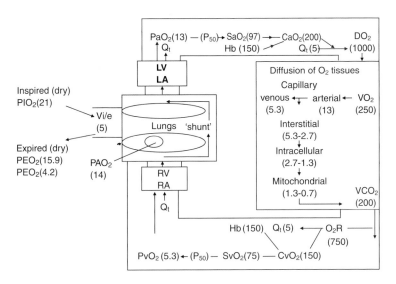

Figure 22.1 *Oxygen transport from atmosphere to mitochondria. Values in parentheses for a normal 75-kg individual (body surface area: 1.7 m²) breathing air (FiO₂: 0.21) at standard atmospheric pressure (P_B: 101 kPa). Partial pressures of O₂, CO₂ in kPa; saturation in %; contents (CaO₂, CvO₂) in mL L⁻¹; Hb in g L⁻¹; blood/gas flows (Q_t, Vi/e) in L min⁻¹; oxygen delivery return (DO₂,O₂R), VO₂ and VCO₂ in mL min⁻¹. P_{50} defines position of O₂–haemoglobin dissociation curve; it is the PO₂ at which 50% of haemoglobin is saturated (normally 3.5 kPa). SO₂, O₂ saturation (%); PO₂, O₂ partial pressure (kPa); PIO₂, inspired PO₂; PEO₂, mixed expired PO₂; PECO₂, mixed expired PCO₂; PAO₂, alveolar PO₂; PaO₂, arterial PO₂; SaO₂, arterial SO₂; SvO₂, mixed venous SO₂; Q_t, cardiac output; Hb, haemoglobin; CaO₂, arterial O₂ content; CvO₂, mixed venous O₂ content; VO₂, O₂ consumption; VCO₂, CO₂ production; O₂R, O₂ return; DO₂, O₂, O₂ delivery; Vi/e, insp/exp minute volume; LV, left ventricle; LA, left atrium; RV, right ventricle; LV, left ventricle.*

Table 22.2 provides a practical illustration of the impact on global O_2 delivery (DO_2) of correcting hypoxaemia, anaemia and a low cardiac output. This emphasizes that:

- global DO_2 may be reduced by anaemia, O_2 desaturation or a low cardiac output, either singly or in combination;
- global DO_2 depends on O_2 saturation rather than partial pressure and, due to the sigmoid shape of the oxyhaemoglobin dissociation curve, little extra benefit derives from increasing PaO_2 above the value (~9 kPa) that ensures that over 90% of haemoglobin is saturated with O_2. However, this does not apply to the diffusive component of O_2 transport that does depend on the gradient of O_2 partial pressure (Fig. 22.3).

Blood transfusion to polycythaemic levels may seem an appropriate way to increase DO_2 and mitigate the impact of a low PaO_2 because this is the response seen in other conditions associated with chronic hypoxaemia such as cyanotic heart disease

and COPD. However, blood viscosity increases markedly above 100 g L⁻¹, which adversely affects regional and microcirculatory blood flow, particularly if perfusion pressure is reduced, resulting in an exacerbation of tissue hypoxia.[42] Recent evidence suggests that even the traditionally accepted haemoglobin concentration for critically ill patients of approximately 100 g L⁻¹ may be too high, because an improved outcome was observed if haemoglobin was maintained between 70 and 90 g L⁻¹, with the exception of patients with coronary artery disease in whom a level of 100 g L⁻¹ remains appropriate.[43] With the chosen haemoglobin concentration achieved by transfusion and with an O_2 saturation (SaO_2) maintained at >90%, further increases in PaO_2 will have little impact on global DO_2, which will then be determined by the cardiac output.

However, increased levels of global DO_2 cannot compensate for disordered regional distribution of DO_2, for impaired diffusion between capillary and cell or for primary metabolic failure within the cell as occurs in sepsis and in cyanide poisoning.

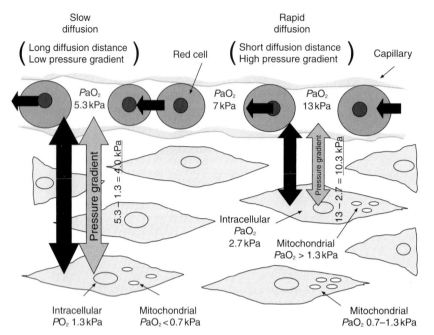

Figure 22.2 *Diagram to show the importance of local capillary oxygen tension and diffusion distance from capillary to cell in determining the rate of oxygen delivery and the intracellular and mitochondrial PaO_2. On the left there is a low capillary PO_2 with a reduced pressure gradient for oxygen diffusion and an increased diffusion distance resulting in a low intracellular and mitochondrial PaO_2. By contrast, on the right the higher PaO_2 partial pressure gradient and the shorter diffusion distance results in significantly higher intracellular PaO_2 values.*

Factors influencing oxygen transport from capillary blood to individual cells

The delivery of O_2 from capillary blood to the cell depends upon:

- factors that influence diffusion: capillary PO_2, tissue oedema, capillary density,
- the rate of O_2 delivery to the capillary (DO_2),
- the position of the O_2 – haemoglobin dissociation relationship (P_{50}),
- the rate of cellular O_2 utilization and uptake (VO_2).

The position of the O_2–haemoglobin dissociation curve – defined as the PaO_2 at which 50% of the haemoglobin is saturated (P_{50}) and which is normally ~3.5 kPa – is influenced by various physicochemical factors. An increase in P_{50} or rightward shift of this relationship reduces the haemoglobin saturation (SaO_2) for any given PaO_2, thereby increasing tissue O_2 availability. This is caused by pyrexia, acidosis, hypercapnia and an increase in intracellular phosphate, notably 2, 3-diphosphoglycerate (2, 3-DPG), and explains in part the benefit derived from hyper-

Table 22.2 *Relative effects of changes in PaO_2, haemoglobin and cardiac output on oxygen delivery*

	FiO$_2$	PaO$_2$ (kPa)	SaO$_2$ (%)	Hb (g L^{-1})	Dissolved O$_2$ (mL L^{-1})	CaO$_2$ (mL L^{-1})	Q$_t$ (mL min^{-1})	DO$_2$ (mL min^{-1})	DO$_2$ % change
Normal[a]	0.21	13.0	96	130	3.0	170	5.3	900	0
Patient[b]	0.21	6.0	75	70	1.4	72	4.0	288	−68
↑ FiO$_2$	0.35	9.0	92	70	2.1	88	4.0	352	+22
↑↑ FiO$_2$	0.60	16.5	98	70	3.8	96	4.0	384	+9
↑ Hb	0.60	16.5	98	105	3.8	142	4.0	568	+48
↑ Q$_t$	0.60	16.5	98	105	3.8	142	6.0	852	+50

[a]Normal 75-kg subject at rest.
[b]Patient with hypoxaemia, anaemia and reduced cardiac output and evidence of global tissue hypoxia.
$DO_2 = CaO_2 \times Q_t$ mL min^{-1}.
$CaO_2 = (Hb \times SaO_2 \times 1.34) + (PaO_2 \times 0.23)$ mL L^{-1}.
Where FiO$_2$ is the fractional inspired O_2 concentration, PaO_2, SaO_2, CaO_2 are, respectively, the partial pressure, saturation and content of O_2 in arterial blood, and Q$_t$ is the cardiac output.
1.34 mL is the volume of O_2 carried by 1 g of 100%-saturated haemoglobin and PaO_2 (kPa) × 0.23 is the amount of O_2 in physical solution in 1 L blood, which is less than 3% of total CaO$_2$ for normal PaO_2 (i.e. < 14 kPa).

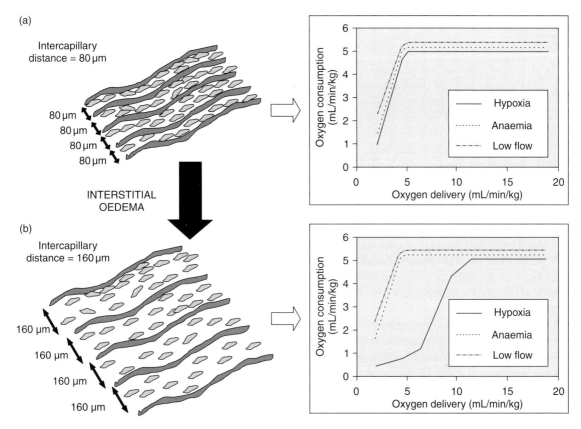

Figure 22.3 *Diagram illustrating the influence of intercapillary distance on the effects of hypoxia, anaemia and low flow on the relationship between oxygen delivery and consumption. With a normal intercapillary distance, as shown in (a), the DO_2/VO_2 relationship is the same, irrespective of whether the reduction in DO_2 is produced by progressive hypoxia, anaemia or reduction in cardiac output. However, in (b) there is an increased intercapillary distance as occurs with tissue oedema, and in this situation progressive reduction in arterial PaO_2 does alter the DO_2/VO_2 relationship, with VO_2 falling at much higher levels of global DO_2. This effect is not seen when DO_2 is reduced by progressive reduction in haemoglobin concentration or cardiac output.*

capnia and why it is important to correct hypophosphataemia.

Mathematical models of tissue hypoxia demonstrate that the fall in intracellular PO_2 resulting from an increase in intercapillary distance is more severe if the reduction in tissue DO_2 is due to 'hypoxic' hypoxia (a fall in PaO_2) rather than due to 'stagnant' (a fall in flow) or 'anaemic' hypoxia (Fig. 22.3). Thus, severe arterial hypoxaemia, particularly in the presence of increased tissue oedema, will result in reduced O_2 diffusion and cellular hypoxia. These observations suggest that the extent of tissue oedema and the level of PaO_2, independent of DO_2, will affect tissue oxygenation and potentially the development of organ dysfunction in critically ill patients.

Therefore, the following strategies directed at improving global O_2 delivery and preventing pulmonary O_2 toxicity are not without potential risk of exacerbating tissue hypoxia:

- reducing FiO_2 to prevent O_2 toxicity,
- giving fluids to increase intravascular volume, particularly in patients with increased endothelial permeability,
- giving vasoactive agents that alter the regional distribution of DO_2.

Improvement in the prognosis for the patient with severe hypoxaemia and incipient or established organ failure awaits the development of technologies and therapies that allow the measurement and manipulation of both the regional distribution of blood flow and other 'downstream' factors in the O_2 cascade.[44]

How tolerant are the tissues of hypoxia?

There is considerable variation in the tolerance of individual organs and cells to hypoxia.[45] Cortical neurons are exquisitely sensitive to sudden reductions in O_2 supply and do not survive sustained periods of hypoxia. Following complete cessation of cerebral perfusion, nuclear magnetic resonance (NMR) studies have shown a 50% decrease in neuronal adenosine triphosphate (ATP) within 30 s and irreversible damage occurring within 3 min. Other tissues can survive anoxia for longer periods: kidneys and liver for approximately 20 min, skeletal muscle for about 75 min and vascular smooth muscle for up to 72 hours. Hair and nails provide the most extreme example of anoxic tolerance because they continue to grow for several days after death.

There is a difference in the tolerance to severe hypoxia and the response to complete anoxia and this also differs in health and disease. In sepsis, inhibition of enzyme systems and O_2 utilization reduces hypoxic tolerance.[46] Methods aimed at enhancing metabolic performance including the use of alternative substrates, techniques to inhibit endotoxin-induced cellular damage and drugs to reduce oxidant intracellular damage are all currently under investigation. Progressive or repeated exposure to hypoxia enhances tissue tolerance to O_2 deprivation in a similar way to altitude acclimatization. An acclimatized mountaineer at the peak of Mount Everest can tolerate a PaO_2 of 4–4.5 kPa for several hours, and patients with severe COPD can survive with a PaO_2 <5 kPa for several years, both of which are degrees of hypoxaemia that, if produced acutely, would result in confusion and a reduced level of consciousness within a few minutes in a normal subject.

So, what is the critical level of tissue oxygenation below which cellular damage will occur? The answer depends predominantly on the co-morbid factors and the duration of hypoxia. For example, young, healthy individuals with the acute respiratory distress syndrome (ARDS) can make a complete recovery following prolonged periods of severe hypoxaemia with PaO_2 as low as 6 kPa and O_2 saturations below 85%. The older patient with widespread atheroma may not survive prolonged hypoxaemia at such levels.

The foregoing analysis might suggest that it would be beneficial to increase the level of FiO_2 to improve tissue oxygenation and so potentially reduce organ failure and lead to an improved outcome. Current practice is to reduce FiO_2 as far as 'reasonably' possible, with the aim of limiting the risk of pulmonary O_2 toxicity. This assumes that the risk is significant, but should we be unduly concerned about pulmonary O_2 toxicity?

Pulmonary oxygen toxicity

The demonstration that ventilation with low tidal volumes reduces ventilator-induced lung injury and improves outcome makes it important to consider whether other lung-protective strategies such as avoiding high levels of inspired O_2 may produce additional benefit. Hyperoxia increases the levels of reactive radicals, hydrogen peroxide and hydroxyl and superoxide ions, which inactivate sulphydryl enzymes thereby disrupting DNA synthesis. This damages the pulmonary capillary membranes and increases interstitial oedema, which reduces lung compliance and further impairs gas exchange. Decreased surfactant levels have also been attributed to high inspired O_2 levels.[47] (See also Chapter 18, p. 239.)

The risk of O_2 toxicity is related to the absolute O_2 tension rather than to FiO_2, as demonstrated by experiments varying the atmospheric pressure at which the gas mixture is delivered. Astronauts suffer no ill-effects from 100% O_2 at one-third atmosphere pressure. Compared to other species, such as rats, humans appear relatively resistant to O_2 toxicity and there is little evidence of significant damage from long-term ventilation with inspired PO_2 (PiO_2) of 50 kPa (FiO_2 of 0.5) at standard atmospheric pressure. However, there is evidence that such levels for long periods may be harmful when there is pre-existing lung damage.[48] One study has shown that an inspired O_2 above 0.6 for over 24 hours does produce reduced diffusion capacity when measured many months after an episode of ARDS.[49] In general, there is an inverse relationship between PO_2 and the safe duration of exposure, i.e. the potential for injury relates to the area under the PO_2– time curve.

It is, of course, difficult in the clinical setting to distinguish lung injury due to O_2 toxicity from that caused by the underlying process and other aspects of management. Nonetheless, on current evidence, prolonged ventilation with PiO_2 60 kPa ($FiO_2 > 0.6$

at 1 atmosphere) may contribute to lung injury and adversely affect both the short-term and long-term outcomes.

Our current practice in selecting the FiO_2 (assuming ventilation at 1 atmosphere or 100 kPa pressure) and corresponding PaO_2 levels that we would consider acceptable can be summarized as follows.

- If $PaO_2 > 10$ kPa with $FiO_2 \leq 0.6$, use lowest FiO_2 up to maximum 0.6 to maintain PaO_2 at 10–12 kPa and continue conventional treatment.
- If $PaO_2 > 10$ kPa with $FiO_2 > 0.6$, target lowest FiO_2 between 0.6 and 0.8 to maintain PaO_2 at 8–10 kPa and start further measures to improve gas exchange, e.g. recruitment manoeuvre.
- If $PaO_2 < 8$ kPa with $FiO_2 > 0.8$, set FiO_2 0.8–1.0 to maintain PaO_2 at 7–8 kPa and urgently start further measures; consider short-term nitric oxide 'rescue' until gas exchange has improved.

It remains uncertain but distinctly possible that the prolonged use of nitric oxide, a highly reactive chemical species, may itself cause lung injury and compound the problems of O_2 toxicity.[50] Because two multicentre trials of the use of nitric oxide in ARDS have demonstrated no survival benefit and also indicate that even the gas exchange benefit may only last for 24 hours, we reduce and stop the nitric oxide as soon as tolerable gas exchange is achieved.

The urgency of correcting severe hypoxaemia requiring FiO_2 of >0.8 is greatly increased if the patient is known to have peripheral vascular disease with coronary and cerebral atheroma, and one would aim to maintain the $PaO_2 \geq 8$ kPa, even if this required an FiO_2 of 1.0, while the further strategies to improve oxygenation were urgently implemented.

Both $FiO_2 > 0.6$ ($PiO_2 > 60$ kPa) and $PaO_2 < 8$ kPa for prolonged (>6 hours) periods may adversely affect outcome in patients with severe lung injury. The need for increasing levels of FiO_2 above 0.6 to maintain $PaO_2 \geq 9$ kPa should prompt consideration of further measures to improve gas exchange and, if necessary, the use of short-term 'rescue' nitric oxide as well as investigations to determine the cause of the decline.

Metabolic considerations in patients with refractory hypoxaemia

Reduction in metabolic rate will reduce tissue O_2 consumption and, if O_2 supply remains constant, will improve cellular oxygenation. This alternative strategy to increasing cellular O_2 delivery may be achieved by:

- ensuring adequate analgesia and sedation to control sympathetic activation from pain, agitation, shivering and various interventions (nursing procedures, physiotherapy, visitors),
- instituting active cooling measures if core temperature exceeds 38 °C: for each °C rise in temperature, O_2 consumption increases by 10–15%,
- avoiding drugs that increase metabolic rate, particularly inotropes such as adrenaline and dobutamine, and other beta-agonists,
- abolishing spontaneous respiratory effort, if necessary using muscle relaxants and thereby eliminating the metabolic costs of breathing.

Fluid management in refractory hypoxaemia

Deciding on fluid therapy for a patient with severe hypoxaemia represents a difficult balance between the risk of increasing extravascular lung water, and further exacerbating the hypoxaemia and potentially the lung injury, and the risk of providing inadequate intravascular volume replacement, resulting in impaired peripheral perfusion and the development of other organ failure. In Chapter 12, 'appropriate' fluid therapy in acute lung injury was summarized as the provision of the minimum intravenous fluid that ensured 'adequate' cardiac output and tissue perfusion. While agreeing with this and that the failure to limit pulmonary vascular pressure and the extent of pulmonary oedema may contribute to ventilator-induced lung injury, such a broad consensus statement leaves the clinician uncertain as to what precisely is meant by 'adequate' cardiac output and tissue perfusion. Conventionally, this decision is based on the atrial filling pressures, which assumes that both pulmonary capillary permeability and the intrathoracic pressure are normal. These assumptions are often not valid in the critically ill, particularly the patient with severe lung injury, in whom atrial filling pressures in excess of 15 or even 20 cmH$_2$O, do not necessarily preclude intravascular depletion.

Measurement of volume pre-load of the left ventricle is more relevant, but has not been possible as part of routine clinical practice, although echocardiography can provide valuable information on the adequacy of filling of the left ventricle and, if performed serially, on the response to volume loading. Techniques for determining intrathoracic blood volume and extravascular lung water are discussed in Chapter 8, but are still being refined and, as yet, are not widely available. However, there are useful bedside signs that should alert the clinician to the possibility of inadequate intrathoracic blood volume:

- Hypotension precipitated by sedation, analgesia or postural change.
- Fluctuation in the arterial pressure trace during positive pressure ventilation and hypotension when increasing levels of PEEP are applied. Indeed, a formal recruitment manoeuvre with the application of PEEP to over 30 cmH$_2$O represents an imposed Valsalva manoeuvre. Intrathoracic volume depletion is indicated by a marked reduction in pulse pressure and mean arterial pressure (as illustrated in Fig. 22.3a), whereas a raised intrathoracic blood volume produces a 'square-wave' response (Fig. 22.3b).
- Brief disconnection from the ventilator causes the blood pressure to rise and venous pressure to fall: the atrial pressure measurement 'off' the ventilator more accurately reflects the ventricular end-diastolic *transmural* pressure. This manoeuvre is, however, relatively contra-indicated in patients with ARDS because any procedure that reduces tracheal pressure will cause de-recruitment, with alveolar collapse and a further exacerbation of the hypoxaemia.

The difficulty of interpreting the absolute levels of the atrial filling pressures (RAP/LAP) may also be resolved by a fluid challenge, although this must be performed with caution in the patient with radiological evidence of increased lung water. We would give a maximum of 200 mL of colloid and observe the impact on blood pressure, flow and atrial filling pressures. In the volume-depleted patient, blood pressure and flow will increase with only a small, transient increase in filling pressures. While pulmonary gas exchange remains satisfactory, there is less anxiety about giving further colloid. Sufficient volume will have been given when either the target pressures are achieved and the evidence of poor peripheral perfusion and organ dysfunction has resolved, or when there is a sustained rise in filling pressures with either deterioration in gas exchange or chest X-ray appearances.

SETTING THE TARGET FLUID BALANCE

The crystalloid and colloid balance over the previous 24 hours and the intravascular and extravascular compartments should be individually reviewed twice a day. The crystalloid balance should include the planned enteral intake, fluid for central lines and drug infusions, urine output and correction for both 'insensible' losses (sweat, diarrhoea) and the state of hydration of the extravascular tissue space. A daily target balance from −1.5 L to > +1 L may be appropriate, but, typically in the patient with severe lung injury, it will be between −1.0 L and +0.5 L. The more robust the circulation and the greater the evidence of tissue oedema, the more negative the crystalloid balance should be.

If the assessment of the extravascular space shows gross peripheral oedema with dense alveolar fluid infiltrates and the presence of pleural effusions, then, while the circulation remains robust, negative fluid balances of 2 L or more per 24 hours would be appropriate, using either forced naturesis if renal function is maintained or haemofiltration if necessary. The potential benefits of achieving such a negative crystalloid balance apply not only to lung function and improving oxygenation, but also to the peripheral tissues, which are frequently oedematous in this setting. Resolution of this tissue oedema will improve O$_2$ diffusion from capillary to cell, as already discussed. During the worst excesses of goal-directed therapy, in grossly oedematous patients referred to our unit with severe acute lung injury, negative crystalloid balances of over 10 L were achieved within 72 hours without any apparent adverse effects on the circulation or critical organ perfusion, but resulted in a marked improvement in lung compliance and gas exchange. It should be remembered that both pulmonary and chest-wall compliance improve with the resolution of pulmonary interstitial and alveolar oedema and the reduction of oedema in the tissues of the chest wall.

If the intravascular space is under-filled, and particularly if the patient is already on vasopressor agents (which increase the risk of compromised regional perfusion, particularly to the splanchnic bed), fluid should be given. The rate of crystalloid infusion should be increased but, acutely, the extra volume required to reach the pre-load target should be given as colloid, as described. After appropriate blood transfusion, synthetic colloid rather than albumin should be used. A much-debated meta-analysis comparing the use of albumin with crystalloid or synthetic colloid concluded that, in the critically ill, albumin was associated with an increased mortality.[51] Certainly, attempting to correct a low serum albumin in such patients with a significant inflammatory response is futile because their vascular endothelium will be freely permeable to albumin. There is relatively little evidence on which to base the choice of synthetic colloid (starch or gelatin), but the increase in intravascular volume is sustained for longer with the starch solutions, which also provide a wider range of molecular weight products and a sodium-free option.

Three final observations are relevant with regard to the cardiorespiratory interactions in this group of patients with refractory hypoxaemia. The first is that, if excessive fluid is once given and a marked increase in lung water occurs, it requires a far greater negative crystalloid balance to remove that fluid than the volume originally given. Secondly, correction of intravascular volume depletion with subsequent improvement in cardiac output and O_2 delivery will increase mixed venous O_2 saturation, which, in the context of a large pulmonary shunt, must increase the arterial O_2 tension if the shunt remains unchanged. Finally, further advances in fluid management in patients with severe lung injury will depend on the development of bedside technology that provides reliable measurements of both extravascular lung water and regional tissue perfusion.[44]

Further strategies in the treatment of refractory hypoxaemia

The range of further strategies that have been evaluated in the treatment of severe acute lung injury with refractory hypoxaemia are discussed in Chapter 12. Before embarking on any escalation of treatment, it is important to be sure that the basic ventilatory strategy and general management are optimum. If such measures improve oxygenation and the hypoxaemia index is above 125 mmHg (16.7 kPa), most clinicians would not feel it necessary to introduce additional strategies. However, if the hypoxaemia index does fall below this level, which strategies should be considered? Daily chest X-rays will be performed on such patients and obviously any gas or fluid collection should be drained. It can be difficult to identify the loculated or anterior pneumothorax on antero-posterior chest X-ray and, as discussed in Chapter 10, a computed tomography scan should be considered before embarking on further therapy.

RECRUITMENT MANOEUVRES

The different lung recruitment manoeuvres that can be used are described in Chapter 12, and Figure 8.1 (see Chapter 8) gives an example of such a manoeuvre using a high-frequency oscillator.

The manoeuvre is usually performed in a paralysed patient who is ventilated using low tidal volume (Vt 5–7 mL kg^{-1}), inverse ratio pressure-controlled ventilation with at least 10 cmH$_2$O PEEP already applied. By increasing the PEEP level, the patient is 'held' at end-inspiration at an inflation pressure of 30–45 cmH$_2$O for 30 s to 2 min, after which ventilation is resumed with PEEP set at 15–18 cmH$_2$O, depending on the circulatory response. The blood pressure will frequently fall during the manoeuvre due to the increase in intrathoracic pressure and this will determine the pressure level and the length of time for which it is applied. Extra fluid administration should be avoided and, if necessary, a temporary increase in vasopressor therapy should be used to support the blood pressure.

It is important to remember that de-recruitment readily occurs in these patients secondary to any cause of a fall in tracheal pressure, which include:

- disconnection from the ventilator,
- suctioning down the endotracheal tube, particularly if high pressures are used and despite using a 'closed' suction system,
- bronchoscopy,
- spontaneous inspiratory effort opposing the effect of PEEP and reducing end-expiratory volume,

- chest-wall compression during physiotherapy – this partly explains the hypoxaemia that is often seen in these patients after physiotherapy, which should only be given by an experienced practitioner after careful discussion with the clinical team.

HIGH-FREQUENCY OSCILLATION

This is a mode of ventilation that is conceptually simple and that achieves an 'open lung' and, by eliminating the biphasic swing of tidal breathing, avoids the potential problem with conventional ventilation of cyclical over-inflation and collapse in different parts of the lung. Figure 22.2 illustrates the principles involved. A continuous distending pressure of up to 55 cmH$_2$O is applied by adjusting the gas flow and expiratory valve; this effectively applies super-PEEP and, as it is increased, alveoli are recruited and the functional residual capacity increases. The frequency (180–900 min^{-1}) and amplitude or power of the oscillator determine the resulting tidal volume. This is only in the range 0.1–5 mL kg^{-1}, barely exceeding the physiological dead space, and produces alveolar pressure swings of less than 5 cmH$_2$O. The enhanced gas exchange (both oxygenation and CO$_2$ clearance) that results relies on a combination of different gas transport mechanisms, including Taylor dispersion, molecular diffusion and cardiogenic mixing in addition to convective ventilation.[52] It differs from high-frequency jet ventilation in the mechanism of delivery (oscillator versus jet), and in that expiration is active rather than passive and the alveolar distending pressure is directly set. Unlike jet ventilation, a standard humidifier can be used with high-frequency oscillatory ventilation (HFOV) and nitric oxide can be delivered through the system.

We resort to using HFOV when gas exchange has not responded to other therapies, and have observed striking improvements in gas exchange in most cases. It is generally well tolerated, but problems can arise with hypotension, which may require an increase in vasopressor therapy: any extra fluid should be given with great caution. There is obviously a risk of pneumothorax, but our experience is that it is no more frequent than with conventional ventilation.

Outcome benefit has yet to be demonstrated, but a pilot study involving ARDS patients showed improved oxygenation,[53] and a recent prospective study involving patients with severe ARDS (mean hypoxaemia index <100 mmHg) concluded that it was a safe and effective rescue therapy in severe oxygenation failure.[54]

NITRIC OXIDE

Most clinicians now try to avoid the long-term use of nitric oxide because two large multicentre, randomized studies failed to demonstrate any outcome benefit and suggested that the improvement in oxygenation only lasted for 24 hours. Our practice is to use it as a short-term agent for the transport of patients with otherwise refractory hypoxaemia and also as a rescue therapy while alternative therapies (prone, oscillation) are instituted. There is evidence that it may produce additive benefit when used with almitrine and prone positioning.[55] Concerns remain that longer term use may exacerbate the lung injury and, if used in further randomized studies, it will be important to collect long-term follow-up data on lung function.

POSTURAL THERAPY

Prone positioning produces an impressive improvement in gas exchange in about two-thirds of patients with refractory hypoxaemia and it has become an increasingly popular therapy despite the logistic problems presented in the heavily instrumented patient. A multicentre Italian study confimed such an improvement in gas exchange without any increase in complications in the treatment group, but no outcome benefit could be demonstrated.[56] However, the numbers enrolled (304) may have been inadequate, the treatment group was only 'proned' for 7 hours per day, for a total of 10 days, and there were varying degrees of non-compliance with the study protocol due to staffing shortage.

We believe that it remains a promising therapy and that the imminent production of a 'bed' that will automatically rotate the patient into the prone position with all lines attached promises to eliminate the labour-intensive issues for the staff. It will also allow greater standardization of the precise positioning of the patient when prone, as well as the opportunity to intervene earlier in the disease process and to investigate the impact of different 'proning' intervals and even the effect of continuous rotation in the prone position.

There are a number of other therapies, including surfactant therapy, liquid ventilation and extracorporeal techniques, that are still under investigation but are not, at this stage, either proven or practical alternatives to the therapies discussed.

Future advances will depend on carefully designed, randomized, controlled, multicentre studies that characterize patients precisely and demonstrably execute the agreed protocol, as the ARDSnet group showed in their study of tidal volumes in acute lung injury.

REFERENCES

1. Goldhill, DR, Worthington, L, Mulcahy, M, Sumner, A. The patient-at-risk team: identifying and managing seriously ill ward patients. *Anaesthesia* 1999; **54**: 853–60.

2. Hourihan, F, Bishop, K, Hillman, KM, Daffurn, K, Lee, A. The medical emergency team: a strategy to identify and intervene in high risk patients. *Clin Int Care* 1995; **6**: 269–72.

3. Schein, MH, Hazday, N, Pena, M, Ruben, BH, Sprung, CL. Clinical antecedents to in-hospital cardiac arrest. *Chest* 1990; **98**: 1388–92.

4. Goldhill, DR, White, A, Sumner, A. Physiological values and procedures in the 24 hours before ICU admission from the ward. *Anaesthesia* 1999; **54**: 529–34.

5. *Comprehensive critical care*. London: Department of Health, 2000.

6. Tobin, MJ. *Essentials of critical care medicine*. New York: Churchill Livingstone, 1989.

7. Aubier, M, Muriciano, D, Fournier, M, *et al*. Central respiratory drive in acute respiratory failure of patients with chronic obstructive pulmonary disease. *Am Rev Respir Dis* 1980; **122**: 191–9.

8. Dunn, WF, Nelson, SB, Hubmayr, RD. Oxygen induced hypercarbia in obstructive pulmonary disease. *Am Rev Respir Dis* 1991; **144**: 526–30.

9. Mador, MJ, Tobin, MJ. Acute respiratory failure. In *Chronic obstructive pulmonary disease*. Calverley, P, Pride N, eds. London: Chapman & Hall, 1995; 461–94.

10. Brochard, L, Moncebo, J, Wysocki, M, *et al*. Non invasive ventilation for acute exacerbations of chronic

11. Plant, P, Owen, J, Elliott, M. A multi centre randomised control trial of the early use of non invasive ventilation for acute exacerbations of chronic obstructive pulmonary disease. *Lancet* 2000; **355**: 1931–5.

12. Soo Hoo, GW, Hakiman, I, Santiago, SM. Hypercapnic respiratory failure in COPD patients. Response to therapy. *Chest* 2000; **117**: 169–77.

13. Plant PK, Owen JL, Elliott, MW. Non-invasive ventilation in acute exacerbations of chronic obstructive pulmonary disease: long term survival and predictors of in-hospital outcome. *Thorax* 2001; **56**: 708–12.

14. Carlucci, A, Richard, JC, Wysocki, M, *et al*. Noninvasive versus conventional mechanical ventilation. An epidemiological survey. *Am J Respir Crit Care Med* 2001; **163**: 874–80.

15. British Thoracic guidelines on the use of acute non-invasive ventilation. *Thorax* 2001.

16. Evans, TW. International Consensus Conference in Intensive Care Medicine: non-invasive positive pressure ventilation in acute respiratory failure. *Int Care Med* 2001; **27**: 166–78.

17. *Withholding and withdrawing life prolonging treatment. Guidance for decision-making*. London: BMJ Publishing, 2001.

18. Dales, RE, O'Connor, A, Hebert, P, *et al*. Intubation and mechanical ventilation for COPD: development of an instrument to elicit patient preferences. *Chest* 1999; **116**: 792–800.

19. Vasilyev, S, Schaap, RN, Mortensen, JD. Hospital survival rates of patients with acute respiratory failure in modern respiratory intensive care units. *Chest* 1995; **107**: 1083–8.

20. Connors, AF, Dawson, NV, Thomas, C. Outcomes following acute exacerbations of severe chronic obstructive pulmonary disease. *Am J Respir Crit Care Med* 1996; **154**: 959–67.

21. Wagner, MG, Wagner, DP, *et al*. Hospital and 1 year survival of patients admitted to intensive care units with acute exacerbations of chronic obstructive disease. *JAMA* 1995; **274**: 1852–7.

22. Stauffer, JL, Fayter, N, Graves, B, *et al*. Survival following mechanical ventilation for acute respiratory failure in adult men. *Chest* 1993; **104**: 1222–9.

23. Gracey, DR, Naessens, JM, Krishan, I, *et al*. Hospital and post-hospital survival among patients with COPD who require mechanical ventilation for acute respiratory failure. *Chest* 1989; **101**: 211–14.

obstructive pulmonary disease. *N Engl J Med* 1995; **333**: 817–22.

24. Bardi, G, Pierotello, R, Desideri, M, *et al*. Nasal ventilation in COPD exacerbations: early and late results of a prospective controlled study. *Eur Respir J* 2000; **15**: 98–104.

25. Confalonieri, M, Perigi, P, Scartabellati, A, *et al*. Non invasive mechanical ventilation improves the immediate and long term outcome of COPD patients with acute respiratory failure. *Eur Respir J* 1996; **9**: 422–30.

26. Meecham-Jones, DJ, Paul, ESA, Jones, PW, *et al*. Nasal pressure support ventilation plus oxygen compared with oxygen therapy alone in hypercapnic COPD. *Am J Respir Crit Care Med* 1995; **152**: 538–44.

27. Jones, SE, Packham, S, Hebden, M, Smith, AP. Domicilary nocturnal intermittent positive pressure ventilation in patients with respiratory failure due to severe COPD: long term follow up and effect on survival. *Thorax* 1998; **53**: 495–8.

28. Ely, EW, Baker, A, Dunagan, D, *et al*. Effect of the duration of mechanical ventilation of identifying patients capable of breathing spontaneously. *N Engl J Med* 1996; **335**: 1864–9.

29. Vitacca, M, Vianello, A, Colombo, D, *et al*. Comparison of two methods for weaning patients with chronic obstructive pulmonary disease requiring mechanical ventilation for more than 15 days. *Am J Respir Crit Care Med* 2001; **164**: 225–30.

30. Nava, S, Ambrosino, N, Clini, E, *et al*. Non invasive mechanical ventilation in the weaning of patients with respiratory failure due to chronic obstructive pulmonary disease. A randomised controlled trial. *Ann Intern Med* 1998; **128**: 721–8.

31. Girault, C, Daudenthoni, S, Chevron, V, *et al*. Non invasive ventilation as a systematic extubation and weaning technique in acute on chronic respiratory failure. *Am J Respir Crit Care Med* 1999; **160**: 86–92.

32. Vitacca, M, Ambrosino, N, Clini, E, *et al*. Physiological response to pressure support ventilation delivered before and after extubation in patients not capable of totally spontaneous autonomous breathing. *Am J Respir Crit Care Med* 2001; **164**: 638–41.

33. Carlucci, A, Gregoretti, C, Squadrone, V, *et al*. Preventative use of non-invasive mechanical ventilation (NIMV) to avoid post-extubation respiratory failure: a randomised controlled trial. *Eur Respir J* 2001: **18** (Suppl. 33): 29s.

34. Jaber, S, Carlucci, A, Bourssarsar, M, *et al*. Helium – oxygen in the post extubation period decreases inspiratory effort. *Am J Respir Crit Care Med* 2001; **164**: 633–7.

35. Hamid, S, Noonan, YM, Williams, AJ, Davidson, AC. An audit of weaning from mechanical ventilation in a UK weaning centre. *Thorax* 1999; **54**: 86.

36. Pilcher, D, Hamid, S, Williams, AJ, Davidson, AC. Outcomes, cost and long term survival of patients referred to regional centres for weaning from mechanical ventilation. Presentation at World Congress ICM, Sydney, 2001.

37. Scheinhorn, DJ, Chao, DC, Stearn-Hassenpflug, M, *et al*. Outcomes in post ICU mechanical ventilation. Treatment of 1123 patients at a regional weaning centre. *Chest* 1997; **111**: 1654–9.

38. Bernard, GR, Artigas, A, Brigham, KL, *et al*. and the Consensus Committee of the American European Conference on ARDS. Definitions, mechanisms, relevant outcomes and clinical trial coordination. *Am J Respir Crit Care Med* 1994; **149**: 818–24.

39. Leach, RM, Treacher, DF. The pulmonary physician in critical care 2. Oxygen delivery and consumption in the critically ill. *Thorax* 2002; **57**: 1–7.

40. Wilson, J, Woods, I, *et al*. Reducing the risk of major elective surgery: randomized, controlled trial of preoperative optimisation of oxygen delivery. *BMJ* 1999; **318**: 1099–103.

41. Rivers, E, Nguyen, B, Havstad, S, *et al*. Early goal-directed therapy in the treatment of severe sepsis and septic shock. *N Engl J Med* 2001; **345**: 1368–77.

42. Harrison, MJG, Kendall, BE, Pollock, S, Marshall, F. Effect of haematocrit on carotid stenosis and cerebral infarction. *Lancet* 1981; **ii**: 114–15.

43. Hebert, PC, Wells, G, Blajchman, M, *et al*. A multicenter, randomized, controlled clinical trial of transfusion requirements in critical care. *N Engl J Med* 1999; **340**: 409–17.

44. Consensus Conference. Tissue hypoxia: how to detect, how to correct, how to prevent. *Am J Respir Crit Care Med* 1996; **154**: 1573–8.

45. Robin, ED. Of men and mitochondria: coping with hypoxic dysoxia. *Am Rev Respir Dis* 1980; **122**: 517–31.

46. Bradley, SG. Cellular and molecular mechanisms of action of bacterial endotoxins. *Ann Rev Microbiol* 1979; **33**: 67–94.

47. O'Connor, BS, Vender, JS. Oxygen therapy. *Crit Care Clin* 1995; **11**: 67–78.

48. Denke, SM, Fanburg, BL. Normobaric oxygen toxicity of the lung. *N Engl J Med* 1980; **303**: 726.

49. Elliott, CG, Rasmusson, BY, Crapo, RO, *et al*. Prediction of pulmonary function abnormalities after adult respiratory distress syndrome (ARDS) *Am Rev Respir Dis* 1987; **135**: 634.

50. Pryor, WA. The chemistry of peroxynitrite: product from reaction of nitric oxide with superoxide. *Am J Physiol* 1995; **268**: 699–722.

51. Cochrane Injuries Group Albumin Reviewers. Human albumin administration in critically ill patients: systematic review of randomised controlled trials. *BMJ* 1998; **317**: 235–40.

52. Chang, HK Mechanisms of gas transport during ventilation by HFOV: a brief review. *J Appl Physiol* 1984.

53. Fort, P, Pharma, C, Westerman, J, *et al.* High frequency oscillatory ventilation for adult respiratory distress syndrome, a pilot study. *Crit Care Med* 1997; **25**: 937.

54. Mehta, S, Lapinsky, SE, Hallett, DC, *et al.* Prospective trial of high-frequency oscillation in adults with acute respiratory distress syndrome. *Crit Care Med* 2001; **29**: 1360–9.

55. Borelli, M, Lampati, L, Vascotti, E, Fumagalli, R, Pesenti, A. Hemodynamic and gas exchange response to inhaled nitric oxide and prone positioning in acute respiratory distress syndrome patients. *Crit Care Med* 2000; **28**: 2707–12.

56. Gattinoni, L, Tognoni, G, Pesenti, A, *et al.* and the Prone–Supine Study Group. Effect of prone positioning on the survival of patients with acute respiratory failure. *N Engl J Med* 2001; **345**(8): 568–73.

Index